FREE Study Skills Vide

Dear Customer,

Thank you for your purchase from Mometrix! We consider it an honor and a privilege that you have purchased our product and we want to ensure your satisfaction.

As a way of showing our appreciation and to help us better serve you, we have developed Study Skills Videos that we would like to give you for FREE. These videos cover our *best practices* for getting ready for your exam, from how to use our study materials to how to best prepare for the day of the test.

All that we ask is that you email us with feedback that would describe your experience so far with our product. Good, bad, or indifferent, we want to know what you think!

To get your FREE Study Skills Videos, you can use the **QR code** below, or send us an **email** at studyvideos@mometrix.com with *FREE VIDEOS* in the subject line and the following information in the body of the email:

- The name of the product you purchased.
- Your product rating on a scale of 1-5, with 5 being the highest rating.
- Your feedback. It can be long, short, or anything in between. We just want to know your impressions and experience so far with our product. (Good feedback might include how our study material met your needs and ways we might be able to make it even better. You could highlight features that you found helpful or features that you think we should add.)

If you have any questions or concerns, please don't hesitate to contact me directly.

Thanks again!

Sincerely,

Jay Willis
Vice President
jay.willis@mometrix.com
1-800-673-8175

SCAN HERE

Mometrix
TEST PREPARATION
The World's #1 Test Preparation Company

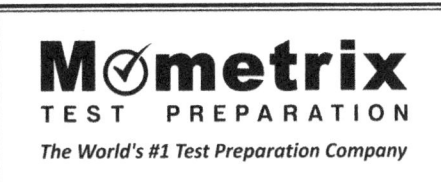

Mometrix
TEST PREPARATION

CBIC®

Exam Secrets Study Guide

Review and CIC Practice Test for the Certification Board of Infection Control and Epidemiology, Inc. (CBIC®) Examination

Written and edited by Mometrix Test Prep

Printed in the United States of America

This paper meets the requirements of ANSI/NISO Z39.48-1992 (Permanence of Paper).

Paperback
ISBN 13: 978-1-5167-1633-3
ISBN 10: 1-5167-1633-7

Ebook
ISBN 13: 978-1-5167-1542-8
ISBN 10: 1-5167-1542-X

Hardback
ISBN 13: 978-1-5167-1856-6
ISBN 10: 1-5167-1856-9

DEAR FUTURE EXAM SUCCESS STORY

First of all, **THANK YOU** for purchasing Mometrix study materials!

Second, congratulations! You are one of the few determined test-takers who are committed to doing whatever it takes to excel on your exam. **You have come to the right place.** We developed these study materials with one goal in mind: to deliver you the information you need in a format that's concise and easy to use.

In addition to optimizing your guide for the content of the test, we've outlined our recommended steps for breaking down the preparation process into small, attainable goals so you can make sure you stay on track.

We've also analyzed the entire test-taking process, identifying the most common pitfalls and showing how you can overcome them and be ready for any curveball the test throws you.

Standardized testing is one of the biggest obstacles on your road to success, which only increases the importance of doing well in the high-pressure, high-stakes environment of test day. Your results on this test could have a significant impact on your future, and this guide provides the information and practical advice to help you achieve your full potential on test day.

Your success is our success

We would love to hear from you! If you would like to share the story of your exam success or if you have any questions or comments in regard to our products, please contact us at **800-673-8175** or **support@mometrix.com**.

Thanks again for your business and we wish you continued success!

Sincerely,
The Mometrix Test Preparation Team

Need more help? Check out our flashcards at:
http://MometrixFlashcards.com/CBIC

TABLE OF CONTENTS

INTRODUCTION 1

SECRET KEY #1 – PLAN BIG, STUDY SMALL 2

SECRET KEY #2 – MAKE YOUR STUDYING COUNT 3

SECRET KEY #3 – PRACTICE THE RIGHT WAY 4

SECRET KEY #4 – PACE YOURSELF 6

SECRET KEY #5 – HAVE A PLAN FOR GUESSING 7

TEST-TAKING STRATEGIES 10

IDENTIFICATION OF INFECTIOUS DISEASE PROCESSES 15
- DIAGNOSTIC, RADIOLOGIC, PROCEDURAL, AND LABORATORY REPORTS 15
- COLONIZATION, INFECTION, AND PSEUDO INFECTIONS 24
- SPECIMEN COLLECTION, TRANSPORTATION, HANDLING, AND STORAGE 34
- CLINICAL SIGNS, SYMPTOMS, AND TEST RESULTS 43
- ANTIMICROBIALS 73
- ASSESSING RISK FACTORS FOR INFECTIOUS DISEASE 79
- MONITORING CURRENT AND EMERGING LOCAL AND GLOBAL THREATS 80

SURVEILLANCE AND EPIDEMIOLOGIC INVESTIGATION 81
- DESIGN OF SURVEILLANCE SYSTEMS 81
- COLLECTION AND COMPILATION OF SURVEILLANCE DATA 95
- INTERPRETATION OF SURVEILLANCE DATA 104
- OUTBREAK INVESTIGATION 117
- KEY COMPONENTS OF SURVEILLANCE AND EPIDEMIOLOGY 134

PREVENTING/CONTROLLING THE TRANSMISSION OF INFECTIOUS AGENTS 138
- DEVELOPING INFECTION PREVENTION POLICIES AND PROCEDURES 138
- INFECTION PREVENTION AND CONTROL STRATEGIES 144
- TRANSMISSION BASED PRECAUTIONS 188
- EMERGENCY PREPAREDNESS AND MANAGEMENT 194

EMPLOYEE/OCCUPATIONAL HEALTH 202
- SCREENING AND IMMUNIZATION PROGRAMS 202
- COMMUNICABLE DISEASES AND EXPOSURES 206
- NEEDLE STICKS AND SPLASHES 213
- IDENTIFYING TRANSMISSION RISKS AND SAFE WORK PRACTICES 215

MANAGEMENT AND COMMUNICATION 217
- PLANNING THE INFECTION CONTROL PROGRAM 217
- COMMUNICATION 227
- QUALITY PERFORMANCE IMPROVEMENT AND PATIENT SAFETY 235

EDUCATION AND RESEARCH 240
- EDUCATION 240
- RESEARCH 248

Environment of Care 255
Environmental Safety 255
Monitoring Elements for a Safe Care Environment 271
Cleaning, Disinfection, Sterilization of Medical Devices and Equipment 277
Cleaning, Disinfecting, and Sterilizing Practices 277
Single-Use and Reprocessed Devices 287
Levels of Disinfection/Sterilization 289
CBIC Practice Test 292
Answer Key and Explanations 318
How to Overcome Test Anxiety 346
Causes of Test Anxiety 346
Elements of Test Anxiety 347
Effects of Test Anxiety 347
Physical Steps for Beating Test Anxiety 348
Mental Steps for Beating Test Anxiety 349
Study Strategy 350
Test Tips 352
Important Qualification 353
Tell Us Your Story 354
Additional Bonus Material 355

Introduction

Thank you for purchasing this resource! You have made the choice to prepare yourself for a test that could have a huge impact on your future, and this guide is designed to help you be fully ready for test day. Obviously, it's important to have a solid understanding of the test material, but you also need to be prepared for the unique environment and stressors of the test, so that you can perform to the best of your abilities.

For this purpose, the first section that appears in this guide is the **Secret Keys**. We've devoted countless hours to meticulously researching what works and what doesn't, and we've boiled down our findings to the five most impactful steps you can take to improve your performance on the test. We start at the beginning with study planning and move through the preparation process, all the way to the testing strategies that will help you get the most out of what you know when you're finally sitting in front of the test.

We recommend that you start preparing for your test as far in advance as possible. However, if you've bought this guide as a last-minute study resource and only have a few days before your test, we recommend that you skip over the first two Secret Keys since they address a long-term study plan.

If you struggle with **test anxiety**, we strongly encourage you to check out our recommendations for how you can overcome it. Test anxiety is a formidable foe, but it can be beaten, and we want to make sure you have the tools you need to defeat it.

Secret Key #1 – Plan Big, Study Small

There's a lot riding on your performance. If you want to ace this test, you're going to need to keep your skills sharp and the material fresh in your mind. You need a plan that lets you review everything you need to know while still fitting in your schedule. We'll break this strategy down into three categories.

Information Organization

Start with the information you already have: the official test outline. From this, you can make a complete list of all the concepts you need to cover before the test. Organize these concepts into groups that can be studied together, and create a list of any related vocabulary you need to learn so you can brush up on any difficult terms. You'll want to keep this vocabulary list handy once you actually start studying since you may need to add to it along the way.

Time Management

Once you have your set of study concepts, decide how to spread them out over the time you have left before the test. Break your study plan into small, clear goals so you have a manageable task for each day and know exactly what you're doing. Then just focus on one small step at a time. When you manage your time this way, you don't need to spend hours at a time studying. Studying a small block of content for a short period each day helps you retain information better and avoid stressing over how much you have left to do. You can relax knowing that you have a plan to cover everything in time. In order for this strategy to be effective though, you have to start studying early and stick to your schedule. Avoid the exhaustion and futility that comes from last-minute cramming!

Study Environment

The environment you study in has a big impact on your learning. Studying in a coffee shop, while probably more enjoyable, is not likely to be as fruitful as studying in a quiet room. It's important to keep distractions to a minimum. You're only planning to study for a short block of time, so make the most of it. Don't pause to check your phone or get up to find a snack. It's also important to **avoid multitasking**. Research has consistently shown that multitasking will make your studying dramatically less effective. Your study area should also be comfortable and well-lit so you don't have the distraction of straining your eyes or sitting on an uncomfortable chair.

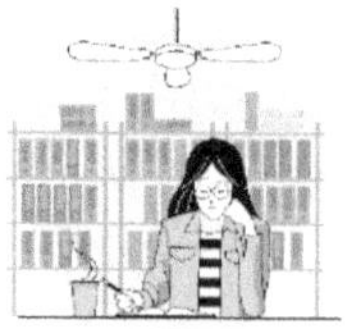

The time of day you study is also important. You want to be rested and alert. Don't wait until just before bedtime. Study when you'll be most likely to comprehend and remember. Even better, if you know what time of day your test will be, set that time aside for study. That way your brain will be used to working on that subject at that specific time and you'll have a better chance of recalling information.

Finally, it can be helpful to team up with others who are studying for the same test. Your actual studying should be done in as isolated an environment as possible, but the work of organizing the information and setting up the study plan can be divided up. In between study sessions, you can discuss with your teammates the concepts that you're all studying and quiz each other on the details. Just be sure that your teammates are as serious about the test as you are. If you find that your study time is being replaced with social time, you might need to find a new team.

Secret Key #2 – Make Your Studying Count

You're devoting a lot of time and effort to preparing for this test, so you want to be absolutely certain it will pay off. This means doing more than just reading the content and hoping you can remember it on test day. It's important to make every minute of study count. There are two main areas you can focus on to make your studying count.

Retention

It doesn't matter how much time you study if you can't remember the material. You need to make sure you are retaining the concepts. To check your retention of the information you're learning, try recalling it at later times with minimal prompting. Try carrying around flashcards and glance at one or two from time to time or ask a friend who's also studying for the test to quiz you.

To enhance your retention, look for ways to put the information into practice so that you can apply it rather than simply recalling it. If you're using the information in practical ways, it will be much easier to remember. Similarly, it helps to solidify a concept in your mind if you're not only reading it to yourself but also explaining it to someone else. Ask a friend to let you teach them about a concept you're a little shaky on (or speak aloud to an imaginary audience if necessary). As you try to summarize, define, give examples, and answer your friend's questions, you'll understand the concepts better and they will stay with you longer. Finally, step back for a big picture view and ask yourself how each piece of information fits with the whole subject. When you link the different concepts together and see them working together as a whole, it's easier to remember the individual components.

Finally, practice showing your work on any multi-step problems, even if you're just studying. Writing out each step you take to solve a problem will help solidify the process in your mind, and you'll be more likely to remember it during the test.

Modality

Modality simply refers to the means or method by which you study. Choosing a study modality that fits your own individual learning style is crucial. No two people learn best in exactly the same way, so it's important to know your strengths and use them to your advantage.

For example, if you learn best by visualization, focus on visualizing a concept in your mind and draw an image or a diagram. Try color-coding your notes, illustrating them, or creating symbols that will trigger your mind to recall a learned concept. If you learn best by hearing or discussing information, find a study partner who learns the same way or read aloud to yourself. Think about how to put the information in your own words. Imagine that you are giving a lecture on the topic and record yourself so you can listen to it later.

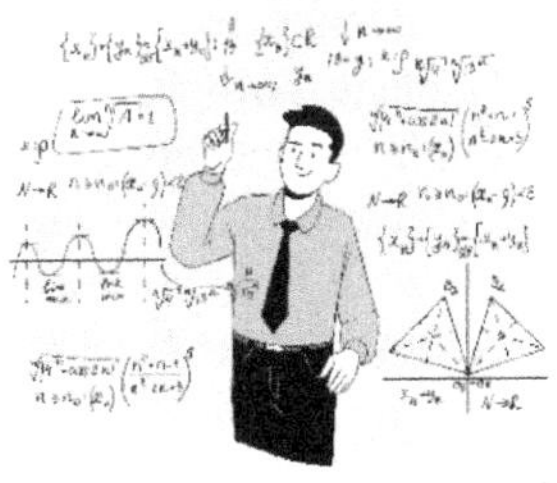

For any learning style, flashcards can be helpful. Organize the information so you can take advantage of spare moments to review. Underline key words or phrases. Use different colors for different categories. Mnemonic devices (such as creating a short list in which every item starts with the same letter) can also help with retention. Find what works best for you and use it to store the information in your mind most effectively and easily.

Secret Key #3 – Practice the Right Way

Your success on test day depends not only on how many hours you put into preparing, but also on whether you prepared the right way. It's good to check along the way to see if your studying is paying off. One of the most effective ways to do this is by taking practice tests to evaluate your progress. Practice tests are useful because they show exactly where you need to improve. Every time you take a practice test, pay special attention to these three groups of questions:

- The questions you got wrong
- The questions you had to guess on, even if you guessed right
- The questions you found difficult or slow to work through

This will show you exactly what your weak areas are, and where you need to devote more study time. Ask yourself why each of these questions gave you trouble. Was it because you didn't understand the material? Was it because you didn't remember the vocabulary? Do you need more repetitions on this type of question to build speed and confidence? Dig into those questions and figure out how you can strengthen your weak areas as you go back to review the material.

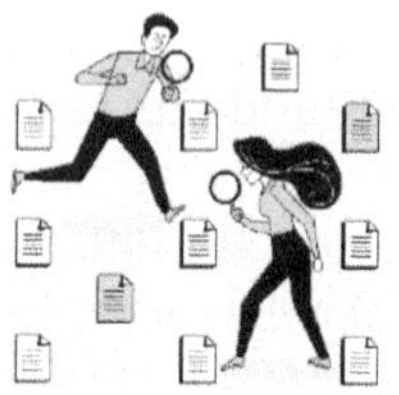

Additionally, many practice tests have a section explaining the answer choices. It can be tempting to read the explanation and think that you now have a good understanding of the concept. However, an explanation likely only covers part of the question's broader context. Even if the explanation makes perfect sense, **go back and investigate** every concept related to the question until you're positive you have a thorough understanding.

As you go along, keep in mind that the practice test is just that: practice. Memorizing these questions and answers will not be very helpful on the actual test because it is unlikely to have any of the same exact questions. If you only know the right answers to the sample questions, you won't be prepared for the real thing. **Study the concepts** until you understand them fully, and then you'll be able to answer any question that shows up on the test.

It's important to wait on the practice tests until you're ready. If you take a test on your first day of study, you may be overwhelmed by the amount of material covered and how much you need to learn. Work up to it gradually.

On test day, you'll need to be prepared for answering questions, managing your time, and using the test-taking strategies you've learned. It's a lot to balance, like a mental marathon that will have a big impact on your future. Like training for a marathon, you'll need to start slowly and work your way up. When test day arrives, you'll be ready.

Start with the strategies you've read in the first two Secret Keys—plan your course and study in the way that works best for you. If you have time, consider using multiple study resources to get different approaches to the same concepts. It can be helpful to see difficult concepts from more than one angle. Then find a good source for practice tests. Many times, the test website will suggest potential study resources or provide sample tests.

Practice Test Strategy

If you're able to find at least three practice tests, we recommend this strategy:

Untimed and Open-Book Practice

Take the first test with no time constraints and with your notes and study guide handy. Take your time and focus on applying the strategies you've learned.

Timed and Open-Book Practice

Take the second practice test open-book as well, but set a timer and practice pacing yourself to finish in time.

Timed and Closed-Book Practice

Take any other practice tests as if it were test day. Set a timer and put away your study materials. Sit at a table or desk in a quiet room, imagine yourself at the testing center, and answer questions as quickly and accurately as possible.

Keep repeating timed and closed-book tests on a regular basis until you run out of practice tests or it's time for the actual test. Your mind will be ready for the schedule and stress of test day, and you'll be able to focus on recalling the material you've learned.

Secret Key #4 – Pace Yourself

Once you're fully prepared for the material on the test, your biggest challenge on test day will be managing your time. Just knowing that the clock is ticking can make you panic even if you have plenty of time left. Work on pacing yourself so you can build confidence against the time constraints of the exam. Pacing is a difficult skill to master, especially in a high-pressure environment, so **practice is vital**.

Set time expectations for your pace based on how much time is available. For example, if a section has 60 questions and the time limit is 30 minutes, you know you have to average 30 seconds or less per question in order to answer them all. Although 30 seconds is the hard limit, set 25 seconds per question as your goal, so you reserve extra time to spend on harder questions. When you budget extra time for the harder questions, you no longer have any reason to stress when those questions take longer to answer.

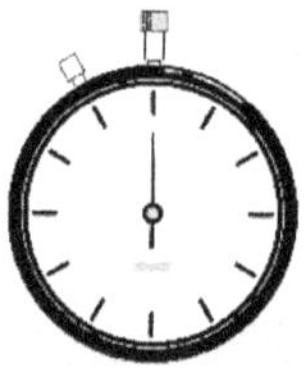

Don't let this time expectation distract you from working through the test at a calm, steady pace, but keep it in mind so you don't spend too much time on any one question. Recognize that taking extra time on one question you don't understand may keep you from answering two that you do understand later in the test. If your time limit for a question is up and you're still not sure of the answer, mark it and move on, and come back to it later if the time and the test format allow. If the testing format doesn't allow you to return to earlier questions, just make an educated guess; then put it out of your mind and move on.

On the easier questions, be careful not to rush. It may seem wise to hurry through them so you have more time for the challenging ones, but it's not worth missing one if you know the concept and just didn't take the time to read the question fully. Work efficiently but make sure you understand the question and have looked at all of the answer choices, since more than one may seem right at first.

Even if you're paying attention to the time, you may find yourself a little behind at some point. You should speed up to get back on track, but do so wisely. Don't panic; just take a few seconds less on each question until you're caught up. Don't guess without thinking, but do look through the answer choices and eliminate any you know are wrong. If you can get down to two choices, it is often worthwhile to guess from those. Once you've chosen an answer, move on and don't dwell on any that you skipped or had to hurry through. If a question was taking too long, chances are it was one of the harder ones, so you weren't as likely to get it right anyway.

On the other hand, if you find yourself getting ahead of schedule, it may be beneficial to slow down a little. The more quickly you work, the more likely you are to make a careless mistake that will affect your score. You've budgeted time for each question, so don't be afraid to spend that time. Practice an efficient but careful pace to get the most out of the time you have.

Secret Key #5 – Have a Plan for Guessing

When you're taking the test, you may find yourself stuck on a question. Some of the answer choices seem better than others, but you don't see the one answer choice that is obviously correct. What do you do?

The scenario described above is very common, yet most test takers have not effectively prepared for it. Developing and practicing a plan for guessing may be one of the single most effective uses of your time as you get ready for the exam.

In developing your plan for guessing, there are three questions to address:

- When should you start the guessing process?
- How should you narrow down the choices?
- Which answer should you choose?

When to Start the Guessing Process

Unless your plan for guessing is to select C every time (which, despite its merits, is not what we recommend), you need to leave yourself enough time to apply your answer elimination strategies. Since you have a limited amount of time for each question, that means that if you're going to give yourself the best shot at guessing correctly, you have to decide quickly whether or not you will guess.

Of course, the best-case scenario is that you don't have to guess at all, so first, see if you can answer the question based on your knowledge of the subject and basic reasoning skills. Focus on the key words in the question and try to jog your memory of related topics. Give yourself a chance to bring the knowledge to mind, but once you realize that you don't have (or you can't access) the knowledge you need to answer the question, it's time to start the guessing process.

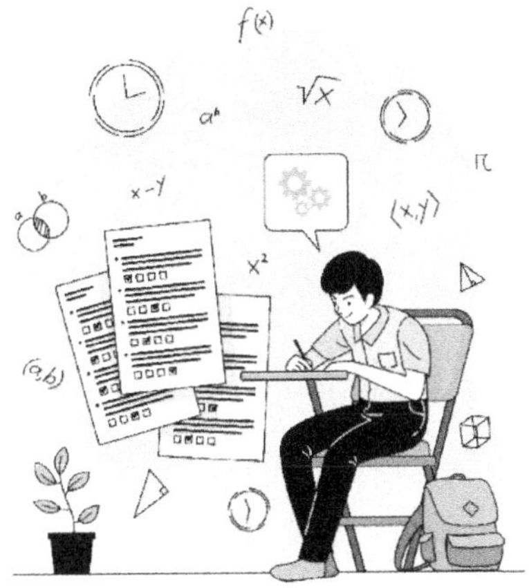

It's almost always better to start the guessing process too early than too late. It only takes a few seconds to remember something and answer the question from knowledge. Carefully eliminating wrong answer choices takes longer. Plus, going through the process of eliminating answer choices can actually help jog your memory.

Summary: Start the guessing process as soon as you decide that you can't answer the question based on your knowledge.

How to Narrow Down the Choices

The next chapter in this book (**Test-Taking Strategies**) includes a wide range of strategies for how to approach questions and how to look for answer choices to eliminate. You will definitely want to read those carefully, practice them, and figure out which ones work best for you. Here though, we're going to address a mindset rather than a particular strategy.

Your odds of guessing an answer correctly depend on how many options you are choosing from.

Number of options left	5	4	3	2	1
Odds of guessing correctly	20%	25%	33%	50%	100%

You can see from this chart just how valuable it is to be able to eliminate incorrect answers and make an educated guess, but there are two things that many test takers do that cause them to miss out on the benefits of guessing:

- Accidentally eliminating the correct answer
- Selecting an answer based on an impression

We'll look at the first one here, and the second one in the next section.

To avoid accidentally eliminating the correct answer, we recommend a thought exercise called **the $5 challenge**. In this challenge, you only eliminate an answer choice from contention if you are willing to bet $5 on it being wrong. Why $5? Five dollars is a small but not insignificant amount of money. It's an amount you could afford to lose but wouldn't want to throw away. And while losing $5 once might not hurt too much, doing it twenty times will set you back $100. In the same way, each small decision you make—eliminating a choice here, guessing on a question there—won't by itself impact your score very much, but when you put them all together, they can make a big difference. By holding each answer choice elimination decision to a higher standard, you can reduce the risk of accidentally eliminating the correct answer.

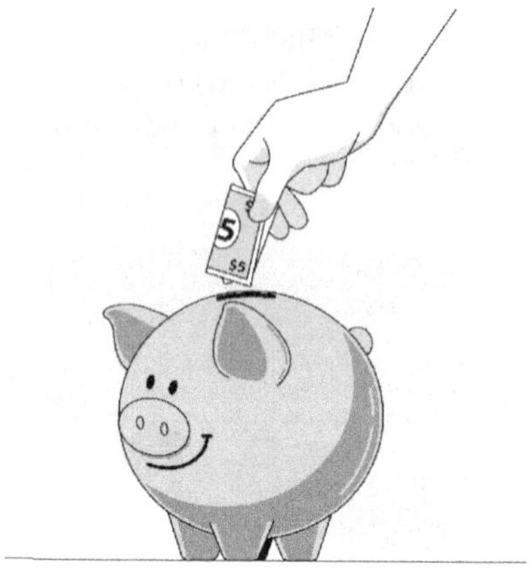

The $5 challenge can also be applied in a positive sense: If you are willing to bet $5 that an answer choice *is* correct, go ahead and mark it as correct.

Summary: Only eliminate an answer choice if you are willing to bet $5 that it is wrong.

Which Answer to Choose

You're taking the test. You've run into a hard question and decided you'll have to guess. You've eliminated all the answer choices you're willing to bet $5 on. Now you have to pick an answer. Why do we even need to talk about this? Why can't you just pick whichever one you feel like when the time comes?

The answer to these questions is that if you don't come into the test with a plan, you'll rely on your impression to select an answer choice, and if you do that, you risk falling into a trap. The test writers know that everyone who takes their test will be guessing on some of the questions, so they intentionally write wrong answer choices to seem plausible. You still have to pick an answer though, and if the wrong answer choices are designed to look right, how can you ever be sure that you're not falling for their trap? The best solution we've found to this dilemma is to take the decision out of your hands entirely. Here is the process we recommend:

Once you've eliminated any choices that you are confident (willing to bet $5) are wrong, select the first remaining choice as your answer.

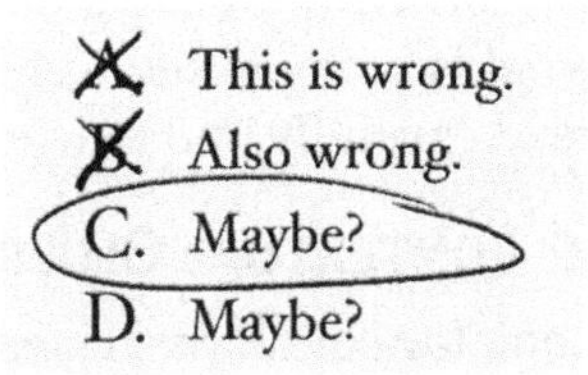

Whether you choose to select the first remaining choice, the second, or the last, the important thing is that you use some preselected standard. Using this approach guarantees that you will not be enticed into selecting an answer choice that looks right, because you are not basing your decision on how the answer choices look.

This is not meant to make you question your knowledge. Instead, it is to help you recognize the difference between your knowledge and your impressions. There's a huge difference between thinking an answer is right because of what you know, and thinking an answer is right because it looks or sounds like it should be right.

Summary: To ensure that your selection is appropriately random, make a predetermined selection from among all answer choices you have not eliminated.

Test-Taking Strategies

This section contains a list of test-taking strategies that you may find helpful as you work through the test. By taking what you know and applying logical thought, you can maximize your chances of answering any question correctly!

It is very important to realize that every question is different and every person is different: no single strategy will work on every question, and no single strategy will work for every person. That's why we've included all of them here, so you can try them out and determine which ones work best for different types of questions and which ones work best for you.

Question Strategies

☑ Read Carefully

Read the question and the answer choices carefully. Don't miss the question because you misread the terms. You have plenty of time to read each question thoroughly and make sure you understand what is being asked. Yet a happy medium must be attained, so don't waste too much time. You must read carefully and efficiently.

☑ Contextual Clues

Look for contextual clues. If the question includes a word you are not familiar with, look at the immediate context for some indication of what the word might mean. Contextual clues can often give you all the information you need to decipher the meaning of an unfamiliar word. Even if you can't determine the meaning, you may be able to narrow down the possibilities enough to make a solid guess at the answer to the question.

☑ Prefixes

If you're having trouble with a word in the question or answer choices, try dissecting it. Take advantage of every clue that the word might include. Prefixes and suffixes can be a huge help. Usually, they allow you to determine a basic meaning. *Pre-* means before, *post-* means after, *pro-* is positive, *de-* is negative. From prefixes and suffixes, you can get an idea of the general meaning of the word and try to put it into context.

☑ Hedge Words

Watch out for critical hedge words, such as *likely, may, can, sometimes, often, almost, mostly, usually, generally, rarely,* and *sometimes.* Question writers insert these hedge phrases to cover every possibility. Often an answer choice will be wrong simply because it leaves no room for exception. Be on guard for answer choices that have definitive words such as *exactly* and *always.*

☑ Switchback Words

Stay alert for *switchbacks.* These are the words and phrases frequently used to alert you to shifts in thought. The most common switchback words are *but, although,* and *however.* Others include *nevertheless, on the other hand, even though, while, in spite of, despite,* and *regardless of.* Switchback words are important to catch because they can change the direction of the question or an answer choice.

✓ Face Value

When in doubt, use common sense. Accept the situation in the problem at face value. Don't read too much into it. These problems will not require you to make wild assumptions. If you have to go beyond creativity and warp time or space in order to have an answer choice fit the question, then you should move on and consider the other answer choices. These are normal problems rooted in reality. The applicable relationship or explanation may not be readily apparent, but it is there for you to figure out. Use your common sense to interpret anything that isn't clear.

Answer Choice Strategies

✓ Answer Selection

The most thorough way to pick an answer choice is to identify and eliminate wrong answers until only one is left, then confirm it is the correct answer. Sometimes an answer choice may immediately seem right, but be careful. The test writers will usually put more than one reasonable answer choice on each question, so take a second to read all of them and make sure that the other choices are not equally obvious. As long as you have time left, it is better to read every answer choice than to pick the first one that looks right without checking the others.

✓ Answer Choice Families

An answer choice family consists of two (in rare cases, three) answer choices that are very similar in construction and cannot all be true at the same time. If you see two answer choices that are direct opposites or parallels, one of them is usually the correct answer. For instance, if one answer choice says that quantity *x* increases and another either says that quantity *x* decreases (opposite) or says that quantity *y* increases (parallel), then those answer choices would fall into the same family. An answer choice that doesn't match the construction of the answer choice family is more likely to be incorrect. Most questions will not have answer choice families, but when they do appear, you should be prepared to recognize them.

✓ Eliminate Answers

Eliminate answer choices as soon as you realize they are wrong, but make sure you consider all possibilities. If you are eliminating answer choices and realize that the last one you are left with is also wrong, don't panic. Start over and consider each choice again. There may be something you missed the first time that you will realize on the second pass.

✓ Avoid Fact Traps

Don't be distracted by an answer choice that is factually true but doesn't answer the question. You are looking for the choice that answers the question. Stay focused on what the question is asking for so you don't accidentally pick an answer that is true but incorrect. Always go back to the question and make sure the answer choice you've selected actually answers the question and is not merely a true statement.

✓ Extreme Statements

In general, you should avoid answers that put forth extreme actions as standard practice or proclaim controversial ideas as established fact. An answer choice that states the "process should be used in certain situations, if…" is much more likely to be correct than one that states the "process should be discontinued completely." The first is a calm rational statement and doesn't even make a definitive, uncompromising stance, using a hedge word *if* to provide wiggle room, whereas the second choice is far more extreme.

⊘ Benchmark

As you read through the answer choices and you come across one that seems to answer the question well, mentally select that answer choice. This is not your final answer, but it's the one that will help you evaluate the other answer choices. The one that you selected is your benchmark or standard for judging each of the other answer choices. Every other answer choice must be compared to your benchmark. That choice is correct until proven otherwise by another answer choice beating it. If you find a better answer, then that one becomes your new benchmark. Once you've decided that no other choice answers the question as well as your benchmark, you have your final answer.

⊘ Predict the Answer

Before you even start looking at the answer choices, it is often best to try to predict the answer. When you come up with the answer on your own, it is easier to avoid distractions and traps because you will know exactly what to look for. The right answer choice is unlikely to be word-for-word what you came up with, but it should be a close match. Even if you are confident that you have the right answer, you should still take the time to read each option before moving on.

General Strategies

⊘ Tough Questions

If you are stumped on a problem or it appears too hard or too difficult, don't waste time. Move on! Remember though, if you can quickly check for obviously incorrect answer choices, your chances of guessing correctly are greatly improved. Before you completely give up, at least try to knock out a couple of possible answers. Eliminate what you can and then guess at the remaining answer choices before moving on.

⊘ Check Your Work

Since you will probably not know every term listed and the answer to every question, it is important that you get credit for the ones that you do know. Don't miss any questions through careless mistakes. If at all possible, try to take a second to look back over your answer selection and make sure you've selected the correct answer choice and haven't made a costly careless mistake (such as marking an answer choice that you didn't mean to mark). This quick double check should more than pay for itself in caught mistakes for the time it costs.

⊘ Pace Yourself

It's easy to be overwhelmed when you're looking at a page full of questions; your mind is confused and full of random thoughts, and the clock is ticking down faster than you would like. Calm down and maintain the pace that you have set for yourself. Especially as you get down to the last few minutes of the test, don't let the small numbers on the clock make you panic. As long as you are on track by monitoring your pace, you are guaranteed to have time for each question.

⊘ Don't Rush

It is very easy to make errors when you are in a hurry. Maintaining a fast pace in answering questions is pointless if it makes you miss questions that you would have gotten right otherwise. Test writers like to include distracting information and wrong answers that seem right. Taking a little extra time to avoid careless mistakes can make all the difference in your test score. Find a pace that allows you to be confident in the answers that you select.

✓ Keep Moving

Panicking will not help you pass the test, so do your best to stay calm and keep moving. Taking deep breaths and going through the answer elimination steps you practiced can help to break through a stress barrier and keep your pace.

Final Notes

The combination of a solid foundation of content knowledge and the confidence that comes from practicing your plan for applying that knowledge is the key to maximizing your performance on test day. As your foundation of content knowledge is built up and strengthened, you'll find that the strategies included in this chapter become more and more effective in helping you quickly sift through the distractions and traps of the test to isolate the correct answer.

Now that you're preparing to move forward into the test content chapters of this book, be sure to keep your goal in mind. As you read, think about how you will be able to apply this information on the test. If you've already seen sample questions for the test and you have an idea of the question format and style, try to come up with questions of your own that you can answer based on what you're reading. This will give you valuable practice applying your knowledge in the same ways you can expect to on test day.

Good luck and good studying!

Identification of Infectious Disease Processes

Diagnostic, Radiologic, Procedural, and Laboratory Reports

Testing Sensitivity and Specificity in Terms of True/False Test Results

Testing results can present as follows:

- **True-positive (TP)**: The test is positive, and the patient has the disease.
- **False-positive (FP):** The test is positive but the patient does not have the disease.
- **True-negative (TN):** The test is negative, and the patient does not have the disease.
- **False-negative (FN):** The test is negative, but the patient does have the disease.

Test sensitivity measures a screening test's ability to correctly identify the presence of a disease. It is the ratio of tests with positive outcomes to the total number of affected (true positive) patients tested. **Test specificity** measures a screening test's ability to correctly identify the absence of disease.

Level of sensitivity	The probability of a **positive** test result when a patient **has** the disease	**Ratio**: TP/(TP+FN)
Degree of specificity	The probability of a **negative** test result when a patient **does not have** the disease	**Ratio**: TN/(TN+FP)
Positive predictive value	The probability that a patient **has** the disease when the patient has tested **positive**	**Ratio**: TP/(TP+FP)
Negative predictive value	The probability that a patient **does not have** the disease when the patient has tested **negative**	**Ratio**: TN/(TN+FN)

Gram Staining

Named after the Danish bacteriologist who devised it in 1882, the **Gram stain** is almost always the first test performed for the identification of bacteria. Both crystal violet and methylene blue are equally effective for staining microorganisms that can commonly be classified as Gram-positive or Gram non-negative. Others that are not stained by crystal violet are referred to as Gram negative and appear red. Some organisms are Gram-non-reactive, either staining poorly or not at all. Others are Gram-variable, staining in an uneven fashion.

Other staining methods are available to visualize components that might otherwise be too difficult to see under a light microscope, used to reveal other microorganisms not readily visualized by the Gram stain, such as mycobacteria, rickettsia, spirochetes, and others.

Use for Diagnosis of Infectious Process

A Gram stain begins with mounting and fixing a specimen on a slide. The specimen is then "stained" as part of a 4-part process that uses dyes to stain Gram-positive bacteria purple and Gram-negative bacteria pink. The process must be done correctly or results can give false positives or negatives. The slide is examined microscopically for white blood cells and bacteria that indicate an infection. The size, shape, and color-stain of the bacteria help to identify it. Gram stains can be done very quickly, usually within an hour. One reason that Gram stains are done prior to cultures is to determine if the specimen is contaminated. For example, if epithelial skin cells are present in a sputum specimen, the specimen may be rejected for culture.

Gram stains during the culture procedure should use young cultures of less than 18 hours as older cultures of some Gram-positive bacteria may give the appearance of Gram-negative organisms.

Ziehl-Neelsen Acid-Fast Stain Testing

Acid-fast bacteria, a type of bacteria that will stain **Gram-positive**, retain the **Ziehl-Neelsen acid-fast stain's** bright red color as a result of the components of their cell walls being thick and composed of approximately 60 percent lipid and less peptidoglycan than other organisms. The stain is used to detect tuberculosis-causing and leprosy-causing organisms (genus *Mycobacterium*).

Complete Blood Count (CBC)

The complete blood count with differential and platelet (thrombocyte) count provides information about blood and other body systems and is an important part of the diagnosis of infectious processes. Red blood cell (erythrocyte) counts and concentrations may vary with anemia, hemorrhage, or various disorders but are not usually an indicator of infection. Platelets may increase from a normal of 150,000-400,000 to over a million during acute infection.

White Blood Cell Count

White blood cell (leukocyte) count is an important indicator of bacterial and viral infection. An increase in WBCs above 10,000 mm^3 (leukocytosis) is typical of acute infections, with the amount of increase related to the severity of the infection, the age of the person, and the amount of resistance. Pregnancy can also increase the white blood count to up to 15,000 mm^3.

WBC is reported as the total number of all white blood cells.

- Normal WBC for non-pregnant adults: 4,800-10,000
- Acute infection: 10,000+; 30,000 indicates a severe infection
- Viral infection: 4,000 and below

Differential

The differential provides the percentage of each different type of leukocyte. An increase in the white blood cell count is usually related to an increase in one type and often an increase in immature neutrophils, known as bands, referred to as a "shift to the left." The increase is described according to the type of cell with the primary increase, so a primary increase in lymphocytes is lymphocytosis. Before computerized reports, when laboratory slips were written by hand, the practice was to write the values for the differential from left to right in this order:

- Bands (immature neutrophils)
- Segs (mature segmented neutrophils)
- Eosinophils
- Basophils
- Lymphocytes
- Monocytes

When one value increases, another decreases. With infection, the percentage of bands (the first on the left) often increases, thus resulting in the **shift to the left** because as the percentage of bands increases, the percentage of segs decreases.

Normal Values

The differential report for immature neutrophils, segmented neutrophils, eosinophils, basophils, lymphocytes, and monocytes are expressed for each as a percentage of the total white blood cell count.

Cell Type	Influencing Factors
Immature Neutrophils Normal: 1-3%	Increase without leukocytosis but with massive infection is a degenerative shift. The prognosis with this type of shift is poor because immature cells are overwhelming the blood. Increase with leukocytosis and with infection is a regenerative shift. The prognosis for this type of shift is good.
Segmented Neutrophils Normal: 50-62%	Increase with acute, localized, or systemic bacterial infection. Decrease with acute bacterial infection (poor prognosis) and viral infections. *Additional factors that affect results*: Stress, exercise, and obstetric labor can increase neutrophils. Steroids can affect the levels of neutrophils for up to 24 hours. Increases or decreases in eosinophils can affect percentage rate of neutrophils.
Eosinophils Normal: 0-3%	Increase than greater than 5% with allergic response and parasitic diseases. Decrease with bodily stress and acute infection. *Additional factors that affect results*: Eosinophil counts are lowest in the morning with rates rising until after midnight, so repeat tests should be done at the same time each day. Stress-inducing burns, surgery, or labor can decrease the count. Some drugs, including steroids, epinephrine, and thyroxine affect levels. Increases or decreases in basophils, monocytes, and lymphocytes affect percentage rate of eosinophils.
Basophils Normal: 0-1%	Increase with blood histamines, infection. Decrease during acute stage of infection.
Lymphocytes Normal: 25-40%	Increase in some viral and bacterial infections, such as TB. Decrease with AIDS.
Monocytes Normal: 3-7%	Increase during recovery stage of acute infection.

Magnetic Resonance Imaging (MRI) and Endoscopic Procedures

Magnetic resonance imaging (MRI) may be done with or without contrast material. It uses radio waves and magnetic fields to create images of internal structures, providing information about infections that may not be obvious with x-rays, CT scans, or ultrasounds. It is especially helpful for assessing infection of the abdominal and pelvic areas. MRIs are more expensive than x-rays, CTs, or ultrasounds so they are often done after other testing has been inconclusive.

Endoscopic procedures using a flexible endoscope inserted through the mouth (for the esophagus, stomach, and small intestine), anus (for the rectum and colon), vagina (for the vagina, cervix, and uterus), or urethra (for the urethra, bladder, and ureters), are used to visualize internal structures, such as the lining of the GI tract and the urinary tract. Endoscopes are equipped with small clippers that allow for biopsies of tissue so that it can be evaluated for infection or mutations indicative of cancer. Endoscopes pose the risk of spreading infection.

X-RAYS, ULTRASOUNDS, AND COMPUTED TOMOGRAPHY (CT) SCANS

X-rays are commonly used to detect infections in the lung. Chest x-rays show areas of consolidation (indicated by dense areas of white) that are often indicative of infection with purulent material present (pneumonia), especially in those with cough and fever.

Ultrasounds are especially helpful for the evaluation of cellulitis of soft tissue to determine if there is an abscess that may not be clinically evident.

Computed tomography (CT) scans may be done with fluoroscopy or contrast material, such as iodine dye, to evaluate for infections. CT scans can differentiate between cellulitis and the formation of abscesses better than a routine x-ray. Chest scans can evaluate the organs and tissues of the chest for infection, abdominal scans can detect abscesses and infection, and urinary tract scans can detect infection in the kidney or bladder. A CT scan can also be used to determine the best insertion point for a needle into an abscess to affect drainage.

NEEDLE ASPIRATIONS AND TISSUE BIOPSIES

Needle aspirations, which may be completed with ultrasound or CT scan guidance, are done to aspirate serous or purulent material to relieve pressure and for culture and evaluation of infection. Needle aspirations are less invasive than biopsies and may be used with puncture wounds where there is little surface tissue loss. Multiple samples may need to be aspirated or the needle position changed, resulting in discomfort for the patient. Premedicating for pain management is recommended when possible. Fine needle aspiration may be used to biopsy infected tissue.

Biopsy of infected tissue may be done under a local anesthetic with a small amount of tissue excised to be examined microscopically, tested, and cultured. Some antiseptics like ethyl alcohol might kill the bacteria and affect resultant cultures. Biopsies may be done because visual inspection alone may not always be effective in determining if infection is present, as infection may be present even without classic signs of infection, such as erythema and swelling.

CULTURES

Cultures in which a sample is grown on a nutrient-rich media may be done with oxygen (aerobic) or without (anaerobic), as indicated or ordered by the physician. After the organism is cultured, sensitivity tests are usually completed to determine which anti-infective agents are most successful in treating the particular pathogenic microorganism. A Gram stain is usually done initially, and then the culture is checked every 24 hours for colonization. Colonies are checked again with Gram stains and also transferred to a separate media for further observation and testing. Cultures are usually negative if there is no growth in 48-72 hours unless there is a very slow growing bacterium or fungus, which may need 4-6 weeks before final results are available. If antibiotics are begun prior to taking a sample for a culture, this can alter the results, making it very difficult to isolate the infective agent, so it is advised to obtain the culture first and then begin antibiotics.

Culture Media

Culture media come in different types:

- **Differential medium**: With this type of medium, an investigator may distinguish types of bacteria because of traits displayed in their growth patterns in that medium.
- **Selective, differential medium**: Used in the isolation of *Staphylococcus aureus,* the most common virulent bacterial agent attacking humans. The medium contains a very high concentration of a material that the pathogen being tested will tolerate but that inhibits most other bacteria. A fermenting material is then chosen that will further allow differentiation of the microorganism by the way it reacts.
- **Enrichment medium**: This uses a medium with a selective growth component, something that selectivity resembles a nutrient from their own environment that only the microorganism in question can process.

Selective Culture Media

A selective medium has components added to it which will inhibit or prevent the growth of certain types or species of bacteria in the lab. In addition, or as an alternative, it may promote the growth of desired species. One can also adjust the physical conditions of a culture medium, such as pH and temperature, to render it selective for organisms that are able to grow under these certain conditions.

Newer selective culture media with enhanced selectivity are under constant development around the world. Tergitol-4 in XLT-4 Agar, for example, enables easier and faster diagnosis of salmonellosis, a task which is often complicated by the presence of background flora and other Enterobacteriaceae on an agar plate. Chemical and pH changes within the medium allow *Salmonella* spp. (black colonies) to be differentiated from organisms such as *E. coli* (yellow colonies) and *Shigella* spp. (red colonies).

Culture Plate Media and Incubation

USP recommends conducting sampling using the appropriate non-selective medium based on the test requirements. Examples include malt extract agar or trypticase soy agar (TSA). When using malt extract for fungi culture, incubate at 20-25 °C for up to 7 days; for bacteria, yeast, and mold, incubate at 22.5 °C (± 2.5 °C) or 32.5 °C (±2.5 °C) for 48-72 hours. TSA media should be incubated at 30-35 °C for 48 hours.

Most importantly, the plate media, incubation temperature, and sample time should be consistent to ensure accurate comparison of data. The decision to change culture media should be phased in gradually and include side-by-side plate sampling for data comparison. Media may also be selected to assess specific microbiological species (e.g., Gram-negative or Gram-positive bacteria).

Sputum Cultures

Sputum cultures are done to determine if there is a bacterium or fungus infection of the lungs or respiratory passages. Sterile specimen containers must be used, and people must be cautioned to avoid mouthwashes that could have antiseptic properties. It is important to make sure that the specimen is coughed up and does not consist of just saliva. A sample may be obtained with a bronchoscopy as well, or via endotracheal tube suction for patients that are intubated. Viruses are frequent causes of respiratory infections, so special viral cultures, in which the sputum is mixed in a test tube with specially prepared animal cells, are often done, requiring days to weeks for final results. Various special culture procedures may be done with sputum to isolate infective agents. Cultures are not effective diagnostic tools for all types of organisms; for example, *Pneumocystis jirovecii*, a common cause of pneumonia in those with depressed immune system, cannot be isolated and grown in culture and must be identified by special stains.

Blood and Wound Cultures

Blood cultures, using a small sample of blood, are done to determine if an infection has invaded the bloodstream from the original site of infection, causing the infection to spread. It is also used to determine the type of bacterium or fungus and sensitivity to anti-infective agents so that proper treatment can be initiated. In many cases, if infection is present, treatment may be started before the culture results and then reevaluated and changed as necessary when the sensitivities are complete. It is important that the skin be carefully cleansed so that the sample is not contaminated by microbes on the surface of the skin.

Wound swab cultures are done by taking swabs of wound exudate from infected tissue. The swab technique usually results in the smallest sample size so the infective agent may not grow in the culture. It is also easy to contaminate the specimen with normal bacterial skin flora or foreign materials in the case of dirty wounds.

Stool Cultures

Stool cultures are done to detect bacteria or other organisms in the stool, resulting from infection of the gastrointestinal tract. Stool samples are collected in a sterile container and must not be contaminated by toilet water or other materials, such as urine; therefore, stools cannot be retrieved from the toilet. Stool specimens are often obtained on three separate days. Most intestinal infections are the result of bacteria, but fungi and viruses may also be implicated. Stool cultures are important to diagnose *Shigella, Salmonella, Campylobacter, Yersinia,* and *Clostridium difficile. Clostridium difficile* may result from treatment with certain antibiotics. In the case of some bacteria, such as *Clostridium difficile*, the stool culture is done to identify the particular toxin produced by a bacterium. Fungal infections, such as *Candida*, may occur in those who are immune-suppressed; additionally, these same patients are also susceptible to infection with viruses, such as cytomegalovirus, so fungal and viral cultures must be done.

Antigen and Antibody Detection Tests

Antigens are proteins of a virus or bacteria while antibodies are compounds that develop in response to antigens. Antigens are found on the surface of infective agents and antibodies in serum. A typical example of a test is the enzyme-linked immunosorbent assay (ELISA), which has an enzyme that is linked to a particular antigen or antibody so that it can detect a specific type of protein associated with the infective agent. The direct fluorescent antibodies (DFA) test uses antibodies tagged with fluorescent dye, to detect antigens. These tagged antibodies are added to a specimen and the antibodies attach to particular antigens, allowing for indirect identification when fluorescence is found upon microscopic examination. Each type of antigen has a particular shape, and only the antibodies that match that shape can attach to it, causing the fluorescent reaction and indicating that infection is present. However, some antigens have similar structure, and antibodies may attach to the wrong antigen, giving a false positive.

Urine Testing

Urinalysis

Urinalysis evaluates the following properties of a urine sample:

- **pH** usually ranges between 4.5-8 with the average 5-6. Medications, such as Mandelamine, some foods (such as cranberries), and Vitamin C may make urine acidic (pH of less than 7). An alkaline urine (pH above 7) occurs with bacteriuria, urinary tract infections, as well as kidney and respiratory diseases.
- **Sediment** is examined microscopically: *Red cell casts* indicate acute infections, *broad casts* indicate kidney disorders, and *white cell casts* indicate pyelonephritis. *Leukocytes* >10 per mcL are present with urinary tract infections. Crystals should be absent.
- **Glucose, ketones, protein, blood, bilirubin, and nitrate** should be negative.
- **Urobilinogen** should be 0.1-1.0 units. Urine glucose may increase with infection (with normal blood glucose). Frank blood may be caused by some parasites and diseases but also by drugs, smoking, excessive exercise, and menstrual fluids. Increased red blood cells in the urine may result from infections of the lower urinary tract.
- **Color** is usually pale yellow/amber and darkens when urine is concentrated, but some foods (beets), medications, stress, exercise, or excessive fluid intake may affect color. Abnormal color may be caused by blood (red), bilirubin (yellow-green), fever (dark amber/orange due to dehydration), or diseases (various colors).
- **Appearance** should be clear but may be slightly cloudy. While cloudy urine may indicate infection with pus or blood present, it can also be related to foods, vaginal contamination, and degree of hydration.
- **Odor** should be slight, but foods, such as asparagus and medications, such as estrogen, may affect odor. Bacteria may give urine a foul smell, depending upon the organism.
- **Specific gravity** is usually about 1.015 to 1.025, but may increase if protein levels increase or if there is fever, vomiting, or dehydration present. Radiopaque contrast material as well as dextrose infusions may affect specific gravity.

Urine Culture and Sensitivities

Urine culture and sensitivities are done to identify infective agents. Results should show fewer than 10,000 organisms/mL of urine. Bacteria found are the result of pathogenic microorganisms or contamination from skin. Counts higher than 10,000 are considered diagnostic for infection. Urine is easily contaminated if clean catch procedures (wiping the area with cleansing pads and capturing the urine mid-stream) are not followed carefully and/or if people have poor hygiene. Urine specimens taken from individuals with a urinary catheter can only be taken immediately upon insertion of a new catheter (from the catheter port, not the collection bag), as catheters can begin to collect bacteria within the bag and tubing over time (hence them being a general risk for infection).

Urine may be too dilute for accurate culture if patients have a large fluid intake. Urine left at room temperature may begin to grow organisms so the results are not accurate. Urine should not be refrigerated more than 2 hours before testing. Urine intended for testing for cytomegalovirus must not be refrigerated. When a urinary tract infection is suspected, samples for culture should be collected in a cup with boric acid or stored at 4 °C because either procedure inhibits growth of contaminant bacteria until the specimen gets to the laboratory, avoiding the possibility of giving a false reading. Urinary cultures are positive for urine infection if the organism is found on Gram stain and if two urine cultures isolate the same organism with >102 colonies/mL of urine in catheterized specimens or <105 colonies/mL of urine with patients receiving appropriate antibiotics.

Urine Dipstick Test for Leukocyte Esterase and/or Nitrate

The urine dipstick test for leukocyte esterase and/or nitrate is used as a quick and inexpensive test to identify purulent material or bacteria in urine. However, this test is most predictive if there are high levels of bacteria. The test for nitrate is more accurate than that for leukocyte esterase, and dipsticks that combine the two are the most accurate. While false positives are unlikely, false negatives may occur when testing for nitrates if there is diuresis that has reduced the level of nitrates in the urine, inadequate nitrates in the diet, or infections caused by *enterococci* and *acinetobacter* because these pathogens do not produce nitrates. Therefore, a high nitrate level is usually indicative of a urinary infection but the absence does not preclude a urinary tract infection. Because of false negatives, a negative dipstick check should be confirmed through urinalysis that includes microscopic examination in the presence of symptoms.

Isolating Disease-Producing Microorganisms from Mixed Bacterial Populations

Isolate microorganisms from mixed populations by doing the following:

- Inoculate and streak specimens directly onto agar-coated plates.
- Selectively inhibit them with antimicrobial drugs or aniline dyes, table salt, or other inhibitory agents.
- Use capillary electrophoresis (CE) with narrow-bore fused-silica capillaries.
- Use capillary zone electrophoresis (CZE) to resolve bacteria into discrete electrophoretic bands.
- Employ selective medium containing lactate and inorganic salts when counting *Desulfovibrio* in soil or water.

Isolating and identifying many of the disease producing microorganisms spread through fecally-contaminated water is not always feasible, so indicator organisms, coliforms or streptococci that are generally present in water containing the pathogens, are used to detect the possible presence of enteric pathogens.

Sampling at Regular Intervals

A patient's blood, sputum, urine, or stool samples may be collected at regular intervals over hours or days. This is primarily to recover microorganisms for diagnostic purposes or follow the patient's progress. Likewise, air and water can be sampled for microorganisms in the air or water to check for pathogens and their flow.

Sampling is done at intervals because there may be insufficient colonization at any particular stage of an infection or contamination to collect sufficient microorganisms. Another reason is that periodic collection can build a picture of the stages of disease or contamination based on the changing populations of pathogens revealed. If multiple, periodic samples are taken after treatment has begun, the purpose is to show whether a particular course of action is effective based on the evidence of observable destruction of pathogens.

Difficulties in Obtaining Rapid Confirmation of Communicable Diseases

Positive confirmation of a communicable disease like whooping cough, Legionnaire's, bird flu, tuberculosis or SARS is gained by culturing samples taken from patients who are suspected of being infected. Waiting to see if the bacteria (or virus, in the case of SARS) grow can take weeks. There are now newer, faster ways of **establishing confirmation through sensitive molecular tests**. However, they are in their early stages and too often are providing erroneous results.

Many of the new molecular tests give rapid results but are technically demanding, and each laboratory may do them in its own way; there are no good estimates of their error rates. But their very sensitivity makes false positives likely.

Culture Contamination

Anywhere from 10-60 percent of all cell cultures may be contaminated with Mycoplasma which, because of its miniscule size (0.15 μm), can pass through filters used to sterilize tissue culture reagents. Mycoplasma contamination may never be eradicated, since they are immune to the usual antibiotics that work by attacking cell walls—something which Mycoplasma lacks.

Tissue cultures are vulnerable to contamination through a number of routes:

- Careless handling of pipettes or flasks
- Dust from skin, hair, or clothing
- Aerosols from talking or coughing
- Dirty or ineffectively sterilized storage conditions
- Other instruments

Often the contamination is not immediately apparent, lacking visible turbidity or changes in pH and erroneous data can be the result because prokaryotes change nucleic acid syntheses, membrane antigenicity, growth rate, interferon production, enzyme kinetics, and cellular metabolism.

Limitations and Advantages of Tests for Diagnosing Infectious Diseases

Though imaging may be used to research the effects of a given pathogen or toxin on the human body, for clinical studies or in response to an outbreak, laboratory tests of blood, stool, or sputum samples are the investigations of choice. Most responses are rapid, though in some cases (particularly with bacterial and fungal infections) incubation becomes necessary, slowing down the process of establishing the source of illness.

However, testing often fails to contribute to the diagnostic process while increasing patient risk and the expense of medical care. Modern laboratory tests and imaging studies are often mistakenly stressed while history and physical examination are downgraded as effective tools of clinical assessment.

Colonization, Infection, and Pseudo Infections

Colonization

Colonization occurs when a pathogenic microorganism invades tissue or the surface of a different species but causes either no reaction or only a slight reaction. Colonization is the first step in the infective process and usually begins with tissue in contact with the external environment and is often associated with the normal flora found on the skin. In colonization, replication does not usually occur or does not occur enough to cause infection. Colonization is present in almost all multi-cellular organisms. Colonization may be temporary or long-term and may result in the host becoming a carrier and shedding the microorganism, and thus infecting others (such as with Methicillin-resistant *Staphylococcus* infections [MRSA]). Colonization frequently occurs in portals of entry, such as the respiratory tract, the genitourinary tract, or the gastrointestinal tract. Other common sites for colonization include the nares and axillae as well as tissues that are compromised, such as open wounds.

Routes of Colonization of Upper Respiratory Tract

There are several ways microbes can reach and colonize the **upper respiratory tract**, including the following:

- **Gastropulmonary route:** Endogenous pathogens travel through the stomach to colonize the oropharynx and trachea.
- **Rectopulmonary route**: Intestinal microorganisms travel externally from the patient's anus to the upper respiratory tract, usually transmitted by the patient's or a healthcare worker's poor sanitary practices.
- **Exogenous (Cross-colonization):** Pathogens transferred through exogenous sources, such as nurses or doctors handling the catheters of ventilation equipment, directly into the tracheobronchial tree.

Colonization of Indwelling Vascular Catheters

Vascular catheters factor into the majority of nosocomial (healthcare-associated) cases of septicemia from *Staphylococcus epidermidis, Staphylococcus aureus,* and *Candida* species, septicemia being the most frequent life-threatening complication of vascular catheters.

Such infections may be the result of colonization, the multiplication of microorganisms at a specific site, in this case, an indwelling vascular catheter on the endo-luminal surface or the external surface of the catheter under the skin. But colonization, rather than leading directly to infection, could just as well be a means for transmitting the infection, so catheter colonization should be confirmed by a semi-quantitative culture of catheter segments growing at least 15 colony-forming units or, by quantitative culture, of at least 100 colony-forming units.

Infection

Infection occurs when a microorganism (virus, bacterium, parasite, viroid, fungus, prion, or other species foreign to the host) passes into a host, then invades, colonizes, and multiplies. Transmission occurs via carriers (people infected with the agent), water, food, airborne inhalation, vectors, or other species.

Immunity normally produces an adequate response to repel invading agents by producing antibodies. If, despite this, the host contracts the disease, it could be because defenses were weakened by deficiencies in immune factors; alternatively, a microorganism's inherent properties might overwhelm a host's defenses through cell destruction or toxin release.

Equation of Infection

The equation of infection is one of several predictive tools used in disease control to calculate interactions between an agent, host, and environment to determine the probability of infection. With quantitative values assigned to each of these factors, the equation looks at the size of the toxic dose that must be transmitted to a host, the host's site of contact with the toxic agent, the duration of contact, the degree of virulence of the agent (the fundamental element of a microorganism that permits infection), and all defenses marshaled by the host to block the invasion to produce an estimate of how probable an infection will be.

Types of Infection

In order for an infection to occur, it must invade the host, which can be done in various means depending on the type of infection:

- **Airborne infections** result from inhalation of pathogenic microorganisms (such as from dust particles) into the respiratory system.
- **Droplet/Aerosol infections** result from inhalation into the respiratory system of pathogenic microorganisms carried in droplets exhaled by others who are already infected (such as from coughing).
- **Endogenous infections** result from dormant pathogenic microorganisms reactivating within the host body (such as from tuberculosis).
- **Subcutaneous/tunnel infections** result from invasion by pathogenic microorganism of the subcutaneous tissue of an artificial opening (such as a stoma or wound).
- **Opportunistic infections** result from pathogenic microorganisms that usually cause no infection but overgrow and invade tissue in response to suppression of the immune system from a variety of conditions, including chemotherapy, antibiotic therapy, and autoimmune disorders (such as AIDS, HIV infection).

Causes of Infection

Everyone will contract some kind of infection at some time, but various factors elevate the probability at any point:

- **Exposure**: For most diseases, brief exposure to a pathogen is all that's needed for an infection to develop.
- **Sufficiency**: Quantities and strength of the pathogen necessary to cause infection vary with the nature of the agent and characteristics of the host.
- **Setting**: In a hospital a mild exposure may be enough to cause infection as the patient is probably already in a weakened state, plus hospitals are full of sick people with plenty of disease agents to be transmitted.
- **Risk factors**: For example, women have a greater risk of developing kidney infection, in part because of their anatomy.

Conditions Necessary for the Survival of an Infectious Agent

A microorganism must possess certain **genetic properties for survival**:

- Defenses against environmental hazards threatening its life
- The capability for reproducing itself
- The ability to compete with enemies who are intent on their own survival

It must remain viable until it has made sufficient contact with a host to bring about infection, and its survival and effectiveness are dependent upon how it is programmed to achieve those goals. A "hit and run" virus evades destruction by jumping from host to host. "Hit and stay viruses" survive through programming for sequestration blockading antigens, evading natural killer cells, escaping from apoptosis, and undergoing antigenic change.

Reservoirs

A reservoir is anywhere than an infectious agent can take up residence and be safe from enemies. It is a friendly habitat in which the agent can live, grow, and multiply before infecting a host. Whatever proves welcoming to the agent (be it human, animal, plant, soil, or substance), may serve as a reservoir, harboring the infectious agent, sometimes with little or no injury to itself. Even a host can serve as a reservoir if it can somehow transfer the agent to another host. Primary reservoirs in healthcare include medical workers, patients, and even operational hospital units like food service.

Medical instruments like dialysis machines, catheters, and Ommaya reservoirs (a type of intraventricular catheter system) can harbor agents. Infections from such instruments usually appear rather quickly, and late onset of infection from devices are rare; however, a case of *Staphylococcus aureus* was reported in a patient seven years after the use of an Ommaya reservoir.

Pathogenesis

Pathogenesis, the mechanism by which a certain agent causes disease, consists of two stages: early pathogenesis, an incubation period that sometimes finishes with *prodrome*, after which the second stage kicks in with discernible early lesions or other specific symptom complexes that enable diagnosis of the clinical disease via laboratory or other tests.

During **early pathogenesis**, the agent becomes established and physiological changes begin. The time between the exposure to an agent and the first appearance of clinical symptoms is the **incubation period** when, although there are no symptoms, the organism may be causing substantial damage. There may a period when non-specific signs and symptoms appear such as headache, fever, and lethargy; this is known as the **prodrome**. Illness, disability, defect, chronic state, complete recovery, residual defect/disability, and/or death may follow. If the infection abates, a **period of resolution** occurs, where the severity of the symptoms gradually decreases.

Prepathogenesis

Prepathogenesis (literally, "before disease is generated") is that period which immediately proceeds the moment when a disease infects the host, this usually (unless the host is suffering some other illness) being a period of health. During **prepathogenesis**, there is usually equilibrium between host, agent, and environment, which is broken when the agent invades the host.

- **Susceptibility**: During this first stage of prepathogenesis, the disease has not developed, but factors favor an uninterrupted march to the full disease.
- **Period of adaptation**: The host has either had a successful (for the host) or unsuccessful response to the pathogen; if successful, no disease will occur and the process will stop.
- **Incubation**: Should disease occur, there will be this period during which the microorganism multiplies to the point of producing a reaction in the host.
- **Clinical symptoms**: The last stage of prepathogenesis. The incubation period ends with either the death of the pathogen or the disease being detected, either clinically or through experience.

STAGES OF PATHOGENESIS

Pathogenesis is the cellular responses and other pathological events involved in the infectious process. A pathogenic organism must find a means of **transmission** from a reservoir to gain access to the host. Once entry is achieved, in order to grow and replicate, the microorganism must attach, through a mechanism called **adherence**, so that it can become established within the host. Some will then use adhesions to attach to a cell for the purpose of entering inside of the cell. This can cause infection in just one type of cell or, in some cases, generalized infection. Microorganisms can cause localized infection, but some emit toxins that can cause disseminated or distant infection or cell damage. Microorganisms produce a variety of **chemicals**, including toxins, to help them gain control. The invading microorganism must **evade** the immune system, which mounts a defense to protect the body. Once entrenched, the microorganism then **transmits** to a new host.

IMPACT OF BIOFILM ON PATHOGENESIS

A **biofilm** is a community of a variety of bacteria and other pathogens that have banded together to form a structure held together by polysaccharide "glue." The biofilm protects the bacteria, providing increased resistance to antibiotics. Additionally, the lack of available nutrients in the biofilm forces the microorganisms to grow more slowly, making them less sensitive to antibiotics that target cells that grow fast. The stress involved in living in the biofilm causes bacteria to release acids and proteins that counteract the antibiotics and confuse the host's immune system. Biofilms have free-roaming bacteria that emerge and circulate, and these are susceptible to antibiotics, but once the drugs stop, new free-roaming bacteria emerge and the infection flares up again. Once a biofilm is established in the body, it is very difficult to treat. Many chronic infections are related to biofilms, especially with gum disease, urinary and bone infections. Invasive medical devices, such as central venous catheters and prosthesis, are common sites for biofilms.

IMPACT OF HUMORAL IMMUNITY ON PATHOGENESIS

Immune host defenses are more specific than innate and are directed against a specific pathogen or its byproducts. This inducible defense system develops resistance and immunity. **Antibody-mediated (humoral) immunity** begins when a microorganism invades a host and carries antigenic substances, which can be components of the cell wall, structures such as fimbriae, toxins, or enzymes. When a macrophage encounters a pathogen, it phagocytizes and destroys it. Then the macrophage displays fragments of the antigen on its surface to activate T cells, which in turn activate B cells, which divide and form plasma cells, which release antibodies that are specific to the antigens. Antibodies are immunoglobulins, of which there are 5 types. The macrophage also forms memory cells, which become part of the permanent immune system. The antibodies bind to antigens, creating what is referred to as the antigen-antibody complex, and destroying the antigen, leading to destruction of the pathogen.

IMPACT OF CELL-MEDIATED IMMUNITY ON PATHOGENESIS

Cell-mediated immunity is a delayed-type hypersensitivity response (DTH) that activates cells rather than antibodies to fight pathogens. This same system is activated against transplants, causing rejection. After macrophages phagocytize antigens, proteins are encoded by a major histocompatibility complex (MHC) so they can display antigenic fragments, alerting T-lymphocyte cells, which are coated with clusters of differentiation (CD), chemical molecules. The thymus releases cytotoxic T killer cells (CD8+) that can recognize the MHC carrying foreign antigen, from bacteria, viruses, tumors, or transplanted tissue. In an activation phase, T cells with the correct receptors for the pathogen divide and multiply. In the effector phase, these cytotoxic T cells release lymphotoxins that destroy the pathogenic cells. T helper (TH) cells (CD4+) secrete lymphokines that stimulate both T cells and B cells to multiply. Suppressor T-cells deactivate the immune response. Cell-mediated immunity is especially effective for viral, fungal, and protozoan infections as well as tumor cells and intracellular bacteria.

Impact of Innate Defenses on Pathogenesis

Innate defenses are those that are common to healthy hosts and provide protection from pathogens. These include the following:

- **Resistance**: Species resistance includes lack of receptors for adhesins, inhospitable temperature or environment, lack of necessary nutrients, and lack of target cells for toxins. Individual resistance may be a factor of age, sex, health, medications, or many other elements.
- **Anatomical barriers**: Bacteria are not able to invade intact skin and the mucus and/or cilia in the mucous membranes make adherence difficult for many bacteria. Acids in the gastrointestinal tract kill many pathogens. The natural acidity of urine is not compatible with many bacteria.
- **Normal flora**: Flora compete with, inhibit, and destroy other pathogens.
- **Antimicrobial agents**: Body fluids, lymphocytes, and macrophages contain numerous proteins and protein compounds that disrupt, inhibit, or kill invading pathogens.
- **Inflammatory response**: Erythema, increased temperature, and edema aid in the functioning of the immune system.
- **Phagocytes**: Cells that can engulf and destroy pathogens are triggered by inflammation.

Relation of Normal Flora to Pathogenicity

Normal flora gain access to the surface of the body by contact with the skin or the mucous membranes of the gastrointestinal, reproductive, or respiratory tracts. Normal flora is not usually found in internal organs, such as the brain or the blood. There are over 200 organisms that are part of the normal flora (mostly bacteria), which vary according to genetics, age, sex, nutrition, environment, and other factors. Many bacteria, such as *Staphylococcus aureus,* are basically pathogenic and can cause opportunistic infections. The largest numbers of flora inhabit the intestinal tract. Intestinal bacteria, such as *Escherichia coli,* have an active role in digestion and prevent colonization of other pathogens, but can also cause infection. Some floras are transient; others permanent. Flora often have tissue tropism, a preference for some types of tissues. Some have surface components that allow them to bind with host cells in order to colonize. Others build bacterial biofilms, slime glue composed primarily of capsules, or use those built by other bacteria.

Bacteria-Mediated and Host-Mediated Pathogenesis

Infection includes the interplay and imbalance between a microorganism and the host. The virulence factor of the pathogen relates to characteristics of **bacteria-mediated pathogenesis**. Some bacteria produce toxins that damage cells, some have protective coatings that prevent phagocytosis by the body's defense, and others have proteins that allow them to adhere to the cells of the host, often entering the cell, resulting in cell damage or destruction. Once inside a cell, the bacteria is often safe from antibodies the host produces to fight the bacterial invasion.

Host-mediated pathogenesis is related to the immune response in reaction to a bacterial infection. This response may cause as much or more damage than the bacteria. In response to some bacteria, the immune system, including lymphocytes, macrophages, and neutrophils, may release toxic factors that cause so much damage to cells that it allows the proliferation of resistant bacteria. In other cases, the lack of cellular response to some bacteria allows them to multiply rapidly.

Issues of Transmission and Virulence as They Relate to Pathogenesis

Transmission can often be evaded by the host if the skin is intact and the mucosa is healthy. Normal flora usually remains in balance unless disease or medications affect the immune system. Pathogenic microorganisms, however, have developed numerous strategies to invade a host. Some spores can withstand long periods in the environment and are resistant to heat and drying, some organisms thrive on the skin and can easily spread to wounds, some can survive well in contaminated fluids, others thrive in conditions of poor hygiene. Incision, rashes, tubes, or trauma that compromises the integrity of the skin or mucous membranes facilitates transmission.

Virulence is the degree of pathogenicity, the ability to cause infection in the host. When comparing organisms, virulence is often evaluated in terms of the infectious/effective dose (ID50/ED50) that will likely cause infection in 50% of those exposed or the lethal dose (LD50) that will cause death in 50% of those exposed.

Incubation

Incubation periods extend from the time a pathogenic microorganism invades a host until the first signs of tissue compromise or infection occur. If the host is a vector, it is the time from invasion until first transmission to other hosts occurs. Incubation periods vary considerably, from hours to years, depending upon the type of pathogenic microorganism as well as the type of host and the environment. The incubation period can range from minutes to decades.

Agents have incubation periods specific to them (e.g., 1-3 days for cholera, 14-21 days for rubella). Although it can vary somewhat depending upon the dose or the host's immunity or age, the period can still provide the diagnostician with clues to make a diagnosis.

There is a period between acquisition of an agent and the agent then beginning its activity, a period during which the host is in a state of good health in relation to the infection. This is called the **latent period**, which takes place just prior to the incubation period. When the agent becomes infectious is when the incubation period actually begins.

Analysis of Incubation Periods

One tool of descriptive epidemiology, analysis of an incubation period, is quite important because it provides a means for not only identifying a disease, but also the microorganism causing it and the mechanisms of its spread. Predictions may then be made in preparation for possible spread of the disease, both at the present point and into the immediate future. The incubation period is expressed as an average and by its minimum and maximum lengths.

Determining an incubation period is useful in an epidemic with a common source for determining how long antibiotic therapy should be continued in suspected cases, estimating how fast intervention must be launched in future outbreaks, advising the length of time for quarantine for those with a known/possible exposure to the disease, and for estimating the probable number of deaths that may result in the absence of any public health interventions.

Period of Communicability

That period during which an infectious agent can pass, either directly or indirectly, from a source to a victim, is the **period of communicability**, and it is necessarily an average because the period varies by disease. While pertussis, for example, may be highly communicable in its early catarrhal stage and into the beginning of its paroxysmal stage, this is true only for the first two or three weeks before communicability gradually decreases, and the danger becomes negligible after three weeks.

When a disease requires that its pathogen be present in the blood or other tissues of an intermediary before passage to the host, the period of communicability for that intermediating vector must also be noted. For plague, fleas that provide the reservoir for the agent may remain infective for months under suitable conditions. The pneumonic plague they cause, therefore, may be highly communicable, but only under appropriate sanitary and climatic conditions and housing situations. With some types of infections, such as measles, communicability is higher during the incubation period than during the active disease. The periods of communicability may be continuous, as with HIV infection, or intermittent. Communicability/infectivity may depend upon sufficient numbers of pathogenic organisms within the blood or tissue of the host.

Disease Carriers

Hosts infected by the transmittable agent become reservoirs, or carriers. Types of carriers include:

- **Non-apparent carriers:** Carry and transmit an agent while they, themselves, remain free of disease. These can include incubatory carriers who can carry and transmit an agent before they, themselves, contract the disease.
- **Convalescent carriers:** Can carry and transmit the agent for some time after they, themselves, have recovered from the disease. A convalescent carrier who can transmit the agent for more than a year is described as a chronic carrier.
- **Zoonoses:** Agents carried by non-human animal vertebrates that can be passed to humans.

Zoonoses

The World Health Organization defines zoonoses as diseases that originate in animal vertebrates and are naturally transmitted between these vertebrates and humans. Calvin Schwabe, the godfather of veterinary public health, takes a slightly more liberal view of zoonoses, defining them as diseases whose agents are shared in nature with other vertebrate species.

- **Direct zoonoses** such as leptospirosis and anthrax may be perpetuated in nature by a single vertebrate species.
- **Cyclozoonoses** include those vertebrate animals in which the host requires two different animals to complete its life cycle. For example, the influenza virus is commonly passed from birds to pigs to humans.

Emergence of Direct Zoonotic Diseases

Changes elsewhere in the environment can bring on zoonotic diseases. Such change is likely to be produced by **climate changes** or **changes in land use** patterns. These impact reservoir distribution and, in chain reaction fashion, produce changes in animal behavior and population size. For instance, changes in ambient temperature and rainfall patterns will affect populations of bacteria and parasites; drought may affect vegetation that affects populations of rodents carrying hantaviruses.

Climate change also produces changes in human behavior that encourage the emergence of diseases: an increase in warm, sunny days in the Pacific Northwest can lead to more days of hiking and camping. This raises the probabilities of contact between reservoirs of agents and their potential hosts.

Creating maps combining agent survival characteristics with climate variables enables some degree of risk surveillance.

Metazoonoses and Saprozoonoses

A **metazoonosis** is the type of disease wherein an agent multiplies, develops, or does both, within an invertebrate host before being transmitted to a vertebrate host. The emergence of a metazoonotic disease where there was not one before may occur through changes in the distribution of vectors, the numbers of hosts or reservoirs, or their distribution, size, or behavior. Global warming will likely result in a redistribution of such vectors as larval mosquitoes that thrive anywhere there is sufficient warmth for them to develop.

Saprozoonoses transmit infections through non-animal reservoirs such as food plants, soil, or other organic material. Deforestation and agricultural activities affect their spread, but they can be tracked easily through conventional environmental monitoring and GIS mapping techniques. They are not difficult to control.

Factors Influencing Transmission of Disease from Animals to Humans

Several factors may influence the transmission of diseases from animals to humans. Among them are the following:

- Route of transmission
- Length of the animal's incubation period: This is important in some diseases with long incubation periods; animals of this species may be preferred for laboratory investigations, as they may be studied and sacrificed before they become infective for humans.
- The stability of the agent: Most important in direct transmission, where the agent is exposed to environmental changes.
- Population density of the animals in the colony: The more crowded the colony, the better the chances of the disease being passed among them.
- Husbandry practices (animal health and hygiene care): Low risk vs. high risk
- Vector control over wild rodents and insects
- Virulence of the agent
- Length of time that the animal is infective

Contamination

Contamination can have different meanings depending upon its context. Foul detritus in a water supply is, for example, a pollutant frequently described as a contaminant. It may be something offensive or damaging to the environment, even damaging to human beings. But, to the epidemiologist, if it is not infectious, it is not a contaminant.

In epidemiology, a contaminant is any extraneous material, usually a microorganism that has the capacity to render anything infectious, this includes animate or inanimate articles and may be, therefore, a source for transmission of infection.

Contamination as an Infectious Process

Contamination is an invasion of pathogenic microorganisms into the tissue, (such as a surgical site) or onto the surface (skin) of a host or inanimate articles (such as surgical instruments or doorknobs) or substances (such as food or liquid solutions), but in fewer numbers than an infection so that there are usually insufficient numbers to cause serious compromise of tissue although contamination can result in infection. Contamination of food products with *E. coli* have caused major outbreaks of infection, so contamination can be very dangerous, and much of infection control efforts are aimed at reducing contamination of the environment in order to prevent transmission and resultant infections. A wound that is simply contaminated with a pathogenic microorganism may heal without serious problem, but if the microorganisms replicate and invade the tissue, the subsequent tissue damage may interfere with the healing process.

Food Contamination

Phases of Bacterial Growth in Food

Bacterial growth in food generally proceeds through a series of four phases:

- **Lag phase:** The time for microorganisms to become accustomed to their new environment. There is little or no growth during this phase.
- **Log phase:** Bacteria logarithmic, or exponential, growth begins; the rate of multiplication is the most rapid and constant.
- **Stationary phase:** The rate of multiplication slows down due to lack of nutrients and build-up of toxins. At the same time, bacteria are constantly dying so the numbers actually remain constant.
- **Death phase:** Cell numbers decrease as growth stops and existing cells die off.

Requirements for the Survival of Microorganisms in Food

Types of **microorganisms have specific needs** for different levels of oxygen for their growth and survival:

- Obligate aerobes: Require O_2
- Facultative: Grow with or without oxygen
- Microaerophilic: Prefer very low levels of oxygen
- Aerotolerant Anaerobes: Grow with or without oxygen
- Obligate Anaerobes: Oxygen is lethal

Certain biological structures in plants and animals provide physical barriers to microorganisms. These include skin, rinds, feathers, and bark.

Many foods have antimicrobial factors that protect them against colonization. Milk, for example, has several nonimmunological proteins which inhibit the growth and metabolism of many microorganisms:

- Lactoperoxidase
- Lactoferrin
- Lysozyme
- Xanthine

Pseudo Infections and Pseudo-Outbreaks

Pseudo infections should be suspected when an organism is cultured from an unusual body site or an unusual organism is cultured from any site on the body. In both cases, there is colonization of pathogens without clinical signs of infection appropriate to that organism. The colonization may be superficial, the specimen may have become contaminated, or there may have been a laboratory error. When clusters of the same type of colonization occur without infection, it is deemed a **pseudo-outbreak**. There are different types of pseudo infections:

- **Pseudobacteria**, especially *Bacillus, Pseudomonas, and Streptococcus* species, usually as the result of normal flora or contamination of the specimen.
- **Pseudomeningitis**, with bacteria or fungus in cerebrospinal fluid but without expected clinical symptoms matching the organism usually result from contamination of specimen.
- **Pseudopneumonias**, usually related to contaminated bronchoscopes, respiratory equipment of solutions.
- **Pseudobacteriuria** usually results from contamination of external urinary drainage system.

True infections must be differentiated from pseudo infections so that patients can be properly treated.

Benefits of Normal Flora to the Host

The normal flora of the body is necessary and benefit the host in a number of ways.

- **Synthesis and secretion of vitamins**: Bacteria are an important source of Vitamin K and Vitamin B_{12}, which is secreted by enteric bacteria, such as *E. coli.*
- **Resistance to colonization**: The normal flora attaches to host cells, preventing competing bacteria from attaching and colonizing. They also compete for nutrition.
- **Inhibition or destruction of pathogens**: Bacterial flora may produce substances, such as fatty acids or bacteriocins, which destroy invading pathogens.
- **Develops tissue**: In response to normal flora, the walls of some structure, such as the cecum and some lymphatic tissue thicken and strengthen.
- **Stimulation of antibodies**: Normal flora have antigenic properties that stimulate formation of "natural" antibodies in the host. These antibodies can cross-react with the antigens of related pathogens as part of an immune response.

Specimen Collection, Transportation, Handling, and Storage

Transport Media

Common transport media include the following:

Transport Media	Collection Container/Instructions
Biopsy, tissue, or swab	Viral/chlamydia transport media
Blood	An EDTA (lavender top) or heparinized tube (green top)
Cerebral spinal fluid (CSF) or respiratory secretions	Sterile container
Nasopharyngeal wash or throat wash	Dry, sterile specimen container
Sterile body fluids	Sterile leakproof containers
Stool	Leakproof container with no preservatives
Vesicle	Place swab in viral transport media and transport immediately on ice
Urine	Sterile container without preservatives
Anaerobic cultures	Transport media with strong reducing agents, oxygen-free tubes, or plastic oxygen-impermeable envelopes with catalysts that change hydrogen and oxygen to water

Collecting Swab Specimens

Swabs may be used to collect specimens from the nares, the throat, or wounds. If purulent material is being collected from a wound, it is better to send a sample of the pus in a sterile container rather than collecting a specimen with a swab if the drainage is sufficient.

- **Collection** should be done wearing gloves and holding the container that receives the swab as close as possible to the swabbed area to avoid contaminating the environment with droplets. The container should be labeled before collection. The swab is inserted into the container, usually a tube, slowly to avoid contaminating the mouth. Some types require that the end of the swab be broken or cut, which has the potential for spreading infection, so this should be done gently.
- **Handling** the specimen container should occur after the container is bagged.
- **Transport** should be done immediately.
- **Storage** should be in designated areas following guidelines.

Collecting Aspirants

Aspirants include any fluids aspirated from the chest, joints, cerebrospinal area, sinuses, abscesses, cysts, or other.

- **Collection** requires aseptic techniques, including gloves, with needle puncture and then aspiration of fluid. Skin antiseptics are used, but those with a strong residual effect, such as chlorhexidine, should be avoided. The container should be dry, break-proof, and sterile. A protective mask is usually not needed although it may be used when obtaining cerebrospinal fluid with some infectious diseases, such as meningococcal meningitis. The needle should be removed if there is a safety method to prevent needle stick in order to reduce spraying and the fluid gently expelled into the specimen container, which is then bagged.
- **Handling** should be with gloves until the container is bagged.
- **Transport** to the lab should be done immediately.
- **Storage** should be in designated areas following guidelines specific for the type of aspirant. Cerebrospinal fluid degrades quickly and should be tested immediately.

Collecting Sputum Specimens

Sputum specimens can easily contaminate the outside rim of the container as people often cough directly over the container or place their mouths on it, so containers should always be considered contaminated.

- **Collection** should be done wearing gloves if obtaining the specimen directly from the patient and when handling the container. If the patient collects the specimen, the patient should be instructed how to produce and collect the specimen. The container should be wide-mouthed and hold at least 50 mL. If possible, the rim should be wiped before the lid is applied and the tissue placed in the biohazard waste receptacle. Collection should be done outside, at a distance from other people, and not in the laboratory.
- **Handling** should be minimal. The specimen container should be placed inside a Ziploc bag that is labeled with name, date, and time of collection.
- **Transport** to the lab should be done immediately.
- **Storage** should be in designated areas following facility guidelines.

Respiratory Tract Specimens

The following guidelines pertain to the collection and transport of specific respiratory specimens:

Specimen	Volume	Container/Transport Device	Additional Considerations
Nasopharynx	N/A	Use sterile swabs with flexible wire shafts (made of plastic or metal).	Used to search out a number of upper respiratory infection types. Cotton and calcium alginate swabs are no longer recommended by the CDC.
Sinus Aspirate and *Tympanocentesis*	N/A	Anaerobic transport vial	None
Oral Cavity	N/A	Swab	None
Throat	N/A	Swab	Appropriate for tonsillar areas, posterior pharynx and areas of inflammation, exudation, ulceration, capsule formation in search of enteroviruses, adenovirus, herpes simplex virus, or cytomegalovirus
Tracheal Aspirate	N/A	Sterile, screw-capped tube or jar	None
Lung Abscess, Emphysema Fluid	N/A	Anaerobic transport vial	None
Transtracheal Aspirate	3-5 mL	Anaerobic transport vial	None
Tuberculosis	3-5 mL	Clean, wide mouthed, leakproof specimen containers. Single use disposable plastic containers (50 mL capacity) are preferred	Collect and process three specimens, with at least one being an "early morning" specimen collected by the patient upon rising. Sputum analysis is the most dangerous lab procedure and must be done in the open air and at a distance from other people. Never collect sputum in the laboratory itself
Bronchial Washings	N/A	Sterile, screw-capped jar	Not appropriate for anaerobic culture unless obtained with a double-lumen, distally occluded catheter
Mycobacteria	3-5 mL	Sterile, screw-capped jar	Collect three specimens in the early a.m. following a deep cough from the patient. A heated aerosol of 10% glycerin and 15% salt may be used to induce the cough

Collecting Urine Specimens

Urine specimens should be collected following standard procedures.

- **Specimen containers** should hold at least 50 mL and have a wide base. They should be sterile, leak resistant, break proof, and have a secure lid. Containers are used only one time and then discarded with other biohazard material.
- **Collection** may be from straight catheterization, drainage from a Foley catheter, or obtained for urination. The staff handling the container and the patient instructed in proper method for obtaining the specimen should wear gloves. At least 10-20 mL should be collected if possible. The containers should be labeled properly, not on the lid, which might become separated from the container.
- **Transport** should be with the specimen container inside of a second container, such as a Ziploc bag so that urine that might be on the outside of the container does not spread contamination.
- **Storage** should be in a designated area and inside the transport container.

Guidelines for the Collection of Specific Urine Specimens

The following guidelines pertain to the collection and transport of urine specimens for viruses, *C. trachomatis,* and bacteria:

- For routine analysis and microscopic evaluation of urine, a sterile, screw-capped tube or jar is the container/transport device, and the volume of collection is 1-10 mL.
- Instruct the patient to discard the first portion of urine stream when voiding and, before voiding is complete, to collect the remaining portion of urine (the "midstream" portion) in the sterile container provided, as a clean-catch or midstream specimen is preferred.
- Cap and label the specimen.
- Place the specimen in the refrigeration until courier pickup. 24-hour specimens must not be collected.
- The specimen is not appropriate for anaerobic cultures.
- For *C. trachomatis*, the specimen is appropriate only for men.

The following guidelines pertain to the collection and transport of urine specimens for mycobacteria, fungi, suprapubic aspirate, and voided urine for parasites:

- Suprapubic aspirate is collected and transported in an anaerobic vial
- Clean-voided midstream urine or urine obtained by catheterization or cystoscopy for mycobacteria, fungi, suprapubic aspirate, and voided urine for parasites go into a sterile, screw-capped tube or jar.
- Though the volume of a sample for detecting suprapubic aspirate is not important, care in handling is, as analyzing this sample is the only certain method for establishing a diagnosis of *anaerobic bacteriuria*.
- More than 20 mL should be sent to the laboratory immediately upon collection or refrigerated for the detection of mycobacteria and fungi, but not held for more than 24-hours, as specimens that old are not usable.
- For detection of *Schistosoma haematobium* eggs, embryonated eggs of human schistosomus (blood flukes), or miracidia (all very uncommon in North America), submit a 24-hour collection of voided urine.

Collecting Genitourinary Tract Specimens

The following guidelines pertain to the collection and transport of genitourinary tract specimens:

Specimen	Volume	Container/Transport Device	Additional Considerations
Herpes Simplex Virus	N/A	Swab	Calcium alginate should be avoided; the specimen should be refrigerated for storage.
Cervical, Vaginal Discharge	N/A	Swab	The specimen is not appropriate for anaerobic culture.
Culdocentesis Fluid	N/A	An anaerobic transport vial	None
Abscess (Pelvic, Tubal, Ovarian)	N/A	An anaerobic transport vial	None
Prostatic Secretion	N/A	Sterile, screw capped bottle	None

Collecting Blood Specimens

Blood should always be considered hazardous and potentially infectious.

- **Collection** should be done using antiseptic techniques and sterile equipment with the person collecting wearing gloves. Collection should be done using vacuum tube blood collection devices. Avoid the use of needle syringes if possible, or if blood must be transferred from the syringe, care should be used to avoid spraying blood or leaking droplets. In some cases, protective eyewear may be used. Blood should not be collected from an arm into which IV fluids are being administered as this can dilute the sample. Blood is drawn in a particular order if multiple tubes are used so that there is no cross-contamination with additives.
- **Handling** should include mixing the additive with the blood by gently rotating the tubes.
- **Transport** to the laboratory should be done immediately.
- **Storage** should be in designated areas following guidelines for the type of testing that is to be done.

Collection and Transport of Specific Infectious Elements in Blood Specimens

The following guidelines pertain to the collection and transport of blood specimens for specific infectious elements:

Specimen	Volume	Container/Transport Device	Additional Considerations
Viruses	5-10 mL; 30-50 mL for HIV	Heparinized tube or clot tube	None
Bacteria	20-30 mL for adults; 1-3 mL for infants and children	Blood culture bottle containing broth or lysis-centrifugation tube	Collect 2 separate blood samples during a 24-hour period, with intervals between cultures determined by the urgency of the clinical situation

Specimen	Volume	Container/Transport Device	Additional Considerations
Leptospires	1 mL	Sterile, heparinized tube	Collect 2 separate blood samples during a 24-hour period, with intervals between cultures determined by the urgency of the clinical situation
Brucellae and Fungi	20-30 mL for adults; 1-3 mL for infants and children	Lysis centrifugation tube or biphasic blood culture bottle	Collect 2 separate blood samples during a 24 hour period, with intervals between cultures determined by the urgency of the clinical situation
Borrelia	N/A	Peripheral smear	The wet mount should be examined by darkfield microscopy or via a smear stained with aniline dyes.
Malaria	N/A	A thick and thin film on clean glass slide	None
Filaria and Trypanosomes	5 mL	Sterile tube containing anticoagulant (citrate, oxalate, heparin)	A drop of blood should be collected on a wet mount, or it should be concentrated, hemolyzed blood rather than stained thick and thin films.

Collecting Fluid Specimens

The following guidelines pertain to the collection and transport of fluid specimens:

Specimens	Volume	Container/Transport Device	Additional Considerations
Exudates, Transudates, Drainage, Pus	1-5 mL	Anaerobic transport vial	None
Abdomen, Chest	1-5 mL for bacteria; less than 10 mL for mycobacteria or fungi	Anaerobic transport vial	None
Synovial	1-5 mL for bacteria; less than 10 mL for mycobacteria or fungi	Anaerobic transport vial	In instances of suspected gonococcal arthritis, use a Thayer-Martin medium modified as an inoculate
Cerebrospinal	1-2 mL for bacteria or viruses; less than 2 mL for mycobacteria or fungi	A sterile, screw capped tube	Immediately forward to the laboratory

Collecting Gastrointestinal Tract Specimens

The following guidelines pertain to the collection and transport of gastrointestinal tract specimens:

Specimen	Volume	Container/Transport Device	Additional Considerations
Stool for Bacteria	N/A	A sterile, screw capped tube or transport medium swab	None
Stool for Ova and Parasites	N/A	A stool carton sealed in a plastic bag with polyvinyl alcohol preservative	None
Anal Swab for Pinworm	N/A	A sterile plastic swab in a tube (SWUBE)	Collection is accomplished by a swab of the peri-anal area, preferably in the morning upon rising and prior to bathing or defecation
Stool for Viruses	N/A	A sterile, screw-capped jar or transport medium swab	None

Collection, Handling, Transport, and Storage for Fecal Specimens

Fecal specimens should not be contaminated with urine, paper, or toilet water, especially if they are to be examined for microorganisms.

- **Collection** should be done after the patient has urinated, if possible. The specimen can be collected in a clean bedpan. Plastic wrap is sometimes placed over the back part of the toilet to catch the feces, but the plastic can become easily contaminated. The fecal specimen is placed in a sterile container, preferably one with a scoop in the lid to facilitate transfer. About 10 mL should be collected for viral or bacterial testing. Testing for parasites requires a larger specimen. The person handling the container and specimen should wear gloves. Swabs of fecal material are almost never sufficient for adequate testing.
- **Handling** should be done after specimen container is bagged with label indicating, name, date, and time of collection.
- **Transport** should be done as quickly as possible.
- **Storage** should be in designated areas following guidelines.

Collecting Catheter Specimens

The following guidelines pertain to the collection and transport of catheter specimens:

Specimen	Volume	Container/Transport Device	Additional Considerations
Borrelia	N/A	A sterile, screw-capped tube or culturette (with swab removed)	For collection, the skin entry site should be disinfected, the catheter removed, and the end going into the tube should be clipped off
Suction, Drainage	N/A	A sterile, screw-capped tube	None
Cultures	N/A	A swab or anaerobic transport vial	None
Scrapings for Dermatophytes	N/A	Sterile Petri dish	None

Collecting Sexually Transmitted Disease Specimens

The following guidelines pertain to the collection and transport of sexually transmitted disease specimens:

Specimen	Volume	Container/Transport Device	Additional Considerations
Treponema Pallidum	N/A	Serous exudates on a clean glass slide or in a capillary pipette	The lesion should be abraded with a clean dry sponge and the preparation examined by darkfield microscopy immediately upon collection
Chlamydia trachomatis	N/A	A swab held in a sucrose-phosphate solution (2 SP)	The urethral or cervical material should be extracted on a swab in solution, then, if stored, refrigerated.
Ureaplasma urealyticum	N/A	A swab held in a sucrose-phosphate solution (2 SP)	The urethral or cervical material should be extracted on a swab in solution, then, if stored, refrigerated.
Trichomonas vaginalis	N/A	Swab	None

The following guidelines pertain to the collection and transport of sexually transmitted disease specimens:

Specimen	Volume	Container/Transport Device	Additional Considerations
Neisseria gonorrhoeae	N/A	Swab or a Petrie dish with a modified Thayer-Martin medium containing antibiotics and nutrients which facilitate the growth of *Neisseria* species while inhibiting the growth of Gram-positive organisms and most bacilli	For women, collection is accomplished by taking a cervical culture; if the cervix is not accessible, the sample is taken by inserting the swab via the urethral or vaginal canal. For men, collect material for a smear and culture with a swab or sterile bacteriologic loop inserted via the urethra.
Haemophilus ducreyi	N/A	Swab	None

Collecting Eye Specimens

The following guidelines pertain to the collection and transport of eye specimens:

Specimen	Volume	Container/ Transport Device	Additional Considerations
Corneal Lesion or Scraping	N/A	N/A	The specimen should be inoculated directly onto proper media and applied directly to clean microscope slides for staining and microscopic examination.
Conjunctiva Examination for Prostatic Secretion	N/A	N/A	The specimen should be inoculated directly onto proper media and applied directly to clean microscope slides for staining and microscopic examination.
Neisseria gonorrhoeae	N/A	A modified Thayer-Martin medium	The swab should be inoculated directly onto the medium.
Chlamydia trachomatis	N/A	A sucrose-phosphate solution (2 SP) or swab for a direct smear	The specimen material should be extracted on the swab in solution, and then refrigerated for storage.
Bacteria, Fungi, Viruses	A representative sample	Sterile, screw capped bottle	The specimen collected must be an adequate portion to ensure recovery of sufficient organisms.

Selecting and Collecting Specimens During Infection Control and Outbreak Investigations

When selecting and collecting specimens during infection control procedures and outbreak investigations, these guidelines should be followed:

- Follow protocols set down for collection for each type of disease; collect in amounts sufficient to allow effective and complete analysis
- Obtain written consent from patients if specimens will be stored
- Complete collection before dosing the patient with antimicrobial agents
- Collection in viral infections should occur near the start of the acute phase to improve virus recovery
- Avoid contamination, particularly by organisms from skin and mucous membranes
- Keep specimens at required temperatures
- Label all specimens: Name of patient, date and time taken, location where taken, and who collected the specimen
- Take care with biohazardous specimens that require special containment
- Do not delay sending specimens to the laboratory

Clinical Signs, Symptoms, and Test Results

Patient Assessment for Exposure to Communicable Disease

Patient exposure to communicable disease can be difficult to assess as the person may not be aware of exposure or may be reluctant to discuss it because of privacy issues. Doing a careful and thorough history and physical assessment can provide information that suggests exposure. Questioning people about symptoms rather than diseases may elicit more information: "Have you had contact with anyone with a rash?" or "Have you experienced night sweats?" Exposure to a communicable disease can occur outside of the hospital as well as inside. Exposure to communicable disease can be endogenous (self-infection) or exogenous (cross-infection). Endogenous infections, for example, can result from the normal body flora or an area of infection (such as a boil) contaminating a surgical wound. Exogenous infections can occur by contact with someone who is infected, such as another patient or a staff member, or by airborne particles. Both types of infection can occur in the hospital.

Signs and Symptoms of Infection

Signs and symptoms of infection in patients should be assessed continually. Common infections involve the wound or surgical site, the lungs, and the urinary system, so particular attention should be paid to these areas. Assessment will vary according to diagnosis:

- Wound or surgical site should be checked and evaluated for erythema, edema, and discharge.
- Systemic indications of infection, such as an increase in temperature or changes in vital signs should be monitored regularly.
- Lungs should be evaluated by spirometer and auscultation. Cough, shortness of breath, or sputum production should be noted. Patient should receive instruction in deep breathing and coughing exercises to prevent atelectasis.
- Urine should be monitored for amount, color, and consistency and any burning or other dysuria should be evaluated. Discomfort in the bladder area, flanks, or lower back could indicate infection. Ensuring adequate fluid intake and monitoring intake and output can help to prevent urinary infections.

Classification of Microorganisms

Bacteria

Clinical classification of bacteria takes into account those characteristics that are helpful in identifying infectious processes:

- **Gram-positive or Gram-negative status**: Most bacteria are Gram-negative or Gram-positive although a few cannot be identified by staining. While Gram stain is not used to identify the specific bacteria, it is frequently referred to clinically.
- **Taxonomic status**: Taxonomy is based on the genera and species of a bacterium, but this can be confusing because some names have changed or two names are used. Genome sequencing should standardize identification.
- **Anaerobic/aerobic status**: Some bacteria are strictly anaerobic, but very few are strictly aerobic. Those that have flexibility and can grow in either aerobic or anaerobic conditions are called facultative.

- **Usual environment**: Bacteria are classified according to where they usually reside as flora or where they usually cause infection.
- **Virulence factor**: Bacteria vary widely in virulence. Some are actively invasive but others only cause opportunistic infections.

Bacterial Infections

Bacterial infections can be described by the following characteristics:

- **Subclinical** infections cause no obvious symptoms
- **Latent** infections occur when people have no symptoms of infection but can be carriers.
- **Accidental** infections occur outside of the normal transmission mode, such as from needle sticks or acts of bioterrorism.
- **Opportunistic** infections occur when normal flora overgrows, usually in the presence of immunosuppression.
- **Primary** infections include clinical symptoms.
- **Secondary** infections follow a primary infection because of host compromise.
- **Mixed** infections occur when more than one pathogen is the causative agent.
- **Acute** infections present rapidly with obvious symptoms that may persist for days or weeks.
- **Chronic** infections persist for long periods of time, months or years.
- **Localized** infections remain in a circumscribed area.
- **Systemic** infections are generalized, may involve many different areas of the body, and often spread through the blood stream.
- **Retrograde** infections are those in which the bacteria are able to ascend a structure, such as a duct.
- **Fulminant** infections are severe, rapid, acute infections.

Virulence Factors

Virulence factors, which allow the microorganism to invade a host and multiply, vary from one microorganism to another, with some much more virulent than others because of inherent characteristics:

- **Adherence:** Some bacteria are more readily able to adhere to mucosal surfaces, such as those that develop fimbriae that facilitate adherence, making them more able to colonize and multiply.
- **Invasiveness:** Some bacteria have chemical components on their surfaces, either on the plasmids or chromosome, which facilitate invasion of host cells.
- **Structure:** Some bacteria are encapsulated, effectively protecting them from phagocytosis or destruction.
- **Toxins:** Many bacteria produce lipopolysaccharide, protein, or enzyme toxins (endotoxins and exotoxins) that are extremely poisonous to the host and can cause severe systemic reactions, acute infection, sepsis, shock, and death.
- **Iron-biding factors (siderophores):** Some bacteria are able to use the host's supply of iron to multiply and grow, competing with the host and facilitating infection.

Gram-Negative Bacteria

The cell walls of Gram-negative bacteria are characterized by red staining. The cell wall is thinner than that of Gram-positive bacteria; however, there are two separate layers to the wall: a thin inner layer of peptidoglycan (carbohydrate polymers bound by proteins), an intervening periplasmic space, and the outer membranous layer (the lipopolysaccharide layer), which produces endotoxins, making Gram-negative bacteria extremely pathogenic. A component of the outer layer is called the S-layer; it aids in adherence and protection from pathogens. The outer layer serves to protect Gram-negative organisms from antibiotics or detergents that would disrupt the inner peptidoglycan layer and provides resistance to penicillin and other compounds. Ampicillin is able to penetrate the exterior wall although many bacteria have become resistant.

Common **Gram-negative cocci (round) bacteria** include:

- *Neisseria gonorrhoeae*
- *Neisseria meningitides*
- *Moraxella catarrhalis*

Common **Gram-negative bacilli (rods)** include:

- *Haemophilus influenzae*
- *Legionella pneumophila*
- *Pseudomonas aeruginosa*
- *Escherichia coli*
- *Helicobacter pylori*

GRAM-POSITIVE BACTERIA

thick cell wall → Peptidoglycan wall

Gram-positive bacteria are characterized by purple staining; the cell walls tend to be thicker than those of Gram-negative bacteria. About 90% of the cell wall of Gram-positive bacteria is made of peptidoglycan (carbohydrate polymers bound by proteins). The number of peptidoglycan layers varies, but can be more than 20, making a thick-walled cell. An S-layer is attached to the peptidoglycan layer to protect the cell and aid in adherence. Gram-positive organisms tend to be easier to kill than Gram-negative because they lack the outer wall of Gram-negative organisms, and they are more sensitive to penicillin although there are resistant strains. Peptidoglycan does not occur naturally in the human body, so it is easily recognized by the immune system as an invading organism.

Common **Gram-positive cocci bacteria** include:

- *Streptococcus pneumoniae*
- *Staphylococcus aureus*
- *Enterococcus*

Common **Gram-positive bacilli bacteria** include:

- *Corynebacterium diphtheriae*
- *Listeria monocytogenes*
- *Bacillus anthracis.*

ENTERIC BACTERIUM AND NON-FERMENTATIVE GRAM-NEGATIVE BACILLI

Technically, and by tradition, an **enteric bacterium** is one that is found in the intestinal tract of both healthy and diseased warm-blooded animals. However, as bacteriologists now use the word, it refers only to *E. coli* and its relatives, even if some relatives of *E. coli* do not make their homes in the gastrointestinal tract. It represents one of the most closely related and cohesive groups of bacteria, which is probably why *E. coli* are the bacteria that are the subject of most studies, with a name that has the greatest recognition among the public.

Among the many bacteria classified in the family *Enterobacteriales* are *Citrobacter, Edwardsiella, Enterobacter, Erwinia, Escherichia, Klebsiella, Proteus, Providencia, Salmonella, Serratia, Shigella,* and *Yersinia* (along with several other genera, including *Hafnia, Morganella, Photorhabdus,* and *Xenorhabdus*).

A variety of microorganisms comprise the group known as **non-fermentative Gram-negative bacilli**. With their reservoirs of infection being aquatic environments (including several commonly found in medical facilities) these bacteria include *Pseudomonas* species, *Stenotrophomonas, Acinetobacter, Burkholderia, Flavobacterium,* and *Achromobacter* species. Differing greatly in their levels of virulence, all are resistant to the usual antibiotics. As a result, the non-fermentative Gram-negative bacteria represent important healthcare-associated infection pathogens.

Protozoa

Protozoa are single-cell microorganisms with a nucleus that live primarily off of bacteria. They share similarities to animals, but (except for Myxozoa) they are neither animals nor plants. Many protozoa are free living and are ubiquitous in soil and water. They are often divided according to their method of locomotion: flagellates, amoeboids, sporozoans, and ciliates. Some protozoa are able to form protective cysts, which can survive outside the host, sometimes for long periods, before transmission to another host. Protozoa are parasites to humans and cause a wide range of infections. Enteric protozoa, such as *Giardia intestinalis* and *Entamoeba histolytica,* can cause severe diarrhea. Other diseases caused by protozoa include malaria, Chagas disease, babesiosis, toxoplasmosis, Trichomonas infection, and amoebic dysentery. Protozoa take a huge toll of life, especially in developing countries, but some diseases, such as Chagas disease, are becoming more common in the United States as people emigrate from endemic areas of Latin America.

Viruses

Viruses (virions) are sub-microscopic and generally considered non-living because they lack cell structures. Viruses consist of nucleic acid, single or double-strand DNA and/or RNA (the genome), encapsulated in a protein coating called a capsid. Some have a lipid envelope about the capsid with glycoprotein spikes. The purpose of viruses is to reproduce, but they require a host cell with a protein receptor to which a virus must bind to penetrate the cell membrane. The viral genome carries encoding that allows it to use the cell to replicate in a *lytic* or *lysogenic* cycle. In the lytic cycle, the virus forces the cell to manufacture proteins and new genomes. After new viral particles form, the cell ruptures, releasing the viruses. In a lysogenic cycle, the virus integrates the DNA of the host and as the cell replicates, the virus replicates with it. The virus remains dormant until it activates and begins a lytic cycle. Viruses that infect bacteria are *bacteriophages* (or *phages).*

Review Video: Viruses
Visit mometrix.com/academy and enter code: 984455

Retroviruses

Retroviruses are a sub-category of viruses. Retroviruses must have three characteristics: a genome that contains ribonucleic acid (RNA), the enzyme reverse transcriptase, and a protein body surrounding by a protein envelope. While some viruses contain DNA, retroviruses do not. After the virus enters the cell of a host, the reverse transcriptase uses the RNA genome to make DNA copies of the genome. Since genetic information was previously believed to transmit from DNA to RNA, this process was considered backward "retro," thus the name retrovirus. After the DNA copy is made, it invades one of the host cell's chromosomes and becomes part of the genetic makeup of the cell. To date, two retroviruses are known to infect human hosts: HTLV-1, which causes adult T-cell leukemia and HIV (human immunodeficiency virus). By invading T-helper lymphocyte cells, HIV attacks and disrupts the immune system that should detect and destroy pathogens.

Satellite Viruses and Prions

Satellite viruses are essentially parasitic viruses that coinfect with a helper virus, which allows the satellite to use helper protein to replicate along with the helper virus. Hepatitis B may have a coinfection with the satellite virus, Hepatitis Delta, increasing the virulence of the infection.

Prions (derived from "Proteinaceous" and "infection") are proteins that cause infection, casting some doubt on the long-held belief that DNA and RNA were the molecules required for life. Originally described as a "slow virus," a prion is not bacterial, viral, or fungal, and it can cause genetic, infectious, or sporadic disorders. In all of these disorders, prion proteins (PrP) are modified. Prion diseases are rare, but neurodegenerative and often have long incubation periods. The CDC recognizes the following prion diseases: Fatal familial insomnia, Kuru, Creutzfeldt-Jakob Disease, Variant Creutzfeldt-Jakob Disease, and Gerstmann-Straussler-Scheinker Syndrome.

Fungi

Fungi were originally classified as plants, but they do not produce their own food through photosynthesis and must, like animals, get the food from another source. Fungi vary widely, from one-celled microorganisms to multi-celled chains that are miles long. Fungi are used to make antibiotics, but they can also cause infection and disease. Two common classifications of fungi are molds (including mushrooms) and yeast. Fungi are not motile, but some produce spores, which can be inhaled. Some, such as the yeast *Candida albicans*, are part of the normal flora of the skin but can overgrow in an opportunistic infection. As microorganisms, fungal infections can invade the sinuses, the mouth, the respiratory system, and the vagina. Antibiotics may affect the balance between bacteria and yeast, causing infection. Fungal infections include histoplasmosis, blastomycosis, and coccidioidomycosis. Fungal infections, such as *Pneumocystis jirovecii (*formerly *carinii)* pose a serious problem for the immunocompromised. Antifungal drugs are available, but systemic fungal infections are difficult to treat.

Dermal Microorganisms

There are three groups of dermal microorganisms:

- **Resident flora**: Microorganisms found within body cavities. These may consist of several hundred different types. Diet, sanitary conditions, air pollution, and hygienic habits all influence what species make up resident flora; more often than not, they are essential to the body's function and they even protect the body, though sometimes they cause disease.
- **Transient flora**: Colonize the host for hours or weeks but do not establish permanent residence; they may be benign or disease-causing, but they do not reproduce themselves.
- **Infectious flora**: Found within various populations:
    - Children attending day care
    - Prison inmates
    - Men who have sex with other men
    - Players of competitive sports

Skin flora can be transmitted easily from person to person, not simply through direct contact sports but also sports that involve little skin to skin contact among players. This is probably because competitive sports participants might more readily develop abrasions and other skin trauma that could facilitate entry of pathogens.

Classifications of Communicable Diseases

Communicable diseases can be classified a number of ways, and the classifications are not necessarily mutually exclusive; for example, pubic lice may be classified as a contact disease or a sexually-transmitted disease:

- **Sexually transmitted:** Transmitted through vaginal, oral, and/or anal sex and includes HIV/AIDS, syphilis, gonorrhea, and chlamydia.
- **Contact:** Transmitted through direct body contact or contact with personal belongings, such as clothing, and includes scabies, bedbugs, fungal skin/nail infections, trachoma, and pediculosis as well as contaminated environmental surfaces or hands, such as with MRSA and *Clostridium difficile.* Contact may also include diseases caused by inhalation of droplets (>5 μm), such as influenza and upper respiratory infections.
- **Airborne:** Transmitted by small suspended droplets (<5 μm) and includes tuberculosis, rubella, and leprosy.
- **Vector-borne:** Transmitted by particular vectors, usually insects, and includes yellow fever, plague, Lyme disease, West Nile disease, and leishmaniasis.
- **Fecal-oral:** Transmitted by oral-fecal contact and includes bacillary dysentery and enterohemorrhagic *Escherichia coli.*
- **Helminthic:** Transmitted by ingestion or invasion of helminths and includes pinworms, hookworms, ascariasis, and strongyloidiasis.
- **Zoonotic:** Transmitted by animals/animal products and includes anthrax, rabies, tetanus, and brucellosis.

Wound Classifications According to Risk of Infection

The **traditional wound classification system** classifies surgical wounds according to wound type and risk of infection:

Class	Wound Type	Risk for Infection	Description
Class I	Clean wounds	<2%	Clean wounds (risk <2%) do not enter an area of the body that is usually colonized by normal flora, such as the urinary or gastrointestinal tracts. There is primary closure and closed drainage, if necessary, with no break in aseptic technique.
Class II	Clean-contaminated wounds	<10%	Clean-contaminated wounds (risk <10%) enter into colonized parts of the body, such as the respiratory or urinary tract, but surgery is elective and controlled rather than emergency. There is no indication of infection or break in aseptic technique.
Class III	Contaminated wounds	20%	Contaminated wounds (risk 20%) have obvious inflammation but no purulent discharge. They may involve spillage of the gastrointestinal tract, penetrating wounds (<4 hours), and/or substantial break in aseptic technique.
Class IV	Dirty-infected wounds	40%	Dirty-infected wounds (risk 40%) show obvious inflammation and purulent discharge. There may be perforation of viscera prior to surgery and/or penetrating wounds (>4 hours).

Healthcare-Associated Infections (HAIs)

Using the definition of the National Healthcare Safety Network (NHSN), a healthcare-associated infection is a localized or systematic condition resulting from adverse reactions to an infectious agent (or a toxin generated by the agent) not present before a patient's admission to a medical facility. The infection can be caused by endogenous or exogenous sources.

The Centers for Disease Control have set up a coding system, containing definitions for healthcare-associated infections and breaking the infections down by the various sites at which they occur.

Of note, colonization that does not cause untoward signs and symptoms, or injury that results in inflammation is not considered a healthcare-associated infection. Infections that are present on admission and latent infections that have reactivated are not healthcare-associated infections.

HAIs Among Children

Primary bloodstream infections (28%), pneumonia (21%), and urinary tract infections (15%) are the most frequent healthcare-associated infections among children found in ICUs and high-risk nurseries. An invasive device, such as a catheter, almost invariably has a role in the infection. Infection sites and pathogens involved are not uniform but are of several types of infections distributed over various sites in patterns related to age. The illnesses also are not, in general, the same as those reported for the occupants of adult ICUs.

In addition to an association with intrinsic risk factors such as low birth weight and gestational age, outbreaks of *Klebsiella pneumoniae* BSIs in high-risk nurseries have been associated with extrinsic factors. These include procedures necessary to intravenous therapy, use of antimicrobials, and cross-transmission. Bloodstream healthcare-associated infections (BSIs) are a leading cause of morbidity and mortality for neonates in high-risk nurseries.

Staphylococcus Aureus

Staphylococcus aureus is a Gram-positive aerobic coccus that grows in clusters. *S. aureus* is commonly found on the skin, and the most common reservoir is the anterior nares. *S. aureus* is often also found in the axillae, the perineum, irritated skin, and mucous membranes. *S. aureus* attaches with surface proteins that promote colonization. *S. aureus* is not susceptible to complement protein cascade although there are antibodies that can block some receptors, preventing adhesion. However, once attached, the bacteria are coated with proteins from the host cell wall, and this shields the bacteria. *S. aureus* produces a number of exotoxins and endotoxins, including enterotoxins, toxic shock syndrome toxins, and epidermolytic toxins. *S. aureus* can become extremely virulent and can spread quickly through compromised tissue. It can spread though contact with purulent material and close contact with someone infected. *S. aureus* is a major cause of healthcare-associated infection post-operative infections, both localized and systemic, and infections from indwelling tubes and devices. There are increasingly resistant forms.

Methicillin-Resistant Staphylococcus Aureus (MRSA)

Methicillin-resistant *Staphylococcus aureus (*MRSA*)* poses a serious problem. Penicillin was first introduced in 1942, and shortly thereafter, penicillin-resistant bacteria arose. In 1959, methicillin was introduced to combat penicillin-resistant *S. aureus,* but within 2 years, methicillin-resistant forms were identified. Since that time, MRSA has spread throughout the world. In the United States, it is estimated that approximately 5% of hospitalized patients have MRSA in their nares or on their skin. Many MRSA forms are resistant to multiple antibiotics and respond only to vancomycin or other investigational drugs, and there are now vancomycin-resistant forms. People who have had invasive procedures or are immunocompromised are most often infected. MRSA has numerous hospital-associated strains (HA-MRSA) that have adapted well to the hospital environment, but community-associated (CA-MRSA) forms, usually skin infections, have been isolated as well. Most HA-MRSA is caused by autoinfection in people who are already carriers with nasal carriage, frequently related to prior antibiotic use and/or prolonged hospitalization.

PRECAUTIONS

MRSA is often colonized on the skin and especially in the anterior nares and can easily spread through contact with contaminated surfaces or hands. Community-acquired as well as healthcare-associated infections are of grave concern. Precautions include:

- Prompt diagnosis and treatment with vancomycin or other antibiotics
- Standard and contact precautions with use of gloves and gown. Masks may also be used, especially if patient has pneumonia.
- Droplet precautions with pneumonia.
- Place patient in private room or cohort.
- Routine surveillance of high-risk patients or those with previous history of MRSA.

VANCOMYCIN RESISTANT ENTEROCOCCI (VRE)

Vancomycin resistant *enterococci* (VRE) was first identified in 1986 but has shown a rapid increase in both intensive care units and medical/surgical units with about 25% of *enterococci* infection now VRE. Patients who are immunocompromised or severely ill are at increased risk as well as those admitted to intensive care units or hospitalized for lengthy periods. VRE is also associated with antibiotic use, including vancomycin and others, such as Clindamycin and Ciprofloxacin. VRE can occur systemically or infect the urinary tract or surgical sites. Some people are colonized but have no symptoms although they may pose a threat to others as it may survive on surfaces for up to 6 days. VRE infections are treatable by other antibiotics, but MDRE infections are increasingly resistant to two or more antibiotics, including vancomycin. Restriction of vancomycin use alone has not proven successful in controlling development of VRE or MDRE because other antibiotics, such as clindamycin, cephalosporin, aztreonam, ciprofloxacin, aminoglycoside, and metronidazole are implicated. Prior antibiotic use is present in almost all patients with MDRE.

PRECAUTIONS:

- Isolation with barrier precautions (gown and gloves) during all patient contact, even entering room.
- Hand hygiene both before and after contact and use of gloves.
- Use of dedicated equipment to reduce transmission.
- Policy to limit vancomycin use.
- Thorough cleaning of isolation room.

STREPTOCOCCUS

GROUP A BETA-HEMOLYTIC STREPTOCOCCI

Streptococcus pyogenes is a Gram-positive coccus that lacks mobility and does not produce spores. It grows in pairs or chains. It is a frequent pathogen of humans, usually causing a secondary infection after a viral infection or disruption of the normal flora. Historically, Group A beta-hemolytic streptococcus (GABHS) has caused puerperal fever and scarlet fever, and there has been a recent increase in invasive GABHS infections, from mild pharyngitis and impetigo to severe invasive infections, including cellulites and necrotizing fasciitis. GABHS infections are concerns for burn wounds as well as puerperal and neonatal infections. GABHS has numerous virulence factors that can cause a number of different diseases. It can colonize and multiply rapidly. GABHS has a hyaluronic acid capsule that contains antigens similar to those of human cells, confusing the immune system and protecting it from phagocytosis. Additionally, it produces exotoxins, such as pyrogenic toxin, which can cause toxic shock syndrome. Sequelae can include rheumatic fever and kidney disease. Most infections involve the skin or the respiratory system.

Group B β-Hemolytic Streptococci

Streptococcus agalactiae or Group B β-hemolytic streptococci (GBS) is a Gram-positive coccus that is part of the normal flora of the gastrointestinal system but may colonize the urogenital system of females although most infant infections are related to healthcare-associated infection rather than maternal transmission. The virulence factor of GBS relates to the protective capsule that prevents phagocytosis, thereby allowing it to colonize and multiply. GBS has been implicated in a wide range of nosocomial infections. GBS has increasingly been a cause of infections in neonatal units, causing pneumonia, meningitis, and sepsis. Meningitis can also occur in later onset, about 3-4 weeks after birth, with severe sequelae. GBS is also implicated in severe puerperal infections, but using cultures to screen women who are infected and administering antibiotics has cut infections. GBS infections may occur as wound infections after Caesarean sections, especially in women who are immunocompromised.

Streptococcus Pneumoniae

Streptococcus pneumoniae is a Gram-positive elongated anaerobic coccus. It may occur singly, in pairs (most common), or in chains. It lacks motility and does not produce spores. It is part of the transient flora of the nasopharynx. *S. pneumoniae* is encased in a polysaccharide capsule that prevents phagocytosis. The cell wall activates the alternative complement cascade (among others), causing an inflammatory reaction and as the *S. pneumoniae* is destroyed, it releases pneumolysin and other cytotoxins that increase inflammation, kill cells, and can cause septic shock. The cell wall is composed of six layers of peptidoglycan and contains choline that allows it to adhere to cells with choline-binding receptors, including almost all human cells. *S. pneumoniae* has a transformation system that allows it to easily mutate and develop resistance to antibiotics. It is the most common cause of lobar pneumonia in adults, and there have been frequent outbreaks in nursing homes. Immunization is the primary method of prevention.

Enterobacteriaceae

Enterobacteriaceae are facultative anaerobic Gram-negative bacilli that are part of the natural flora of the gastrointestinal tract. They are also commonly found in the soil, water, and plants. Most have flagella for motility, and they do not produce spores. *Enterobacteriaceae* comprise numerous genera, including *Escherichia coli, Shigella, Salmonella, Klebsiella, Enterobacter, Proteus,* and *Yersinia.* Virulence varies according to the ability of the organism to metabolize lactose. Those that do not are usually pathogenic. Adherence factors also impact virulence as some genera and species have more effective adhesins than others. *Enterobacteriaceae* produce toxins that can be extremely dangerous. *Enterobacteriaceae* cause less than a third of nosocomial infections, a decreasing number. However, they cause about half of the urinary tract infections and a quarter of the postoperative infections, and increasing resistance to antibiotics increases the risk of sepsis, diarrhea, and meningitis. Many species are able to cause symptoms that are similar, so identifying the pathogen is important.

Escherichia Coli

Escherichia coli, the coliform bacteria most abundant in the colon and normally innocuous can, upon acquiring a virulence factor, cause enteric infections such as traveler's diarrhea. This can then lead to osmotic diarrhea by inhibiting uptake of salt. It can also cause Hemolytic uremic syndrome

(HUS), making possible acute renal failure as well as urinary tract infections like cystitis and pyelonephritis, neonatal meningitis, respiratory infection, and bacteremia.

Escherichia comes in several species:

- *Enteropathogenic Escherichia coli*, a problem in developing nations, especially among children.
- *Enteroinvasive Escherichia coli* has the same virulence factor as Shigella, with plasmid mediated invasion and destruction of the colon.
- *Enterohemorrhagic Escherichia coli* inhabit undercooked meat and causes blood-heavy diarrhea without fever or inflammation but with severe abdominal cramps (a syndrome called hemorrhagic colitis).

Treatment of the GI symptoms brought on by *Escherichia* begins with rehydration. Antibiotics are discouraged, due to the germ's resistance; urinary tract infections can be treated with Bactrim or ampicillin, and meningitis with 3rd generation cephalosporin (ceftriaxone).

Pathogenesis of *E. Coli*

Escherichia coli is a facultative anaerobic Gram-negative bacillus that is part of the normal flora of the intestines. There are hundreds of serotypes of *E. coli*, based on O, H, and K antigens. *E. coli* serves a necessary role in digestion and production of Vitamin K and B-complex vitamins as well as suppressing growth of harmful bacteria that may invade the intestines; however, it is also the biggest cause of urinary infections and some strains, such as 0157:H7 are extremely virulent, causing severe diarrhea, hemolytic uremia, and death. There are five classes of diarrhea-producing *E. coli. E. coli* produces both endotoxins and exotoxins that causes diarrhea, and since death of the organism releases toxins, antibiotic treatment can make some infections and symptoms worse. As a nosocomial infection, *E. coli* primarily causes urinary tract infections (especially related to catheters), diarrhea, and neonatal meningitis but it can also lead to pneumonia, and bacteremia (usually secondary to urinary infection). Endotoxins can cause intravascular coagulation and death.

E. Coli Outbreaks

Undercooked or raw ground beef has been behind many of the documented outbreaks of *E. coli*, but also cited have been alfalfa sprouts, dry-cured salami, lettuce, unpasteurized fruit juices, game meat, and cheese curds. Young victims may develop hemolytic uremic syndrome (HUS); this can produce permanent loss of kidney function. HUS is combined with two other symptoms, fever and neurologic distress, to make up the condition thrombotic thrombocytopenic purpura (TTP), which has a mortality rate in the elderly, as high as 50%.

Salmonellae

Salmonellae, with its hundreds of serotypes, is classified by the Ewing system into three groups: *Salmonella typhi, Salmonella cholerae-suis,* and *Salmonella enteritidis*. There is one serotype for each of the first two and 1,500 for the third.

- Enterocolitis: Caused by *S. enteritidis* or *S. typhimurium.*
- Typhoid Fever (*S.* typhi): Also called enteric fever when caused by similar serotypes.
- Septicemia (*Salmonella cholerae-suis*): Found in 1 of 20,000 uncooked egg whites in the US, according to the CDC.
- Lobar pneumonia: Severe and resistant to multiple antibiotics, caused by *klebsiella pneumoniae*
- Struvite kidney stones: An outcome of infection by *Proteus* species.

The mainstay of treatment is keeping the patient from becoming hypovolemic and keeping electrolytes balanced. In some cases, life-threatening sepsis may occur, requiring treatment with antibiotics; fluoroquinolones are the antibiotics of choice. Antibiotic prophylaxis is usually contraindicated except in children younger than 1 year of age who are at risk for bacteremia or those who are immunocompromised. Patients who handle food as an occupation and those who are healthcare workers should not return to work until symptoms abate.

SHIGELLA

The illness caused by ***Shigella*** (shigellosis) accounts for about 10% of the reported outbreaks of foodborne illness in this country, at an estimated 450,000 cases. Infants, the elderly, and the infirm are susceptible to the severest symptoms of the disease, but all humans are susceptible to some degree. Fatalities may be as high as 10-15% with some strains. Shigellosis is a very common malady suffered by individuals with acquired immune deficiency syndrome (AIDS).

The organism is frequently found in water polluted with human feces. Infection, which requires as few as 10 cells, depending on age and condition of the host, is characterized by abdominal pain, cramps, diarrhea, fever, vomiting, blood, pus, or mucus in stools.

Shigella is transmitted fecal-oral route from contaminated food and water and occurs primarily in children 6-36 months of age. It is characterized by bloody diarrhea, abdominal pain, and fever. Treatment is tailored to cultures but use fluoroquinolones once daily for 3 days while waiting for culture results or trimethoprim-sulfamethoxazole (TMP-SMZ): TMP 160 mg and SMZ 800 mg per day given orally in 2 divided doses every 12 hours for 5 days.

ACINETOBACTER AND BRUCELLA

Acinetobacter baumannii is frequently found in the hospital environment, commonly colonizing irrigating solutions and intravenous solutions. Recently it has become a much more major infectious agent, as previously it was known for colonizing but not infecting. *Acinetobacter* pneumonias occur in outbreaks and are usually associated with colonized respiratory support equipment or fluids. Nosocomial meningitis may occur in colonized neurosurgical patients with external ventricular drainage tubes. It has always been an organism inherently resistant to multiple antibiotics, and because it has the ability to develop resistance, there are now resistant strains that do not respond to any available antibiotics. Empiric antibiotics, prior to C&S returning should be selected based on facility patterns, but in general a broad-spectrum cephalosporin or a carbapenem are good choices. Aggressive control of healthcare-associated infection of these bacteria is crucial.

Brucella is a strictly aerobic, Gram-negative coccobacillus which causes Brucellosis, a disease similar in its symptoms to influenza, though there can be chronic recurrent fever, joint pain, and fatigue. Carried by animals, it causes only incidental infections in humans. Rare in the USA (about 100 cases/year), afflicted individuals with non-focal disease are usually treated with oral doxycycline combined with parenteral streptomycin or gentamicin. Doxycycline combined with rifampin is a more convenient option, as both doses are administered orally, but this combination has had a higher rate of treatment failure than doxycycline with either streptomycin or gentamicin.

ENTEROBACTER

Important nosocomial pathogens responsible for various infections, *Enterobacter cloacae* and *Enterobacter aerogenes* rarely cause disease in a healthy individual and are seldom seen in community outbreaks. Particularly lethal among very young and very old hospitalized patients and those already suffering from serious underlying conditions, the average mortality rate is estimated to be 20-46%, and possibly higher.

Risk factors for nosocomial *Enterobacter* species infections include:

- Extended hospitalization
- An invasive procedure within the last three days
- Treatment with antibiotics in the past month
- A central venous catheter

For infection with nosocomial multidrug-resistant strains, specific risk factors are the recent use of broad-spectrum cephalosporins or aminoglycosides and ICU care. Certain antibiotics, particularly third-generation cephalosporins, should be avoided because resistant mutants can appear quickly, and multiple antibiotic resistances complicate management of the infection. The source of infection may be exogenous or via colonization of the skin, gastrointestinal tract, or urinary tract.

Enterococci

Enterococci are Gram-positive facultative anaerobic (preferring oxygen but able to survive without it) cocci that usually occur in pairs. Only a few of the 21 species cause human infections. *Enterococci* are part of the normal flora of the gastrointestinal tract, which is the reservoir for most nosocomial infections, but they can also be found on skin, wounds, and chronic decubitus ulcers. They were formerly classified as *Streptococci* and look similar. *E. faecalis* causes 60-90% of infections and *E. faecium* causes 5-16%, but *E. faecium* is of increasing concern because it has developed vancomycin resistant strains. *Enterococci* are difficult to treat because they are intrinsically resistant to numerous antibiotics, including penicillins and cephalosporins. Additionally, they have acquired resistance to many others, including tetracyclines and vancomycin. Infections include urinary infections, bacteremia, endocarditis as well as infections in wounds and the abdominal and pelvic areas. Person-to-person transmission is common in nosocomial infections.

Campylobacter Jejuni

While seldom deadly, *Campylobacter*, being the most common cause of diarrhea in the United States, is the cause of considerable misery. Of the approximately 100,000 who contract it yearly in the USA, only about 100 die. It can sometimes occur in outbreaks, and there may be long-term consequences of infection. Some people may have arthritis following Campylobacteriosis; others may develop Guillain-Barré syndrome, a rare autoimmune disease that affects nerves throughout the body beginning several weeks after the diarrheal illness. Paralysis that may last several weeks usually requires intensive care. As many as 40% of Guillain-Barré syndrome cases in this country may be triggered by Campylobacteriosis, usually as a result of eating or handling raw or undercooked poultry meat. An outbreak in 1988 was caused by milk that had been improperly pasteurized.

Campylobacter usually presents with diarrhea with fever, vomiting, and abdominal pain and persists 7-12 days. Treatment (in uncomplicated cases) involves azithromycin 500 mg orally for 3 days or until symptoms improve. Levofloxacin is an acceptable alternative, though this medication has higher rates of resistance.

Clostridium Botulinum

Foodborne botulism is a toxin that is destroyed if heated at 80 °C for 10 minutes. The heat-resistant spores of *Clostridium botulinum*, however, can produce a deadly neurotoxin in poorly processed foods, with most of the outbreaks reported annually in the United States (10-30) associated with home-canned foods. Occasionally, though, commercially produced foods are at fault with canned meat products, canned vegetables, and canned seafood products being the most frequent sources. A victim must be treated immediately upon ingestion with an antitoxin; otherwise, there is an elevated chance of death. The organism and its spores occur widely in soils as well as stream, lake, and ocean sediments, intestinal tracts of fish and mammals, and in the gills and viscera of crabs and other shellfish. It also appears in honey, which is definitively linked to infant botulism but not in any cases involving adults. Foods are not involved in the botulism sometimes found in wounds; it results when *C. botulinum* infects a wound, producing toxins which travel via the blood stream to infect other parts of the body. Treatment includes:

- Gastric emptying of food remaining in stomach
- Antitoxin: Trivalent antitoxin as per CDC
- Supportive care, including mechanical ventilation if necessary
- Infant botulism: *BabyBIG* (botulism immune globulin) is now available

Vibrio Cholerae Serogroup O1

Unsanitary conditions pollute waters providing the breeding grounds for Vibrio cholerae Serogroup O1, the bacterium responsible for epidemic cholera.

Cholera was reported in 1991 in Peru, and grew to epidemic proportions, spreading north to Mexico, infecting 1,099,882 and killing 10,453. It was the only cholera epidemic in the Western Hemisphere in the 20th Century. The last major outbreak in the United States was 1911, but sporadic cases reported between 1973 and 1991 suggest that strains of the organism may now be found in the temperate coastal waters surrounding the USA.

Ingested viable bacteria attach to the small intestine and produce cholera toxin. Dehydration and loss of essential electrolytes can lead to death. Individuals infected with cholera require rehydration, either intravenously or orally, with a solution containing sodium chloride, sodium bicarbonate, potassium chloride, and dextrose (glucose). The illness is generally self-limiting. Antibiotics such as tetracycline have been demonstrated to shorten the course of the illness.

Listeria Monocytogenes

Listeriosis, caused by *Listeria monocytogenes* finds expression in encephalitis, meningitis (or meningoencephalitis), and septicemia.

- It is also a factor in intrauterine or cervical infections in pregnant women. (It can result in stillbirth or spontaneous abortion.)
- It has been associated with consuming raw or badly pasteurized milk, raw meats of all types, ice cream, and uncooked vegetables. Cheeses, raw and cooked poultry, fermented raw meat sausages, and raw and smoked fish are thought to be other sources.
- It can grow in refrigerated foods.
- Listeriosis is effectively treated with penicillin, ampicillin, or gentamicin.

Onset to GI symptoms may take more than 12 hours, whereas the time to serious forms of listeriosis may range from a few days to three weeks. At least 1,600 cases of listeriosis end in 260 deaths per year in the US (CDC). Overall mortality attributed to the bacillus ranges from 50% in septicemia to as high as 70% in listeric meningitis; it may go beyond 80% in perinatal/neonatal infections. For infections during pregnancy, the mother usually survives.

Pseudomonas Aeruginosa

Pseudomonas aeruginosa is an opportunistic pathogen, exploiting breaks in host defenses to initiate urinary tract infections, respiratory system infections, dermatitis, soft tissue infections, bacteremia, bone and joint infections, gastrointestinal infections, and variety of healthcare-associated infections. Particularly active in patients with cancer, cystic fibrosis, severe burns, or immunosuppressed AIDS, this disease has a fatality rate of 50% in these patients.

Accounting for 10% of all healthcare-associated infections, *Pseudomonas aeruginosa* is the fourth most commonly isolated nosocomial pathogen. Only fluoroquinolones, gentamicin, and imipenem are effective against it, and even these drugs are not effective against all strains. The futility of treating *Pseudomonas* infections with antibiotics is most dramatically illustrated in cystic fibrosis patients, virtually all of whom eventually become infected with a strain so resistant that it cannot be treated, and death is the general outcome.

PATHOGENESIS

Pseudomonas aeruginosa is a Gram-negative aerobic bacillus that is ubiquitous in soil and water, favoring moist conditions. It can grow in the absence of oxygen if nitrate is available. *P. aeruginosa* has fimbriae that facilitate adherence to epithelial cells in the respiratory tract. *P. aeruginosa* is encapsulated, providing protection from antibodies, and produces toxins, enzymes, cytotoxins, and hemolysins that resist phagocytosis and destroy cells of the host. *P. aeruginosa* is an opportunistic infection, invading compromised tissue. It can cause severe infections of virtually all systems and is especially dangerous for those with severe burns or with immunosuppression. Additionally, *P. aeruginosa* is resistant to many common antibiotics and some strains have proven resistant to all antimicrobials. Because *P. aeruginosa* has a high virulence factor, it can easily invade the bloodstream, causing bacteremia, which carries a 40% mortality rate. Bacteremia may also result from contaminated liquids and equipment, such as endoscopes.

LEGIONELLA

Legionella is a Gram-negative obligate aerobic bacillus that is motile. *Legionella* is comprised of 48 species, but *L. pneumophila* causes 90% of infections, most often in those who are immunocompromised. *Legionella* is an intracellular pathogenic agent that replicates within monocytic phagocytes (depending on the availability of iron) and alveolar macrophages. Both antibody-mediated (which can result in long-term resistance) and cell-mediated immunity responses occur to combat infection. *Legionella* colonizes water distribution systems because it can survive chlorine treatment. It grows well in hot water tanks. Air-conditioning systems, despite wide belief, have not been implicated in the spread of infection. Nosocomial infections correlate with use of ventilators, intubation, and naso-gastric tubes. Using tap water instead of sterile water to cleanse equipment can lead to infection. The most common infections are Pontiac fever, which is flu-like, and pneumonia, which can lead to dissemination of the pathogen throughout the body, causing multi-organ failure.

LEGIONNAIRE'S DISEASE

At an American Legion convention in 1976, one Legionnaire after another became ill with an acute pneumonia-like illness; 34 of the 221 who were stricken died. A CDC investigation ensued to track down the cause, a bacterium they named *Legionella.* It thrived in the convention hotel's cooling tower from which the bacteria were actively pumped into the hotel through the air conditioning system. (This led to new worldwide restrictions requiring more stringent cleaning for cooling towers and large-scale air conditioning systems.)

Since 1977, 41 species of *Legionella* species containing 62 serogroups have been characterized; one of them, *Legionella pneumophila,* is responsible for more than 80% of Legionnaires' disease cases, and among its 13 serogroups, Serogroup 1 is responsible for 95% of these cases. The *Legionella* bacteria are widely distributed at a low concentration, flourishing in both warm and cold water, from lakes to shower heads. They cause disease only if inhaled.

Neisseria Gonorrhea

Sexually transmitted *Neisseria gonorrhea*, unable to survive dehydration or cool conditions, causes urethritis with dysuria and purulent discharge in the male and, in the female, most commonly infects the endocervix, from whence it produces purulent vaginal discharge and bleeding and, if not treated, can ascend to cause salpingitis (PID). This can lead to sterility, ectopic pregnancy, or Fitz-Hugh-Curtis syndrome.

However, it is often asymptomatic during early infection. One outcome, ophthalmia neonatorum (a purulent conjunctivitis), in the past was passed from mother to infant but is now rare, thanks to the initiation of treatment by prophylactic erythromycin eye ointment (formerly $AgNO_3$ solution) applied at birth.

Though disseminated gonorrhea infections can sometimes lead to endocarditis and meningitis, more often they cause septic arthritis. As the disease is penicillin resistant, it must be countered with ceftriaxone 500 mg to 1 g IM in 1 dose.

Coronaviruses

Coronaviruses are relatively large RNA viruses that appear to have a crown or halo about them when viewed microscopically. They were first identified in chickens in 1937. A number of different coronaviruses have been identified as pathogens of animals, such as dogs, and by 2005, five different human coronaviruses had been identified, but more may exist. Coronaviruses are inhaled or ingested by oral-fecal route into the respiratory system where they cause both upper and lower respiratory infection or into the gastrointestinal system where they cause gastroenteritis. They are believed to be responsible for 10-30% of viruses that cause the common cold; however, they are implicated in more serious infections, such as severe acute respiratory syndrome (SARS) and more recently the COVID-19 pandemic. Coronaviruses replicate in cytoplasm after they enter into the host cell by endocytosis and membrane fusion. Reinfections can occur, suggesting that there are a number of different serotypes.

COVID-19 (SARS-CoV-2)

COVID-19 is an infection caused by a coronavirus (SARS-CoV-2) that is extremely contagious. The incubation period ranges from 10-14 days (average 5 days), and many of those who are infected are asymptomatic carriers. SARS-CoV-2 is able to spread both through droplet and aerosol transmission. The reproduction number (R0) is considerably higher than that of the flu (usually about 1.1) and varies depending on containment efforts. For example, the R0 got as high as 11.6 in March 2020 but stabilized to about 1 in mid-2021, but outbreaks of the Delta variant risked increasing the R0 again. In about 80% of patients, the viral load clears within 10-14 days. In others, the disease progresses. When the coronavirus invades the respiratory system, it attaches to enzyme-2 (ACE-2) receptors of pulmonary alveolar epithelial cells with S1 viral spikes and enters the cell, where viral replication, transcription, and translation take place. Protein biosynthesis occurs within the cytoplasm and new viral particles are released into the extracellular space with apoptosis of host cells. The body reacts with a cytokine storm. CD8 mediated cytotoxicity causes diffuse damage to alveoli and acute respiratory distress syndrome.

COVID-19 has also been proven to attack other body systems, causing clotting issues (leading to the loss of limbs in severe cases), inflammation of the lining of the heart (leading to permanent damage in some cases), and other issues of organ dysfunction or failure that are still being studied.

Signs and Symptoms

The initial signs and symptoms for COVID-19 infection are similar to those of the flu: fever, chills, cough, and myalgia. Up to a third of patients may experience shortness of breath. Loss of taste and smell is often an early symptom. Other symptoms can include nausea, diarrhea, hemoptysis, hallucinations and confusion, hives, rash, and conjunctivitis. Some infected individuals develop "COVID toes," painful itchy inflammation and discoloration of the toes (red to purple), sometimes with petechial macular lesions. The most common complication is bilateral interstitial pneumonia, which usually develops 8-9 days after initial symptoms and can progress to severe respiratory distress within a few hours. Up to 20% of hospitalized patients develop cardiac injury, and up to 30% show signs of kidney failure. Patients are also at risk for blood clots, which can lead to stroke or pulmonary embolus. A multisystem inflammatory syndrome, which is life threatening, may affect both adults and children.

Risk Factors

While people of any age can contract COVID-19/SARS-CoV-2 infection, those at the greatest risk are middle aged and older adults, especially those with preexisting health problems. Other risk factors include those who are immunocompromised and those with lung disorders, such as cystic fibrosis, asthma, COPD, pulmonary fibrosis, and pulmonary cancer as these patients have high rates of interstitial pneumonia. Because COVID may cause cardiac injury, those with existing heart disease (cardiomyopathy, heart failure, coronary artery disease, congenital heart disease, and pulmonary hypertension) are at increased risk. Other disorders that increase risk of developing severe disease include obesity, HIV/AIDS, diabetes mellitus, sickle cell anemia, thalassemia, chronic kidney disease, chronic liver disease, and Down syndrome. While children initially had low rates of symptomatic disease, later variants of the virus, including the Delta variant, have resulted in a larger number of children developing symptoms.

Laboratory Testing for Diagnosis

Numerous tests are FDA approved for COVID-19 (SARS-CoV-2) detection. Sensitivity and specificity vary but range from 90-100% for approved tests. Specimens in the United States were most commonly collected via nasal and nasopharyngeal swabs:

- **Nucleic Acid Amplification Test (NAAT):** Detects COVID-19 genetic material and identifies the virus's RNA sequences. The genetic material obtained in the specimen is amplified, so even a very small amount of the virus in the specimen is detected and false negatives are rare but may occur with rapid tests. Both laboratory and point-of-care tests are available with laboratory tests more sensitive. Different NAAT methods include Reverse Transcription Polymerase Chain Reaction (RT-PCR) (most common) and isothermal amplification methods. NAATs are often used to confirm lower sensitivity tests. NAATs may remain positive for extended periods after active infection has subsided, so the test may not indicate contagiousness.
- **Antigen test:** Detects the presence of viral antigens and are often used for screening because results may be available within minutes (through rapid tests), but antigen tests are less sensitive than NAATs and both false positives and false negative may occur, so confirmatory testing may be necessary.

Mycobacterium Tuberculosis

Mycobacterium tuberculosis is a non-motile obligate aerobic bacillus that forms chains, which are associated with a toxic surface component called cord factor. *M. tuberculosis* is neither Gram-negative nor positive. As an extracellular agent, it needs oxygen, so it is attracted to the upper respiratory tract. It is also a facultative intracellular invader, allowing it to evade the immune system. Humans serve as the reservoir for this pathogen. The virulence is increased because of a unique cell wall composed of peptidoglycan but also complex lipids that provide antibiotic resistance and include acids that protect the cell, cord factor that is toxic to host cells, and Wax-D, which protects the cell envelope. The host immune system attempts to control the spread of *M. tuberculosis* by walling it off with macrophages, causing a positive skin reaction (cell-mediated immune response) but no infection. Resistant strains are an increasing cause of concern. Healthcare-associated infection outbreaks have occurred, often related to failure to identify an infected source.

Drug Resistant Strains of Tuberculosis

Multi-drug resistant tuberculosis (MDR-TB) is resistant to at least two commonly used first-line drugs, isoniazid (INH) and rifampin, while **extensively drug resistant tuberculosis (XDR-TB)** is also resistant to all fluoroquinolones and at least one of the three second-line drugs: Amikacin, kanamycin, or capreomycin.

XDR-TB emerged as a worldwide concern in 2005. In the United States, it is at present most commonly found in foreign-born patients but also occurs in immunocompromised patients. Active TB requires treatment for extended periods of time, usually 18-24 months, with multiple drugs.

Since the 1980s there has been increased need to use second-line drugs to combat infection. There are two primary causes for the increased resistance:

- Failure to complete a course of treatment
- Mismanaged treatment, including incorrect medication, dosage, or duration of therapy.

People who have had previous TB are at increased risk and should be monitored carefully. Drug resistant TB increasingly poses a risk for patients and staff in healthcare facilities.

Clostridium Difficile

Clostridium difficile is an anaerobic Gram-positive bacillus that produces endospores. It is commonly found in healthcare facilities. Normal intestinal flora provide resistance to *C. difficile,* but if the flora is disrupted by antibiotic use (or sometimes chemotherapeutic agents) and the host is an asymptomatic carrier or has acquired the infection during or after treatment, then *C. difficile* can begin to overgrow. *C. difficile* produces a lethal cytotoxin (Toxin B) and an endotoxin with cytotoxic action (Toxin A) that causes fluid to accumulate in the colon and severe damage to mucous membranes. *C. difficile* causes more healthcare-associated infection diarrhea cases than any other microorganism. All antibiotics can cause *C. difficile* infections but Clindamycin and cephalosporins are most-frequently implicated. Symptoms vary widely, from mild diarrhea to lethal sepsis. It can cause diarrhea, colitis, and pseudomembranous colitis, and megacolon. Infection may not be obvious for weeks after completion of antibiotics.

Aspergillus Spp.

Aspergillus spp. are filamentous (having long threads) fungi, which increasingly cause nosocomial infections. They are ubiquitous in the environment and are aerobic, grow as molds, and produce spores that become airborne and can invade the respiratory tract. There are about 180 species, but about 20 are human pathogens. Most healthy people are resistant to *Aspergillus,* but it can invade almost all organs, although rarely infecting the blood. Invasive infections occur in those who are immunocompromised, such as those having transplants or receiving chemotherapy. Mortality rates are as high as 90% for invasive infections and treatment often involves surgical debridement as well as medical treatment. Mold remediation, high efficiency particulate air (HEPA) filtration and laminar airflow rooms have been used to avoid infection, and antifungal prophylaxis may also be indicated. *A. fumigatus* and *flavus* cause most invasive infections. *A. fumigatus* and *clavatus* activate the antigen-antibody immune response, causing a hypersensitivity reaction.

Pulmonary Aspergillus

Caused by the fungus aspergillus and commonly found on dead leaves, bird droppings, and compost piles, pulmonary aspergillosis forms a fungus ball at the site of previous lung disease and becomes invasive pulmonary aspergillosis when the infection spreads. Affecting any organ, including heart, lungs, brain, and kidneys and, as the disease spreads, the nervous system and skin, and difficult to cure, it eventually causes multi-organ system failure. It is treated with antifungal medications. The kind of immuno-suppression and low white blood cell count typical of patients who have had chemotherapy or bone marrow transplantation are major risk factors. Patients with the invasive form of pulmonary aspergillosis are usually critically ill, and prognosis is often not good.

Management of Pulmonary Aspergillosis

The best way to confine pulmonary aspergillosis and treat it is to have a facility equipped to do so. This means constructing new specialized-care units for patients at high risk for infection by ensuring that patient rooms have adequate capacity to minimize fungal spore counts. This is accomplished through:

- High-efficiency particulate air (HEPA) filtration that is 99.97% efficient in filtering particles greater than or equal to 0.3 µm in diameter
- Air-intake and exhaust ports placed such that room air comes in from one side of the room, flows across the patient's bed, and exits on the opposite side of the room
- Positive air pressure maintained continuously; there can be a problem when the patient has a second condition, such as tuberculosis, which requires negative air pressure, in which case an anteroom with a second exhaust system is needed
- Properly sealed rooms in which windows, doors, and intake and exhaust ports are designed to achieve complete sealing of the room against air leaks
- Room-air is cycled at least 12 times per hour

Candida

Candida is a yeast fungal pathogen. *C. albicans* is the most common, but non-*C. albicans* pathogenic forms, some resistant to antifungal medications, have caused healthcare-associated infection outbreaks. Humans and animals are the reservoirs for *Candida*, and *C. albicans* is part of the normal flora of mucous membranes and can cause superficial infections, such as thrush and vaginitis. *Candida* species can adhere to multiple host tissues, but an intact cell mediated immune system can limit infection. If this immune system is defective (as with AIDS) *Candida* can overgrow and lead to mucocutaneous or cutaneous lesions and sepsis. *Candida* multiplies in a bioform structure that provides protection from antifungals. Intact skin is an effective barrier, but lesions, burns, and intravascular tubes can allow invasion. Normal intestinal flora also suppresses *Candida*, but disruption caused by antimicrobials allows infection. *C. tropicalis* can cause invasive candidiasis, particularly in leukemia patients. *C. parapsilosis* is an environmental contaminant and can be transferred on the hands and causes infections of the bloodstream.

Influenza A and B

Influenza A is more virulent and common than **influenza B**, but both have been linked to epidemics and pose threats to those hospitalized, especially the young and elderly populations. Influenza A is an avian virus that has migrated to humans while Influenza B only affects humans, which are reservoirs for both. Influenza viruses are round or filamentous and have an RNA genome, which consists of eight segments inside a protein envelope. The segmented genome allows for new strains to develop easily and quickly, making vaccines short lived. The virus binds to the host cell, allowing entry of the RNA into the host. The genes are copied and the host cell begins producing viral particles. Influenza viruses stimulate the antibody mediated immune response. Influenza infections usually present as fever, chills, myalgia, and cough but can progress to viral pneumonia and secondary bacterial pneumonia. Transmission is by droplet particles directly to mucous membranes or by infected hands making contact with mucous membranes.

HERPESVIRUSES

CYTOMEGALOVIRUS

Cytomegalovirus (CMV) is in the herpesvirus family and contains DNA in its genome. The cell envelope is formed from the cell membranes of budding virions. Outside of the host, the virus is easily destroyed by disinfectants. CMV infections are ubiquitous in humans and are usually asymptomatic but may cause a mononucleosis type illness in some. CMV is much more serious in those who are immunocompromised as it can invade and replicate in any organ in the body and has been implicated in transplant rejection. People may develop pneumonia, liver infection, and anemia. CMV also poses a threat to pregnant women and to the fetus of a newly infected mother. CMV retinitis is a serious complication of HIV infection, increasing as the CD4 count decreases. CMV can be transmitted placentally, in body fluids, and on the hands, a common cause of healthcare-associated infection transmission; therefore, handwashing procedures are extremely important to prevent healthcare-associated infection.

HERPES SIMPLEX VIRUSES

Herpes simplex virus 1 causes herpetic lesions primarily on the lips and face, a "cold sore," and is spread directly by contact with infected lesions, often through kissing or oral sex. **Herpes simplex virus 2** causes lesions primarily in the urogenital area and is spread by sexual contact. Both types can occur in either area or on other areas of the body. Between infections, both viruses remain in a latent state and can be reactivated. Herpes 1 usually migrates to the trigeminal root ganglia while Herpes 2 remains dormant in the sacral plexus. The antibody-mediated immune response controls latency, during which the virus replicates much more slowly, but can reactivate during illness, fever, or times of stress. When the immune system is compromised, the virus can reactivate and spread out of control causing severe, large, painful lesions and may result in encephalitis, pneumonia esophagitis, ocular disease, and proctitis. Patients and staff with active lesions can spread herpes, resulting in healthcare-associated infection outbreaks in infants and adults.

VARICELLA-ZOSTER VIRUS

Varicella-zoster virus (human herpes virus 3) in the herpes virus family causes both chicken pox, and herpes zoster (shingles). The varicella-zoster virus contains double strands of DNA and has a protective envelope. Once it gains entry to a host from airborne droplets, it begins to replicate. A rash, initially red that becomes vesicular, appears about two weeks after initial infection with the infection running its course in 10-21 days. While most chickenpox infections are mild, they can result in viral encephalitis or pneumonia, especially in those who are immunocompromised. After infection, the host's antibody mediated immune response confers immunity to chicken pox; however, the virus remains dormant in the dorsal root ganglia or the cranial nerve ganglia and can become reactivated. Reactivation results in herpes zoster, involving severe pain along the involved nerve and a vesicular rash, usually around the trunk or the head. Pain can persist for weeks or months. Herpes zoster is spread by direct contact with vesicles, causing chickenpox in those who are not immune.

Hepatitis

Hepatitis A

Primarily transmitted person-to-person through contact through fecal contamination, hepatitis A virus (HAV) is most often found in areas of poor sanitation and overcrowding, though epidemics from contaminated food and water also occur. In the latter, water, shellfish, and salads are the most frequent sources. When contaminated foods are the source, infected workers in food processing plants and restaurants are commonly behind it. On rare occasions, HAV has been transmitted in blood transfusions.

Hepatitis A has a worldwide distribution. Outbreaks are common in crowded housing projects, institutions, prisons, and military installations. Major epidemics in foreign countries occurred in 1954, 1961, and 1971. The period of communicability extends from early in the incubation period to about a week after the development of jaundice. Most cases resolve within three weeks and there are seldom fatalities. (Hepatitis E, which has symptoms similar to Hepatitis A, has a fatality rate of 20% among pregnant women.)

Pathogenesis of Hepatitis A

Hepatitis A virus (HAV) is an RNA picornavirus that replicates in the liver, is secreted into the gallbladder, and enters the intestines. The virus triggers an antibody mediated immune response with IgM that confers immunity, so reinfection and chronic infection does not occur. HAV infection is often asymptomatic in children, but adults may develop jaundice, general malaise, pain in the abdomen, nausea, and diarrhea. Because infants are usually asymptomatic, infection with HAV may not be suspected in neonatal units. Healthcare-associated infections have occurred when there has been a break in infection control and HAV from infected stool of infants or adults with diarrhea was transmitted on the hands of staff. Vaccine is available but not routinely administered.

Hepatitis B

Hepatitis B virus (HBV) is a DNA virus of the family *Hepadnaviridae* and is transmitted through contact with blood either. The DNA genome enters the host cell nucleus and then copies and replicates. The cell-mediated immune response that destroys the virus also causes damage to hepatic cells, resulting in acute hepatitis. Chronic infection occurs in 90% of infants and 6% of those over 5 years old, with 15-25% of those with chronic infection developing liver cancer. The virus can remain stable in the environment for a week. Outbreaks in healthcare facilities have occurred because of contaminated blood sampling and hemodialysis equipment as well as from the use of multi-dose vials. Using single-dose vials and disposable equipment as well as proper handwashing techniques are important for prevention of nosocomial infections. Vaccine is available and advised for healthcare workers who may come in contact with blood. Children are now routinely vaccinated for HBV.

Incidence, Risk Factors, and Pathways for Hepatitis B Infection

The contact with the blood or body fluids of an infected person necessary for acquiring **Hepatitis B** can be accomplished through:

- Having unprotected sex with an infected person
- Sharing needles
- An accidental needle stick

It can also be passed from infected mother to her baby at birth. High-risk behavior for HBV infection includes:

- Multiple sex partners
- Male homosexual intercourse
- Sex with an infected partner
- Injecting illegal drugs
- Healthcare and public safety work
- Living with persons with chronic HBV infection
- Hemodialysis

There are about 1.25 million people in the US with chronic Hepatitis B virus; some 80,000, mostly young adults, become infected with it annually, and between 4,000 and 5,000 people die from it each year. Hepatitis B has the same symptoms as Hepatitis A: loss of appetite, jaundice, diarrhea, joint pain, and nausea. But, while Hepatitis A is a short-term illness, HBV can persist, with the dangers of being untreated including cirrhosis, cancer of the liver, and death.

Hepatitis C

Hepatitis C virus (HCV) is a single-strand RNA *Flaviviridae* virus that binds to receptors on hepatic cells and enters to begin replicating. HCV readily mutates, which helps it to evade the host's immune response. There are six genotypes and several subtypes of HCV with some types more virulent and resistive to treatment than others. There is no vaccine. HCV is transmitted directly through blood or items, such as shared needles, contaminated with blood. It can be spread by sexual contact. Prior to 1992, the blood supply was contaminated with HCV, as was clotting factors made before 1987. HCV causes an acute infection (in the first six months), but 55-85% develop chronic infection with 70% of those developing chronic liver disease. HCV is the primary reason for liver transplants. Nosocomial infections are similar to HBV and related to contaminated blood sampling equipment, multidose vials, improperly sterilized equipment, and breakdown in infection control methods.

Human Immunodeficiency Virus (HIV)

Human immunodeficiency virus (HIV) is a slow-acting retrovirus of the genus lentivirus. HIV binds with cells that have CD4 receptors, primarily CD4+ T cells and other cells of the immune system, enters the cells and begins replicating. Host cells are destroyed in a number of ways:

- **Disruption of cell wall** or cellular function may be caused after large numbers of replicated viral cells bud through the cell membrane or build up inside the cell.
- **Formation of syncytia** occurs when cells infected with HIV fuse with nearby cells creating giant cells, thus allowing HIV to spread from one cell to many.
- **Apoptosis**, or cell death, occurs when HIV sends a signal to uninfected cells, causing them to self-destruct.
- **Binding to cell surface** of uninfected cell by HIV gives the appearance that the cell is infected, causing it to be targeted by killer T cells as part of the immune response.

HIV is spread through blood or other bodily fluids and blood contaminated equipment.

Review Video: AIDS Infections and Malignancies
Visit mometrix.com/academy and enter code: 319526

ROTAVIRUSES

Rotaviruses, transmitted by the fecal-oral route, are spread most commonly by dirty hands. Commonly found in day care centers, pediatric and geriatric wards, and family homes, they may also be found in uncooked food contaminated by infected food handlers. Sanitary measures adequate for bacteria and parasites seem to be ineffective in controlling rotavirus; a similar incidence of infection is observed in countries with both high and low health standards.

Sufferers from severe diarrhea who do not get quick access to fluid and electrolyte replacement may die; otherwise, recovery from infections is usually complete. Childhood mortality due to rotavirus is relatively low in the US, with an estimated 20-60 deaths/year, but approaches about 200,000 deaths per year worldwide. Of childhood cases of severe diarrhea that require hospitalization, about half can be attributed to Group A rotavirus. Group B rotavirus is endemic primarily to China.

NORWALK FAMILY OF VIRUSES

Viral gastroenteritis, more commonly known as food poisoning, has at its root a member of the Norwalk family of viruses. It is a preeminent cause of illness in the US. It is estimated that Norwalk viruses are behind about a third of all viral gastroenteritis cases, and the only viral illness reported to a greater extent is the common cold. Though not permanent (people can become reinfected), half the population over 18 develops immunity because it gradually increases with age.

Norwalk gastroenteritis is transmitted through drinking water or foods that have been contaminated with human feces, water being the most common source of outbreaks. Eating raw or insufficiently steamed clams and oysters that come from polluted beds makes for a high risk for Norwalk virus infection. But other foods, not just shellfish, may be contaminated by food handlers. Illness usually comes on about 24 to 48 hours after eating or drinking. The disease is self-limiting, lasting between one day and 60 hours, and is mild. It is characterized by diarrhea, nausea, vomiting, and abdominal pain.

RESPIRATORY SYNCYTIAL VIRUS (RSV)

Infecting nearly all infants by the age of two years, respiratory syncytial virus (RSV) is the most common respiratory pathogen found in young children. Easily spread by physical contact with contaminated secretions, it can live for half an hour or more on hands, five hours on countertops, and several hours on used wipes. RSV is usually a mild respiratory illness for adults because healthy people can and do produce antibodies against the virus.

In infants and young children, RSV can cause pneumonia, inflammation of the small airways of the lungs, and croup, incidence of which is about 125,000 infants yearly with cases serious enough to be hospitalized, of whom 1-2% die. Inflammation of terminal bronchioles marks acute bronchiolitis in small children, leading to hyperinflation of air sacs distal to bronchiole. Complete plugging of bronchiole with air resorption leads to collapse that can be life threatening. Bronchiolitis appears in seasonal epidemics but can also be seen year-round in poorer communities throughout the world. It is usually preceded by coryzal symptoms which later develop into a major pulmonary illness. Clinically there is fever, rapid respiration, exhausting cough, and wheezing.

It is imperative that infants with RSV in a high-risk nursery be isolated from others and that special care be taken that any physical contact does not result in cross-contamination. Premature infants, immunocompromised infants, and infants with either chronic lung disease or certain forms of heart disease are at increased risk for severe RSV disease.

Review Video: Respiratory Diseases
Visit mometrix.com/academy and enter code: 973392

Chagas Disease

Chagas disease, caused by the protozoan parasite *Trypanosoma cruzi,* is endemic to much of Mexico, Central, and South America, and is transmitted when a triatomine insect bites the skin and deposits contaminated feces in the wound. The parasite invades organs and is transmitted through blood and organ donations. Chagas is an emerging disease in the United States where a large Latin American immigrant population has brought many cases. The CDC estimates that approximately 300,000 individuals with Chagas disease currently live in the United States. Chagas has three stages, acute with either no or flu-like symptoms for most people, an intermediate stage that is asymptomatic, and a chronic stage that occurs about 30 years after infection, presenting with severe cardiomyopathy and digestive problems. People are often unaware that they are infected but the disease poses a danger to the blood supply. Treatment is often ineffective after the acute stage. Most blood banks have begun testing for Chagas disease. Only universal precautions are necessary for Chagas disease.

Scabies

Scabies is caused by a microscopic mite, *Sarcoptes scabiei hominis,* that tunnels under the outer layer of skin, raising small lines a few millimeters long. Mites prefer warm areas, such as between the fingers and in skin folds, but can infest any area of the body. As the mites burrow, they cause intense itching and subsequent scratching can result in secondary infections. Scabies is spread very easily through person-to-person contact and has become a problem in nursing homes and extended care facilities where staff spread the infection from one patient to another. Incubation time is 6-8 weeks and itching usually begins in about 30 days, so people may be unaware they are transmitting scabies. Most infestations involve only about a dozen mites, but a severe form of scabies infection, Norwegian or crusted scabies, can occur in the elderly or those who are immunocompromised. In this case, lesions can contain thousands of mites, making this type highly contagious.

Giardia Lamblia

Giardia lamblia is the causative agent of giardiasis, the most frequent source of non-bacterial diarrhea in North America. Ingestion of one or more protozoan cysts may bring on diarrhea within a week, though, for most bacterial illnesses, at least thousands of organisms may have to be consumed to produce illness. Giardiasis most frequently results from drinking contaminated water, though outbreaks have been traced to food contamination, and it is impossible to rule out contaminated vegetables eaten raw as sources of infection. It is more prevalent in children, possibly because many adults seem to have a lasting immunity after infection. This organism is implicated in 25% of the cases of gastrointestinal disease and may be present asymptomatically. Symptoms occur 7 to 14 days after ingestion of one or more cysts and include diarrhea with greasy, floating stools (rarely bloody), stomach cramps, nausea, and flatulence, lasting 2 to 6 weeks. A chronic infection may develop that can last for months or years. Diagnosis is based on three stool specimens, ELISA, or PCR for DNA. Treatment includes correcting fluid and electrolyte issues and antibiotics for symptomatic patients or patients who are food handlers, immunocompromised, or children who attend day care type settings:

- Tinidazole 2 g orally in a single dose **OR** Nitazoxanide 500 mg twice daily for 3 days
- Foods that contain lactose should be avoided for one month after treatment

Cryptosporidiosis

Severe watery diarrhea marks intestinal **cryptosporidiosis**, while tracheal cryptosporidiosis's cardinal symptoms are coughing, mild fever; and sometimes severe intestinal distress. They are both caused by a single-celled obligate intracellular parasite. Herd animals (cows, goats, sheep) and humans may be infected with the *Cryptosporidium parvum* sporocysts, which are resistant to most chemical disinfectants. Drying and the ultraviolet portion of sunlight are deadly to them.

Presumably, one organism in infected food touched by a contaminated food handler can initiate an infection. Incidence is high in child day care centers where food is served. Another possible source of human infection is raw manure that has been spread over garden vegetables, but large outbreaks invariably have contaminated water supplies as their source.

Up to 80% of the population has been infected with cryptosporidiosis. There is no effective treatment and the severe watery diarrhea is often a contributor in the death of AIDS victims; invasion of the pulmonary system may also be fatal.

Entamoeba Histolytica

Amebiasis (or amoebiasis), the infection caused by *Entamoeba histolytica,* can last for up to four years with no symptoms, some gastrointestinal distress, or dysentery, complete with blood and mucus. Potential complications include pain from ulcers or abscesses and, rarely, intestinal blockage.

The amoeba's cysts survive, especially under moist conditions, in water and soils and on foods. They result in infections when they are swallowed; they excyst to the trophozoite stage in the digestive tract, with the possibility of other tissues being invaded. Ingestion of one viable cyst, it is thought, is enough to cause an infection.

Amebiasis is transmitted primarily by fecal contamination of drinking water and foods and also through direct contact with dirty hands or objects. Sexual contact may also transmit the disease. AIDS/ARC patients are especially vulnerable. Fatalities are infrequent.

Anisakis Simplex

Anisakid nematodes (roundworms) are a hazard for those who consume raw or undercooked seafood, as are *Anisakis simplex* (herring worm), and *Pseudoterranova (Phocanema, Terranova) decipiens* (cod or seal worm). Reported encounters are rare in North America, typically less than 20 per year. However, it is suspected that many cases may be suffered after eating sushi or sashimi and go undetected. Symptoms appear anywhere between an hour and two weeks. Anisakids rarely reach full maturity in humans because they are generally expelled from the GI tract spontaneously within three weeks. Severe cases, while rare, are extremely painful and require surgical intervention.

The larvae of *Ascaris lumbricoides*, a large roundworm and a terrestrial relative of anisakids, may sometimes also crawl up into the throat and nasal passages. Symptoms include malnutrition, abdominal discomfort, and passing worms in stool or emesis. Treatment includes albendazole 400 mg orally twice daily for up to 21 days.

Diseases Caused by Anisakis Simples

Seafood is the principal source of human infections from the larval worm *Anisakis simplex*, whose adults are found in the stomachs of whales and dolphins. There their fertilized eggs pass out with the host's feces. The eggs develop into larvae that hatch and infect minute crustaceans. These, in turn, are eaten by fish and squid and infect them. It is believed that nematode larvae move from the viscera to the flesh of the fish they inhabit if the fish (most commonly cod, haddock, fluke, pacific salmon, herring, flounder, and monkfish) are not gutted promptly after being caught.

Shellfish Associated Toxins

Though good statistical data on the occurrence and severity of cases stemming from eating shellfish that feed upon algae that can produce a variety of toxins are largely unavailable, we know that mollusks can pass on four types of poison:

- **Paralytic Shellfish Poisoning (PSP):** Attacks the nervous system, causing tingling, burning, numbness, drowsiness, incoherent speech, and respiratory paralysis; it comes from cockles, mussels, scallops, or clams and is the most serious type of shellfish-related poisoning.
- **Diarrheic Shellfish Poisoning (DSP):** Derived from mussels, oysters, and scallops, leads to no more than a mild gastrointestinal disorder.
- **Neurotoxic Shellfish Poisoning (NSP):** From shellfish harvested along the Florida coast and the Gulf of Mexico; causes dizziness, tingling, and numbness of lips, tongue, and throat, muscular pain, reversal of the sensations of hot and cold, diarrhea, and vomiting.
- **Amnesic Shellfish Poisoning (ASP):** From mussels; produces gastrointestinal disorders and neurological problems (confusion, memory loss, disorientation, seizure, and coma). All fatalities to date have involved elderly patients.

Mushroom and Toadstool Poisoning

Eating raw or cooked fruiting mushrooms or toadstools (another term for poisonous mushrooms) picked in the wild can lead to mushroom poisoning because some mushrooms contain one or more active toxins such as Amanitin (the most toxic), Gyromitrin, Orellanine, Muscarine, Ibotenic Acid, Muscimol, Psilocybin, or Coprine.

There is no simple way of distinguishing in the wild edible mushrooms from poisonous toadstools. The mushrooms that cause human poisoning cannot, by cooking, canning, freezing, or putting them through any other means of processing, render them nontoxic. The normal course of the disease varies with the mushroom species eaten and how much is eaten. Each poisonous species contains one or more toxic compounds unique to few other species. Therefore, cases of mushroom poisoning are also unique one from another. Poisonings in the United States are almost always caused by misidentification of what their hunters mistakenly believe to be edible fungi.

Symptoms

Symptoms of, and prognoses for, mushroom poisoning vary depending upon the species consumed and the amount ingested. The chemistry of many of the mushroom toxins is unknown and positive identification of the mushrooms eaten is often lacking, so it is their physiological effects on the eater that most often form the basis for identifying the mushroom that is the culprit. Mushroom toxins are classed in four categories:

- **Protoplasmic poisons:** Destroy cells, followed by organ failure
- **Neurotoxin compounds:** Bring on copious sweating, hallucinations, and other symptoms possibly leading up to a comatose state
- **Gastrointestinal irritants:** Produce symptoms of food poisoning
- **Disulfiram-like toxins:** Produce no symptoms without alcohol being consumed within 72 hours after eating them, and then a brief case of acute toxic syndrome results.

Much diagnosis is based on symptoms and recent dietary history. Seldom are positive identifications made of the mushroom species involved, and the few clinical tests that exist are too slow to be of clinical value.

Scombroid Poisoning

Its symptoms easily confused with those of other maladies, Scombroid poisoning often goes unreported though being one of the most common forms of fish poisoning in the United States. High levels of histamine and possibly other vasoactive amines and compounds found in some foods favor the growth of certain bacteria in food. This happens either during the production of Swiss cheese and such products or by spoilage of fishery products, tuna and mahi mahi poisoning being prominent. There is nothing that would visually tip one off to the presence of the toxin, and the toxic effect cannot be cancelled out by cooking, canning, or freezing.

Initial symptoms may include a tingling or burning sensation in the mouth, a rash on the upper body, a drop in blood pressure, headaches, and itching which may progress to nausea, vomiting, and diarrhea and may require hospitalization, particularly in the case of elderly or impaired patients. Generally speaking, the illness lasts no longer than three hours.

Aflatoxins

Aflatoxins, toxic compounds found in certain strains of the fungi *Aspergillus flavus* and *A. parasiticus*, grow on select foods and animal feeds when temperature and humidity are favorable. Contamination is most pronounced in tree nuts, peanuts (and thus peanut butter), and other oilseeds, including corn and cottonseed. It can also be found in the milk of dairy cattle that have eaten contaminated feed.

The compounds produce acute necrosis of tissue, cirrhosis, and carcinoma of the liver in a number of animal species, probably including humans, though outbreaks of aflatoxicosis in humans have rarely been reported; however, while such cases *have* happened, but they are not always recognized for what they are. Susceptibility to aflatoxins is not known, and what studies that have been performed on human ingestion of aflatoxins there are have focused on their carcinogenic potential.

Epidemiological studies in Africa and Southeast Asia suggest a connection between aflatoxins consumed in the diet and the incidence of hepatoma, which is high.

Diseases Caused by the Combination of Honey Bees and Rhododendrons

Honey intoxication is caused by human consumption of a substance produced by bees that have collected and processed pollen from rhododendrons. Other names associated with the disease, rare in humans, is rhododendron poisoning, mad honey intoxication, or grayanotoxin poisoning (grayanotoxins cause the intoxication).

Symptoms include dizziness, weakness, excessive perspiration, nausea, and vomiting shortly after the toxic honey is ingested and possibly low blood pressure or shock, bradyarrhythmia, sinus bradycardia, nodal rhythm, Wolff-Parkinson-White syndrome, or complete atrioventricular block. Intervention is seldom required; recovery generally comes about within 24 hours. Severe low blood pressure may be raised with the administration of fluids and correction of bradycardia; vasopressors are rarely needed. Sinus bradycardia and conduction defects usually respond to atropine therapy.

Individuals who get honey from hobby farmers in possession of only a few hives are at increased risk. Massive quantities of honey from different sources are mingled during commercial processing, generally serving to dilute any toxic substance.

Proteus Mirabilis

As a cause of non-nosocomial acquired urinary tract infections, the *proteus mirabilis* is second only to *E. coli*, but also causes wound infections, septicemia, and pneumonia, mostly in hospitalized patients by emitting *urease*, an enzyme that catalyzes the splitting of urea into ammonia and carbon dioxide. This causes the pH of urine to rise, allowing unchecked growth of the bacteria.

The higher pH is also toxic to renal cells, making possible urinary stones that can make *proteus* infections chronic. Over time the stones may grow large enough to cause obstruction and renal failure. In addition, they block the free flow of urine, inhibiting one of the body's natural cleansing mechanisms. Bacteria permeating the stones reinitiate infections even after antibiotic treatment.

P. mirabilis is generally susceptible to most antibiotics apart from tetracycline. However, some strains are resistant to first generation cephalosporins and ampicillins.

Prions

Prions, though disease-producing, are not cellular organisms or viruses, being normal proteins of animal tissues that can misfold and become infectious. They are associated with a group of diseases called transmissible spongiform encephalopathies (TSEs). Both the cattle disease, bovine spongiform encephalopathy (BSE), and the human disease vCJD (a variant of Creutzfeldt-Jakob disease) that results from eating infected beef, are known as "mad cow disease" and appear to be caused by the same agent.

Significant numbers of vCJD cases have occurred only in the United Kingdom; isolated cases have been reported in other countries. The United Kingdom epidemic that began in 1986 and affected nearly 200,000 cattle, has been waning. There is a possibility, however, that large numbers of apparently healthy persons might be incubating the disease. Though government agencies in many countries continue to implement new measures to minimize this and other associated risks, the possibility of "phantom carriers" raises concerns about iatrogenic transmission of the disease through insufficient sterilization of instruments used in surgery and medical diagnostic procedures and through blood and organ donations from unsuspected carriers.

Mad Cow Disease

The disease begins when cattle consume commercial feed containing processed high-risk cattle tissues of cows infected with BSE; this is thought to transfer prions that are absorbed into the steer's body during digestion. There the prions begin a process of changing the animal's normal protein counterparts into abnormal proteins like themselves. The practice of putting animal protein into feed for herbivore farm species has been banned, and the result is a noticeable decline in the number of cases.

After an extended incubation period of years in the human body, the disease results in irreversible neurodegeneration. Cases of vCJD usually present psychiatric problems, with depression being prominent. Problems with gait and muscle coordination, along with other neurologic signs appear, such as chronic forgetfulness. Severe problems with processing information and speaking ensue. Eventually, as victims become increasingly unable to care for themselves, they are hospitalized until death.

Fifth Disease

With fifth disease, a mild rash illness occurring most commonly in children (though adults are also susceptible), the child is usually not very ill, and the rash resolves in 7-10 days. The cause is human parvovirus B19 (animal parvoviruses are different and do not infect humans). It is highly contagious and transmitted through contact with respiratory secretions (e.g., saliva, sputum, or nasal mucus) before the illness moves into its mild rash phase.

Parvovirus B19 infection, however, may cause serious illness in persons with sickle-cell disease, chronic anemia, pregnant women, and people who have problems with their immune systems. People who have leukemia or cancer, who are born with immune deficiencies, who have received an organ transplant, or who have human immunodeficiency virus (HIV) infection are at risk for serious illness due to parvovirus B19 infection and should seek medical attention. They may need to be hospitalized. All others need only rest and reduce activity levels.

Adenoviruses

The 49 distinct types of adenoviruses can cause a number of illnesses such as gastroenteritis, conjunctivitis, and cystitis. Epidemics of febrile disease with conjunctivitis are associated with waterborne transmission of some adenovirus types, often centering on inadequately chlorinated swimming pools and small lakes. But most commonly, adenoviruses cause respiratory illnesses ranging from the common cold to pneumonia. Unusually resistant to chemical or physical agents and adverse pH conditions, they can sustain prolonged survival outside the body.

First encountered by soldiers during World War II, acute respiratory disease (ARD) may be related to a combination of adenovirus infections and conditions of crowding and stress. ARD, an epidemic form of acute pneumonic disease, can be prevented by enteric capsulation of a live vaccine strain activated in the gut.

Rhinoviruses

There are more than 100 serotypes of one virus family of rhinoviruses, *Picornaviridae,* that cause half of all inhalational URIs (referred to as common colds), which helps to explain why colds are so readily spread by droplets from the nose and mouth. It also explains why colds are acquired simply by taking breaths in a poorly ventilated room in which there are cold carriers in the first two days of infectious coryza. Though an infection resolves in about a week, it may temporarily upset the mucosal cilia and predispose to secondary invaders, especially bacterial infections, anything from sinusitis to pneumonia, which may require antibiotic treatment.

A short period of immunity to all colds follows a rhinovirus cold, but a prolonged immunity forms against the specific serotype that caused the most recent infection.

Bloodstream Infections

Bloodstream infections (BSIs) have increased markedly over the last few decades with approximately 350,000 patients infected each year. BSIs are defined as pathogens isolated in the blood of someone hospitalized for >48 hours. There are two basic types:

- **Primary** infections arise in the bloodstream and may be related to intravascular devices.
- **Secondary** infections spread systemically from an infection elsewhere in the body, such as from a urinary or wound infection.

There are a number of issues related to diagnosing a BSIs from blood cultures:

- **Skin preparation** must be adequate to prevent contamination of sample.
- **Blood volume** must be 10-20 mL in order to detect low concentrations of organisms.
- **Timing** should be as soon as possible after symptoms appear.
- **Venipuncture** should be done peripherally rather than obtaining blood from intravascular catheter, which may be contaminated.

Catheter-Related vs. Primary Blood Stream Infections

Intravascular catheters put patients at risk for local and systemic infection. In the United States, only counting specifically central venous catheters and only including ICUs, annually there are about 80,000 central venous catheter-related bloodstream infections. Serious complications may occur to produce considerable annual morbidity, simply because of the great frequency with which such catheters are used. Catheter-related bloodstream infections and general bloodstream infections should be treated as separate entities when accounting for attributable mortality rates between primary and catheter-related bacteremia. A laboratory confirmed bloodstream infection (LCBI) is a bloodstream infection confirmed by positive blood cultures that are not related to an infection at any other site OR the patient has positive symptoms of an infection, laboratory results indicating an infection that are not related to another site, and on two blood cultures drawn from separate areas the same commensal organism is present on culture results. A central line-associated blood stream infection is a LCBI where a central line was in place for more than two days prior to symptoms of infection/positive blood cultures.

Types of Catheter-Related Blood Stream Infections

Types of catheter-related blood stream (CRBS) infections:

- **Central Venous Catheter infection**: Catheters placed in large veins in the neck, chest, or groin occasionally cause *Staphylococcus aureus* or *Staphylococcus epidermidis* sepsis. To prevent infection, some central lines are now coated or impregnated with antibiotics or silver sulfadiazine.
- **Local catheter-related infection**: Though far more common than CVC infection, the outcomes and expenses related to infection are far less serious.
- **Exit-site infection**: Drainage of blood and/or pus from the exit site of a catheter; it may include redness double the size of the catheter diameter, tenderness, overgrown granulated tissue, and swelling. Dressings are unlikely to prevent infections.
- **Tunnel infection**: Cellulitis spreads around a subcutaneous tunnel tract.

Newborns and Infants

Infiltration by microorganisms in young children at IV catheter **sites** is frequent because their veins, small and fragile, may require multiple IV sticks. This can increase the incidence of healthcare-associated infections, especially when IV use is heavy. The most common avenue of infection is migration of floral organisms at the insertion site into a cutaneous catheter tract, thereby leading to colonization of the catheter tip. Frequent hand washing, good hygiene, and careful attention to policy and procedure in starting IVs are necessary.

While practicing good skin antisepsis, alcohol should not be used for initial skin preparation or for removing other compounds, such as chlorhexidine or povidone-iodine, from the skin because alcohol dries the skin and is highly absorbed. The skin is best rinsed with sterile water.

Secure IVs and catheters with tape or steristrips, allowing for continuous visual inspection of the catheter site and requiring fewer changes than standard gauze and tape dressing while reliably securing the catheter.

Identifying Potential Infection Due to Reportable Pathogens

In a small facility or targeted area of the hospital, reviewing all **laboratory reports** may be possible, but in larger facilities with multiple at-risk populations, targeted review is more efficient. Computerized laboratory reporting systems that can flag particular pathogens or threshold rates facilitate the review of laboratory findings. "Alert" pathogens, those that are frequently implicated in healthcare-associated infections, such as *Staphylococcus aureus* and *Pseudomonas aeruginosa* should always be tagged for review. The infection control personnel reviewing laboratory reports should be familiar with microbiology and with typical lab results for the complete blood count with the ability to recognize increases in leukocytes and differential shifts that may indicate infections. This person should also be knowledgeable about common healthcare-associated infections as well as those of particular concern for at risk populations in the facility related to outbreaks or breaches in infection control. Reports should be reviewed for unusual findings or clusters of infection.

Antimicrobials

Modes of Action of Antimicrobial Therapeutic Agents

Antimicrobial therapeutic agents include antibiotics that inhibit the growth of or kill bacteria, antifungals, antiprotozoals, and antivirals. Antibiotics that injure bacterial plasma membranes lead to cell death through leakage of cell contents.

Two of the five different modes of action that antimicrobial therapeutic agents take are **inhibition of cell wall synthesis** and **disruption of cell membrane function**. Bacterial cell walls are chemically and morphologically distinct from any structures found in animal cells. What happens when cell wall synthesis is inhibited is that an agent ruptures the membrane of the microorganism, releasing cell contents. A similar outcome results from disrupting cell-membrane function.

The three additional modes of action by antimicrobial therapeutic agents are as follows:

- **Inhibiting protein synthesis**: One group of antimicrobials works by disrupting ribosomes, thereby inhibiting translation, the synthesis of polypeptides. Antibiotics that inhibit protein synthesis include streptomycin and tetracycline.
- **Interfering with nucleic acid synthesis**: Antimicrobial agents like Flucytosine (an antifungal agent), the rifamycins, and the quinolones can inhibit nucleotide synthesis or interconversion. They can also prevent DNA from functioning properly and interfere with the replication and transcription of DNA.
- **Interfering with the normal functions of cells such as cell division**: Antimetabolites such as Thioguanine, used to treat acute leukemias, affect a cell's metabolites, substances required for normal biochemical reactions to take place. The drugs accomplish this by, among other things, disrupting microbial enzymes. They inhibit cell division and, therefore, stop the growth of tumors by interfering with DNA production.

Selective Toxicity in Antimicrobial Therapy

An antimicrobial agent is a chemotherapeutic agent used in the treatment of infectious disease whose action is inhibiting microbial growth and microbial survival. It is **selectively toxic** if, when administered, it harms an invading species without harming the host species. This is the principle behind chemotherapy, a term coined by Paul Ehrlich around 1900, referring to the use of chemical agents to kill infectious organisms. Ehrlich based his work on the hypothesis that, if microorganisms selectively took up stains, why should they not selectively take up toxic materials?

The maximum tolerable dose per kilogram of body weight, divided by the minimum dose per kilogram body weight that will cure the disease is termed the chemotherapeutic index.

Spectrum of Activity of Antimicrobial Therapy

The spectrum of activity refers to all of the varied microorganisms a particular antimicrobial agent is capable of attacking.

- A **broad-spectrum** antibiotic like tetracycline, having the broadest spectrum of all antibiotics employed, is active against a wider spectrum of microorganisms, including many Gram-positive and Gram-negative bacterial infections.
- An antibiotic that affects only a limited number of microorganisms is said to have a **narrow spectrum** of activity. It does less collateral damage to host microflora while presenting a lower risk of building resistance in the pathogen. It is the agent of choice when attacking a recognized microorganism. Penicillin is one such narrow-spectrum antibiotic. Though broad-spectrum antibiotics do not have these advantages and may produce severe gastrointestinal disorders, there is a clear advantage to using them when pinpoint identification of the infecting pathogen is unavailable at the time treatment must begin.

Side Effects of Antimicrobial Therapeutic Agents

Side effects of antimicrobial therapeutic agents include the following:

- **Allergic reaction**: Penicillin, as an example, can produce anaphylactic shock, a life-threatening reaction.
- **Indigenous microflora may be damaged**: Almost all antibiotics can cause overgrowth of *Clostridium difficile*, which produces a toxin that causes diarrhea, colitis, or overgrowth of *Candida* in the mouth, vagina, or gastrointestinal tract and sometimes produces superinfections with opportunistic pathogens.
- **Cutaneous reactions**: Reported with every class of antimicrobial agent.
- **Hematologic reactions**: Range from possibly fatal blood dyscrasia to hemolytic anemia due to sulfonamides when the patient lacks the enzyme glucose-6-phosphate dehydrogenase.
- **Damage to the liver**: Where some antibiotics are metabolized.
- **Damage to the kidneys**: Can follow the use of aminoglycosides.
- **Neurologic toxicity**: Uncommon, but the aminoglycosides can damage the auditory or vestibular apparatus.

Prophylactic, Empiric, and Therapeutic Uses of Antimicrobials

Prophylactic antimicrobial therapy refers to treatment prior to infection in order to prevent an infection from occurring. Prophylaxis has been over used, has been inconsistent, and has contributed to antibiotic resistance, so duration should be short and the need should be evaluated individually, following guidelines that have been established to provide optimal benefit.

Empiric antimicrobial therapy refers to beginning treatment when an infection appears clinically obvious but the specific causative agent has not yet been identified, such as when a person has pneumonia. Empiric therapy should be given following guidelines and recommendations that consider the site of infection, the most likely causative agents, hospital epidemiology, cost, and susceptibilities.

Therapeutic antimicrobial therapy refers to using treatment that is appropriate for particular microorganisms, following guidelines that have been established in relation to diagnosis, causative agent, cost, and susceptibilities. Treatment should be neither too broad nor narrow and of sufficient duration.

Preoperative Antimicrobial Prophylaxis

The National Surgical Infection Prevention Project has issued recommendations for the use of perioperative antimicrobial prophylaxis. General recommendations include:

- **Timing**: The first dose should be completely administered 1 hour prior to incision. If a fluoroquinolone or vancomycin is indicated, then it should begin being administered 2 hours prior to incision.
- **Duration**: Antimicrobials for most procedures should end within 24 hours of surgery.
- **Limiting additional antimicrobials**: Pre-existing infections should be treated prior to surgery whenever possible. If not, then additional antimicrobial, specific to existing infection, may be necessary.
- **Dosing**: Dosage should be based on age and weight, according to recommendations. Lengthy surgeries may require additional intraoperative dosing.
- **Providing alternatives for those with allergies**: Patients with confirmed allergies to commonly used prophylactic agents would need an alternative antimicrobial. Clindamycin and vancomycin can be considered if data shows the facility does not have a problem with resistance or incidences of infection with *Clostridium difficile* or *Staphylococcus epidermis.*

Antimicrobial Monitoring and Evaluation

Antimicrobial monitoring and evaluation are important aspects of infection control and reduction of antibiotic resistance. A program must be implemented that includes a protocol for use and education for staff. Typical monitoring includes:

- **Antibiotic protocols** for use should include a formulary and guidelines for specific hospital units or patient populations. These protocols must be monitored regularly and updated as needed, with rotation of antibiotics as indicated. Use and effectiveness of antibiotics must be monitored on an ongoing basis. Guidelines should include steps to take if the first line antibiotics are not effective.
- **Laboratory testing** should help to determine the most effective antibiotic control for significant isolates so that treatment is targeted and effective.
- **Stop orders** should be in place in the pharmacy to ensure that antibiotics are ordered for the correct duration of time.
- **Prophylaxis protocols** with specific doses and durations should be established for short-term use of antibiotics in particular circumstances, such as preoperatively.

Antimicrobial Agents for Gram-Positive Staphylococcus Cocci

Gram-positive cocci are several and grouped together based on their Gram-stain reaction, thick cell wall composition, and spherical shape. Most are members of the *Micrococcaceae* family. Although *Micrococcus* is a common human skin contaminant, it is relatively harmless to humans. The most important genus of the *Micrococcaceae* family, clinically, is *Staphylococcus*. It is classified into two major groups: aureus and non-aureus. *S. aureus* and is a leading cause of soft tissue infections, toxic shock syndrome, scalded skin syndrome, food poisoning, acne, pneumonia, meningitis, boils, arthritis, and osteomyelitis (chronic bone infection). The drug of choice for *S. aureus* is penicillin, if the bacteria is not penicillin resistant, however today, most *S. aureus* are penicillin resistant. Empiric treatment that covers methicillin-resistant strains should be started on patients while cultures and sensitivities are pending. Beta-lactam agents such as oxacillin or nafcillin are indicated when the *S. aureus* is penicillin-resistant but methicillin-susceptible. Vancomycin and daptomycin are currently used for methicillin-resistant *S. aureus*, but they have high failure rates and other complications, an infectious disease specialist should be consulted if the patient has MRSA. Those most susceptible to infection by the bacterium *S. epidermis*, an opportunistic pathogen which is a normal resident of human skin, are IV drug users, newborns, elderly, and those using catheters or other artificial appliances.

Antimicrobial Agents for Gram-Positive Streptococcus Cocci

Gram-positive cocci are grouped together based on their Gram-stain reaction, thick cell wall composition, and spherical shape. Most are members of the *Micrococcaceae* family:

One species of ***Streptococcus***, *S. pyogenes*, is responsible for about 90% of all cases of pharyngitis, of which strep throat is one form. Penicillin is usually administered quickly to avoid pneumonia or rheumatic fever. Another species, *S. agalactiae*, also treated with penicillin, is a cause of sexually transmitted urogenital infections in females.

The *Enterococci Streptococci* give rise to such diseases such as septicemia, endocarditis, and appendicitis; one species, *E. faecalis*, causes urinary tract infections, and *E. faecium* is a bacterium resistant to many common antibiotics. *S. pneumoniae* causes pneumonia, meningitis, and otitis media. Patients with penicillin-sensitive *S. pneumoniae* can be treated with a beta-lactam antibiotic.

Antimicrobial Resistance

Those against whom an agent has no activity from the outset are intrinsically **resistant**. Though this may be a significant clinical problem, it is not a major public health issue.

However, when antimicrobial agents are developed, resistance to them is eventually observed in species that were originally fully sensitive. Every use of the antibiotic increases the rate at which bacteria become resistant to it. There is a very high chance that resistance to antibiotics developed in one person gets passed on to others, what is known as acquired antimicrobial resistance, a major public health issue.

Resistance can be acquired through a microorganism's genetic ability to survive a therapeutic agent and then multiply, two possibilities being when chromosomal DNA mutates to become effective against one type of agent or extrachromosomal resistance, and when certain types of resistance R plasmids (R factors) are present.

Mechanisms of Antibiotic Resistance in Bacteria

There are a number of mechanisms by which bacteria are resistant to antibiotics. The antibiotic-bacteria combination, dosage, and duration of therapy all affect the type of resistance. These resistant bacteria have genes in their DNA or plasmids that control protective mechanisms:

- **Inactivation** occurs when the bacteria secrete different enzymes that chemically modify the antibiotics, such as penicillin and chloramphenicol. This is the primary method of antibiotic resistance.
- **Alteration of binding sites** may involve changes or removal of molecules in the cell wall, preventing the antibiotics, such as vancomycin and methicillin, from attaching to the bacteria.
- **Efflux pumps** essentially are mechanisms in the bacteria that serve as pumps to force antibiotics, such as tetracycline and quinolones, out of the cell.
- **Alteration of cell wall** through alterations of proteins eliminates ports of entry into the bacteria cell wall by decreasing permeability.
- **Alteration of a metabolic pathway**, allowing an organism to bypass a reaction impeded by an agent.

Genetic Components of Antibiotic Resistance in Bacteria

Antibiotic resistance is a major area of concern in infection control because of a marked increase in recent years, leading to concern that increasing numbers of microorganisms, especially bacteria, may become resistant to all antibiotics. Antibiotic use can result in **genetic changes** that result in antibiotic resistance. These changes include:

- **Foreign DNA** can be introduced with gene transfers from one type of bacteria to another via plasmids (circular, double strands of DNA that can replicate in a cell but are separate from chromosomal DNA), which carry genes for resistance. Others are able to acquire DNA from the environment.
- **Mutations**, even very minor ones, can select for resistance to antibiotics by altering sensitivity or binding sites.
- **Cross-resistance** occurs when changes in sensitivity to one antibiotic provides resistance to other antibiotics as well.
- **Co-resistance** occurs when multiple mechanisms of resistance are present in the same microorganism.

Controlling and Decreasing Antibiotic Resistance

There are a number of strategies that are employed to attempt to control and decrease antibiotic resistance because poor practice in the administration of antibiotics coupled with inadequate infection control have resulted in increasingly antibiotic-resistant microorganisms. Strategies include:

- **Antibiotic formulary restricting use**: Studies have demonstrated that only about 50% of antibiotic use is appropriate. A formulary lists appropriate antibiotics, including dosage and duration, for different conditions and situations. Usually, a procedure must be followed to justify alternate therapy.
- **Combination antibiotic therapy**: Studies have demonstrated that pairing two antibiotics, such as an older with a newer variety, can treat resistant strains.

Multidrug-Resistant Microorganisms in Respiratory Infections

Antimicrobial resistance is found in such organisms as multidrug-resistant *Mycobacterium tuberculosis*, methicillin-resistant *Staphylococcus aureus* (MRSA), vancomycin-intermediate-resistant *S. aureus* (VISA), vancomycin-resistant enterococci (VRE), and penicillin-resistant pneumococci. Few new antibiotics to replace them are in development.

Concern has been increasing over nosocomial transmission of multidrug-resistant disease, particularly in settings where persons with human immunodeficiency virus (HIV) infection are receiving care. This led in the early 1990s to new guidelines on the isolation of patients with multidrug-resistant tuberculosis. Hospital patients with confirmed or suspected tuberculosis began to be placed in private rooms that had been reengineered to have lower, or negative, air pressure compared with surrounding areas. Ventilating systems which reduced through dilution and filtration mycobacterial contamination of air were installed; and hospital personnel replaced standard surgical masks with particulate respirators when put in contact with infectious tubercular patients.

MULTIDRUG-RESISTANCE ORGANISM AND CLOSTRIDIUM DIFFICILE MODULE

The Multidrug-Resistance Organism and *Clostridium difficile* (MDRO/CDI) Module of the NHSN Patient Safety Component addresses the problem of increasingly resistant organisms because of increased morbidity, length of stay, and costs, as well as difficulty treating the organisms. *Clostridium difficile* has similar properties and is included because of increasing numbers of outbreaks. MDROs that facilities may choose to follow (one or multiple) include MRSA, MSSA, VRE, CephR-Klebsiella, CRE-Ecoli, CRE-Klebsiella, and MDR-Acinetobacter. Surveillance methods for MDROs may be facility-wide by location, selected locations, facility-wide inpatient, or facility-wide outpatient for all specimens or facility-wide inpatient or outpatient with blood specimens only. Surveillance approaches include LabID event for which HAI, POA, and transfer rule do not apply, and infection surveillance with HAI surveillance definitions. LabID event is the easiest method because it does not involve direct examination of the patient but depends solely on lab results from surveillance activities. Surveillance methods for *Clostridium difficile* include facility wide by location, selected locations, facility wide inpatient, and facility wide outpatient.

Assessing Risk Factors for Infectious Disease

Susceptibility

During the period preceding the contracting of a disease, the relative ease or difficulty of contracting a particular infection under given conditions varies from person-to-person because of differences in health, age, gender, and many other variables, and this is known as **susceptibility**. One thing is true of susceptibility for everyone: a host susceptible to infection is one who lacks sufficient immunity to overcome the infecting agent.

Some people may be susceptible to one agent but still resist infection more successfully to others. Genetic factors may help explain why: rare gene disruptions cause fatal vulnerability to specific microbes, even though subtle differences, which are more common, arise from minor variations in many genes. Recently developed medical advances now allow the immune system to be monitored like other organ functions, opening new approaches for therapeutic interventions.

Factors Influencing Susceptibility and the Progress of Infection

Infection is a product of exposure, and many factors can influence exposure:

- A potential host's proximity to reservoirs of agents
- An agent's degree of virulence (its ability to cause an infection)
- Intrinsic host factors like state of health, sex, race, or such immunity factors as prior exposure to the agent. For example, an infection called chorioamnionitis occurs in 0.5 percent to 10 percent of births, sometimes resulting in cerebral palsy. Intrinsic risk factors that could predispose women to the infection might include the genetic makeup of their immune response or stronger bacteria in their genital tracts.

Extrinsic host factors that influence exposure include:

- Contact with infected medical devices
- Immunization
- Access to first aid
- High-risk behaviors
- Being required to come into frequent contact with disease carriers

Assessment of Host Risk Factors

Host risk factors are those conditions or circumstances that put the host at increased risk of developing an infection. Host risk factors include the following:

- **Age**: Those who are very young or very old are often at increased risk. Infants may not have developed antibodies, and the elderly may have decreased immunity.
- **Disease**: Many diseases, such as diabetes and leukemia, increase the risk of infection.
- **Circulatory impairment**: Any decrease in perfusion to an area from disease or injury increases the chance of infection.
- **Medications**: Immunosuppressants and chemotherapy can reduce immunity. Improper use of antibiotics builds resistance.
- **Contact**: Close contact with the source of microorganisms increases the host risk factor.
- **Wounds and instrumentation**: Surgical wounds, ulcers, catheters, or any other thing that allows microorganism's easy access increases risk.
- **Absence of prophylactic antibiotics**: Antibiotics have proven to reduce risk of post-operative infections for some procedures, but guidelines for use are not always followed.

Monitoring Current and Emerging Local and Global Threats

Recognizing Epidemiologically Significant Organisms for Investigation

Epidemiologically significant organisms are those with potential to cause death or serious injury or disease. Some organisms are considered significant because they are invasive and cause outbreaks but also are often resistant to antimicrobials, making control difficult. When epidemiologically significant organisms are identified, usually through active surveillance or cultures, enhanced infection control methods may be needed to control spread of the infection. Microorganisms that are significant include vancomycin-resistant *enterococci* (VRE), *Clostridium difficile* that has caused infection, methicillin-resistant *Staphylococcus aureus (MRSA)* as well as others that can be transmitted directly or indirectly. Antibiotic resistance is increasing among gram-negative bacilli such as *Klebsiella pneumoniae, P. aeruginosa,* and *Enterobacter* spp. Organisms that are deemed significant may vary from one department to another, so that organisms that might prove fatal in the neonatal unit may pose less of a threat to adults, but a facility must be viewed as one unit because of the potential for spread of infection.

Epidemiologic Biomarkers

A biomarker is a measurable event occurring in a biological system, such as that represented by the human body. In epidemiology, a **biomarker** is not a diagnostic test but an indicator that an event has occurred that could later lead to clinical disease. There are three kinds of biologic markers: markers of exposure or dose, markers of effect, and markers of susceptibility. Biomarkers of exposure (or dose) record exposure to a toxic agent, but markers of effect record exposure and response. Markers of susceptibility might be identifying characteristics of persons at increased risk of developing the disease. Biomarker epidemiology is undergoing rapid development and expansion.

Surveillance and Epidemiologic Investigation

Design of Surveillance Systems

General Mission of Epidemiology and Epidemiologic Concerns

The general mission of epidemiology is the prevention of disease and the improvement of the health of the public through excellence in rooting out causes of infection and disease through the applied study of occurrence and distribution of disease in human populations.

A typical program for epidemiologists might be conducting advanced research to discover effective community and policy interventions to reduce alcohol-related social and health problems. Or it might be a program that studies antimicrobial resistance in zoonotic food borne pathogens and commensal bacteria. Other aims might be gaining an understanding of the prevalence of resistance among food borne pathogens, studying the molecular mechanisms that are associated with the development of resistance, and defining the role of commensal bacteria in the development and transfer of resistance.

Steps of a Risk Assessment

A risk assessment is conducted to determine the risk of infection in order to reduce infections by implementing evidence-based preventive measures. Risk assessments may be generalized and include the entire facility or may target specific activities, such as construction and remodeling projects. When completing a risk assessment, patients may be categorized according to risk groups, such as low, medium, high, and highest risk. Steps include:

- Determine the purpose and outline the goals and scope of assessment
- Determine data sources
- Select an assessment tool that meets facility and regulatory requirements
- Select a process to complete the assessment
- Assess such measures as success and failure of prevention activities, isolation activities, policies and procedures, exposure plans, HAIs, employee health and immunization, environmental factors, antimicrobial stewardship, and other factors specific to the facility
- Complete data collection and analysis
- Prepare report and visual presentation of findings (graphs, charts)
- Complete risk management plan with evidence-based preventive measures based on needs identified in the assessment

Standards of Risk Assessments

Outcomes Are Clearly Defined, Properly Measured, and Ascertained in an Unbiased Manner

A standard that all risk assessment studies must meet is that the study outcomes are clearly defined, properly measured, and ascertained in an unbiased manner. Questions to be asked to determine whether a study meets this standard include:

- Was the outcome variable a disease entity, pathological finding, symptom, or a physiological parameter?
- Was variability in the possible outcomes understood and taken into account (e.g., various manifestations of a disease considering its natural history)?
- Was the method of recording the outcome variables reliable? If the outcome was disease, did the design of the study provide for recording the full spectrum of disease?
- Was a standardized classification system, such as the International Classification of Diseases, followed?
- Were the data from a primary or a secondary source?
- Did design and execution of the study minimize the possibility of misclassifying the outcome?
- Was there a review of all diagnoses by qualified medical personnel who were blinded to study exposure?

Procedures Are Described in Sufficient Detail

A second standard that all risk assessment studies must meet is that study procedures are described in sufficient detail to determine whether appropriate methods were used in the design and conduct of the investigation. Questions to be asked to determine whether a study meets this standard include:

- In a cohort study, were the study subjects representative of a larger body of exposed and unexposed persons or, in a case-control study, of diseased and non-diseased persons?
- Was bias minimized, with respect to major risk factors for the disease or condition under study, by having exposed and unexposed persons comparable at baseline in a cohort study, or were cases similar to controls prior to exposure?

Questions regarding procedures include:

- Was bias minimized by having interviewers and data collectors blind to the hypothesis and the case/control status of the subjects?
- Were quality control procedures in use at all stages of the study? What were they?
- Were any effects of nonparticipation, low response rate, or loss to follow-up accounted for in the study results?

NHSN Risk Index Model

The NHSN Risk Index Model was formerly used to assess risk for surgical site infections (SSI) but has been replaced by the risk adjustment process using the SIR with specific models for risk for each procedure based on variables that have been associated with the procedure and infections. These new models may include some aspects of the Risk Index Model, such as the American Society of Anesthesiologists (ASA) score and duration of procedure. The Risk Index Model is based on the sum of scores for three parameters:

- **ASA score:** Includes 6 categories describing physical status. One point is given for any ASA score above 2.
  - 1: Normal patient.
  - 2: Systemic disease, present but mild.
  - 3: Systemic disease, severe but not incapacitating.
  - 4: Systemic disease, life threatening.
  - 5: Moribund patient, likely to not survive without surgical intervention.
  - 6: Brain-dead patient, surgery for the purpose of harvesting organs.
- **Wound class:** One point is given for class C (contaminated) or D (dirty).
- **Duration:** One point for cut point greater than 75th percentile.

T-Point Classification System for Surgical Procedures

The T-point classification system assigns time in hours based on information about average length of surgery. The assigned T point for surgical procedures is the number of hours that equal the 75% percentile. Thus, a T point of 5 means that 75% of these types of surgery are completed within 5 hours. Exceeding the T point increases risk of infection or complications, so this system is used as one aspect of evaluation of surgical site infection risk although time is only one variable and should not be considered in isolation as other risk factors may be of more importance. The following are the T points for common surgical procedures:

- Appendectomy 1
- Hernia repair 2
- Hysterectomy 2
- Hip prosthesis 3
- Vascular repair 3
- Craniotomy 4
- Coronary artery bypass graft 5

CDC/NNIS/NHSN Risk Index System

The Centers for Disease Control and Prevention (CDC)/National Nosocomial Infection Surveillance created the **NNIS Risk Index System** in the early 1990's to standardize reporting of data regarding wound infections. The National Healthcare Safety Network (NHSN) has adopted this system when it absorbed the roles of the former NNIS. This risk index integrates the traditional, T-point, and American Society of Anesthesiologists (ASA) classifications. The Risk Index scores range from 0-3 with a point for each of the applicable variables based on the other classifications:

Points	Associated Risk
0 point	No risk factors
1 point	Score of 3-4 on the traditional classification of wound that is contaminated or dirty
1 point	Score of 3-5 on the ASA preoperative
1 point	Exceeds the T point duration for this type of operation (>75%)

Even with zero point, some risk of infection still exists, but the predictive percentage rate for surgical site infections increases with the Risk Index score:

Score	Chance of Infection
0 score	1.5%
1 score	2.9%
2 score	6.8%
3 score	13.0%

Surveillance Plan

Purpose

The purpose of a surveillance plan should be clearly outlined and may be multifaceted, including the following elements:

- **Decreasing rates of infection**: The primary purpose of a surveillance plan is to identify a means to decrease healthcare-associated infections.
- **Evaluating infection control measures**: Surveillance can evaluate effectiveness of infection control measures.
- **Establishing endemic threshold rates**: Establishing threshold rates can help to enact control measures to reduce rates.
- **Identifying outbreaks**: About 5-10% of infections occur in outbreaks, and comparing data with established endemic threshold rates can help to identify these outbreaks if analysis is done in a regular and timely manner.
- **Achieving staff compliance**: Objective evidence may convince staff to cooperate with infection control measures.
- **Meeting accreditation standards**: Some accreditation agencies require reports of infection rates.
- **Providing defense for malpractice suits**: Providing evidence that a facility is proactive in combating infections can decrease liability.

Steps

The steps to surveillance programs may vary to some degree, but usually contain the following elements:

1. **Establishment of parameters/design** of the survey by determining what will be surveyed, when, and how with clear definitions of events guides the process.
2. **Data collection** should be done consistently, efficiently, and accurately whether by hand or automated system. Sources may include laboratory reports, medical records of targeted patients, interviews, and autopsy reports.
3. **Data summary** must be done so that information is accessible and available for further analysis.
4. **Data analysis** uses statistical measurements appropriate to data and goals. Frequency of analysis varies but must ensure adequate numbers for data to be meaningful.
5. **Analytical interpretation** involves using data to indicate threshold rates, clusters, outbreaks, or other events.
6. **Utilizing results** must include specific steps that will be taken as a result of analytical interpretation. For example, if a threshold for infections is exceeded, clearly defined procedures should be outlined for dealing with that event.

Assessment of the Population

Assessment of the population is a very important component of a surveillance plan because each facility deals with a unique population. In this case, population refers to that segment of patients that will be studied because studying all patients, especially in large facilities, is impractical. Assessing population leads to targeted surveillance where particular areas, procedures, or types of patients are surveyed. Assessment includes:

- **Types of patients** should be evaluated, including whether or not they are medical or surgical and frequent diagnoses.
- **Procedures/treatments** should be assessed to determine those most commonly performed, especially those that are invasive.
- **Liability issues** must be considered in relation to those patients that affect liability and costs.
- **Community health issues**, such as outbreaks, may help to target populations.
- **Risk factors for infection** must be understood and used as part of assessment of needs.
- **Facility resources and support** must be considered because staff assistance is critical.

Resources For Population Assessment

Resources must be utilized to properly assess populations for surveillance. Each facility will have different types of resources available, depending upon the size of the facility, the location, and the types of services it provides. A wide range of resources is often available:

- **Records** include individual medical records as well as summaries and reports from management and different medical units.
- **Risk management** at each facility is a good resource regarding the types of cases that involve liability and costs. Risk management may be able to target areas of concern.
- **Databases** for surgical procedures or other information may be available at institutions and should be analyzed.
- **Community health reports** from both public health and community agencies may have valuable information about community outbreaks and health concerns.
- **Human resources** should have health records and questionnaires regarding health problems and immunization records for staff.

Targeted Surveillance

Site Directed, Unit Directed, Population Directed, and Limited Periodic

Targeted surveillance is limited in scope, focusing on particular types of infections, areas in the facility, or patient population. It is less expensive than hospital wide surveillance and may provide more meaningful data, but clusters of infection outside the survey parameters may be missed. Targeted areas are picked based on characteristics such as frequency of infection, mortality rates, financial costs, and the ability to use date to prevent infections:

- **Site directed** targets particular sites of infection, such as bloodstream, wound, or urine.
- **Unit directed** targets selected service areas of the hospital, such as ICUs or neonatal units.
- **Population directed** targets groups that are considered high-risk, such as transplantation patients and those undergoing other invasive procedures.
- **Limited periodic** combines hospital-wide surveillance of all infections for one month each quarter followed by site directed targets for the rest of the quarter. This increases the chance of detecting clusters of infection, but those that fall outside of the hospital wide surveillance months would still be missed.

Priority Directed and Post-Discharge Surveillance

Priority directed surveillance is also referred to as surveillance by objective. It focuses on prioritizing efforts at infection surveillance in order to meet particular objectives. Serious infections are identified based on morbidity and mortality rates as well as costs and, importantly, the ability to effect preventive measures based on the data, so priority-directed surveillance is often directed at surgical site infections and pneumonia. Other infections are not simply ignored, but most resources are expended in focused areas.

Post-discharge surveillance is conducted in a number of different manners; none standardized, and is more important with the decrease in the length of hospital stays, resulting in missing up to 50% of surgical site infections. Patients may be contacted directly through mailed questionnaires or by telephone. Sometimes physicians are contacted for information. Readmission data is evaluated, and in some cases, patients are followed in clinics or office visits. Data is often insufficient because of difficult with follow-up.

Limitations of Targeted Surveillance

The major problem with hospital wide surveillance is that cost is prohibitive, both in time and money; however, in order to detect all infections and to get a clear idea of the infection control problem of a facility, hospital wide surveillance is necessary. When the CDC National Nosocomial Infections Surveillance system (NNIS) was initiated in 1992, it required hospital wide surveillance but discontinued this in favor of targeted surveillance in 1999 because most hospitals could not afford more comprehensive surveillance. Then in 2004, this surveillance system was discontinued, with the National Healthcare Safety Network taking over the generation of reports on nosocomial infections. It is important that, even with the focus on targeted areas, infection control still does some hospital wide surveillance because only about 20% of healthcare-associated infections occur in the ICU, the main targeted area. Additionally, only about 19% of healthcare-associated infections involve surgical sites. An electronic monitoring program that automatically monitors lab results can easily track all lab work. A rotating system of monitoring different units for specified periods of time can also be used to gain a more comprehensive picture of infections.

Tracer Methodology

Tracer methodology is a method that looks at the continuum of care a patient receives from admission to post-discharge. A patient is selected to be "traced" and the medical record serves as a guide. Tracer methodology uses the experience of this patient to evaluate the processes in place through documents and interviews. For example, if a patient received physical therapy, surveyors may begin with the following:

- **Physical therapists**: How do they receive the orders and arrange patient transport? How is the therapy administered? How is progress noted?
- **Transport staff**: How do they receive requests? How long does transfer take? What routes do they use? How to they transport patients? How do they clean transport equipment? What do they do if emergency arises during transport?
- **Nursing staff**: How do they notify PT of orders? How do they prepare patients? How do they know the therapy schedule? How do they coordinate PT with the need for other treatments? How do they learn about patient progress?

Determining Data Required to Calculate Specific Rates in the Design Phase

The data needed to calculate specific rates when designing a surveillance system depend on the type of rate, but typical required data include the number of target events (such as surgical site infections) and the number of patients at risk (such as all surgical patients). Initial steps include determining what type of data is necessary based on the formula for calculation and where to obtain that data and then to determine the point in time or period of time from which the data will be drawn. Determining the correct numerator and denominator is necessary for results to be valid. A determination must also be made whether to collect data for all patients in the target (denominator) group or to do sampling, but careless sampling may result in selection bias. Once raw figures are obtained, these figures can then be used to do a wide variety of calculations, such as rates, ratios, measures of central tendency, percentages, measures of variability, and frequency distribution.

Establishing Threshold Rates

Threshold rates for infection control require a normal range so that variations below can indicate a decrease in infections or improvement in methods and above can trigger intervention. Establishing threshold rates must be done in each institution because it is extremely difficult to use data from facilities with different populations, different data collection methods, and different testing procedures. Thresholds may relate to particular types of tests or occurrences of infection per number of patients or patient days. The type of threshold to be established must be carefully defined. Establishing threshold rates involves a period of surveillance, which can be facility wide but is often targeted to certain populations or procedures. This period may vary in length depending upon the size of the institution and other factors, but should be sufficient to provide adequate data. The data is compiled and evaluated and outbreak thresholds are then established. At this point, general surveillance is discontinued and surveillance is done related to those that exceed threshold.

Notification Systems for Critical Laboratory Results

A notification system for the reporting of critical laboratory results should be made directly with the laboratory, if possible. Threshold rates should be derived first so that there is clarity about what results to report. If it is not possible to receive notification from the laboratory, then designated staff should be assigned to check lab results and report to the infection control personal. Notification should be done immediately so that intervention can begin. Infection control personnel should be available every day to receive notification. Notification may take various forms, depending upon the institution, staff, equipment, and resources:

- **Telephone**: Reports may be given directly to staff by phone.
- **Fax**: Reports may be faxed to the office of the infection control personnel.
- **Form**: A special form may be provided for notification purposes.
- **Email**: Use of electronic notification is especially useful if software is available that automatically triggers a notification when lab results exceed threshold rates.

Use of Technology

Online Computerized Surveillance Programs

The University of Pittsburgh, in 1999, launched development of the open-source Real Time Outbreak and Disease Surveillance (RODS) system to deploy computer-based outbreak and disease surveillance systems around the nation that would undergo further continuing development by its users. An infrastructure was created, consisting of a website, mailing lists for developers and users, designated software developers, and shared code development tools. By November of 2003, the system was generating heavy usage.

Before RODS system development, several data collection programs had already been available, including the Nolo, NICE, and IDEAS software available through the Centers for Disease Control.

RODS will, it is hoped, through its open-source architecture, extend and enhance the power of those older programs.

Laboratory, Pharmacy, and Radiology Integration

Computer systems in the medical setting have come a long way in the past 10 years. Today, anyone with access to a networked system can, in theory, quickly call up a patient's complete record, including lab data, history, medication regimen, imaging, etc. (Concerns for patient privacy, however, have sometimes made it more difficult to obtain this data.) The most sophisticated systems in hospitals and other health centers can even analyze the data it has stored and returned; this can prove quite helpful in surveillance programs.

Such sophisticated computer systems are now so commonplace that they have spawned a new field, medical informatics, along with its relatives bioinformatics and computational biology, with university training programs leading to degrees in the area. The computer is taking over such functions in epidemiology research as performing more repetitive and time-consuming tasks (e.g., mapping disease genes, analyzing micro-array data); doing knowledge management, such as integration of different knowledge sources; modeling complex, dynamic systems, and processing classical data analysis problems (e.g., gene identification).

Electronic Infection Control Surveillance

Healthcare-associated infection surveillance relies on infection control methods that are time consuming, labor intensive, and relatively inefficient even when the job of compiling and analyzing data is automated through the use of computers. Consequently, given an Infection Control Officer's typical situation of lacking time and person power, available data are more often than not underutilized and the patterns they contain go undiscovered.

A new method, association rule induction, is being tried in an attempt to detect temporal patterns among infection-control surveillance data. This method concentrates on looking for unusual occurrences that might point to associated events rather than frequent, regularly occurring patterns in data. For example, if it is known that healthcare-associated pneumonia frequently follows the admission of homeless alcoholics with upper respiratory infections, a computer algorithm can be programmed to include such information on admission and scan admissions for this data rather than looking for increases in the incidence of pneumonia.

Predesigned Surveillance Software Packages for Infection Control

Managing data by hand can become unwieldy very quickly. Standard spreadsheet software that is packaged with most PCs can be used for simple reporting and data base functions but multiple variables are more difficult to manage. Using these programs often requires extensive programming and development. Utilizing predesigned surveillance software packages can save time and expense and yield more accurate data. Statistical packages, such as SAS, SPSS, and MINITAB are available but have a steep learning curve. The CDC provides a free program, Epi Info, which was originally designed for investigation of outbreaks but can be utilized to manage and analyze data. It consists of four separate modules:

- The **Form Designer module** to design data entry screens
- The **Enter module** to enter data into screens designed with Form Designer
- The **Analysis module** for various types of statistical analysis
- The **Epi Map module** to link data to maps

Commercial software programs specifically designed for infection control, such as AICE and EpiQuest, are also available.

Use of Computerized Systems for Data Analysis

The analysis of data by hand is impractical and time consuming unless the surveyed population is very small. Most statistical analysis is done using computer software programs that automatically analyze the data in a number of different ways and can account for risk factors. Software programs have various other utilizations. They may be used to generate not only numeric data and text reports but also various graphs. The amount and type of data that must be entered into a program varies according to the type of software and the necessary data for reports that will be generated. If different programs are used to collect and analyze data, then the ability to move data from one program to another may be necessary in order to generate reports. Data entry design is important: data to which mathematical calculations are done is entered as numeric data, but some numbers (telephone and Social Security) to which no mathematical calculations are done, are entered as text data.

Screening and Serial Testing Indications and Methods

When designing a surveillance system, screening and serial testing indications and methods must be established:

- **Screening**: With research studies, screening gathers subjects who meet the qualifications for inclusion. In diagnostics, screening refers to the use of various methods such as tests to identify the complaint and go on to its treatment. Mass screening is applied non-selectively to groups or selectively to high-risk groups, generally by public health personnel. Multi-phasic screening consists of a battery of tests and procedures used simultaneously to detect any in an array of diseases.
- **Serial testing**: When a diagnostician has not established the cause of a medical problem, but it does not appear as though time is of the essence, he will probably apply serial testing. One test at a time is done to rule out some causes and indicate what additional tests might be needed to narrow down the possibilities.

Integration of Surveillance Activities Within Affiliated Facilities

Small Acute Hospitals

Because of accreditation requirements and health concerns, most small hospitals have infection preventionists (IPs), but they often have other duties as well. A minimum requirement for a team should include the IP, a physician, an administrator, a pharmacist, and a laboratory representative. Unless laboratory reports are automated, routine review of laboratory findings must be done, but even in small facilities, review may be targeted to high-risk areas or populations. The IP needs to train staff to assist in case finding and train all new hires in infection control procedures as well as giving regular in-service training to review procedures for other staff. Surveillance must take into consideration the population of the facility and the purpose of surveillance so that data collection is meaningful and used for prevention. The IP should maintain contact with the IP from large feeder hospitals in the area and attend conferences and training with them when possible.

Long-Term Care Facilities

Long-term care facilities face many of the same challenges as small acute hospitals in relation to infection control. Often infection control professionals have additional duties, but surveillance data is important to identify problem areas and implement changes. The IP from transferring acute hospitals should provide full information about transfer patients and serve as a resource. The facility IP should check laboratory reports and interview patients and staff at least weekly to facilitate case finding. Incidence rates for targeted infections should be compiled. Education of staff is an important aspect of the IP's duties because staff turnover in long-term care facilities is high.

Staff often begins work with little training or knowledge of infection control, especially nurse aids who may provide the primary patient care. All staff needs to be trained in infection control so that they can assist in case finding and institute preventive measures. Because urinary infections are common, many patients receive antibiotics, so antibiotic review should be ongoing.

Types of Infections Commonly Surveyed in Long-Term Care Facilities

Because people are being discharged early from acute care, many patients in long-term care facilities, especially nursing homes, may suffer from infection at the time of admission or may develop infection that began in the hospital but was undiagnosed. There are a number of infections that are quite common to long-term care facilities and should be targeted for surveillance.

- **Skin and soft tissue infections** can include surgical site infections, decubiti, bacterial or fungal infections, conjunctivitis, and scabies.
- **Respiratory infections** may range from common viral infections to pneumonia.
- **Urinary infections** are frequent because fluid intake is often inadequate and urinary catheters are often used for long-term control of incontinence.
- **Bloodstream infections** may be primary or secondary related to other infections, such as surgical site infection.
- **Gastrointestinal infections** may result in nausea, vomiting, and diarrhea. Bacterial infections can include *Shigella, Salmonella, E. coli,* and *Clostridium difficile.*

Challenges Faced by the Elderly in Long-Term Care Facilities

The elderly population often has decreased antibody mediated and cell mediated immune responses, leaving them less able to combat infections. Additionally, many elderly people suffer from malnutrition, which further impairs cell-mediated immunity. If patients have functional impairment, they may be dependent on staff for toileting and turning, and if not done adequately, patients can develop decubiti, increasing the chance of wound infection. Patients may have medical illnesses, such as circulatory impairment of diabetes that make them prone to infection. Invasive devices, such as feeding tubes and urinary catheters are used frequently, and infection is a common complication. Patients may be too weak to breathe deeply or cough so they are unable to clear bacteria from the respiratory tract. Another problem faced by the elderly is that their inflammatory response to infection is often altered, so they may exhibit fever without other symptoms, or they may exhibit no fever in the presence of infection, so diagnosis can be difficult.

Home Healthcare

There is much that cannot be controlled in the home environment, so staff face challenges in surveillance even while the numbers of home care patients and the severity of illness of these patients is increasing. Many patients have invasive medical devices, sometimes multiple. About 20% of patients already have infections when admitted to home healthcare. The IP, often a staff person with other duties, is dependent on others for much of their data, including the acute hospital, the laboratory, the physician, and the patient. Surveillance in the home often involves weekly reports completed by staff other than the IP. Much of the IP's focus must be on facilitating case finding by training staff and preparing reporting forms. Additionally, the IP must assure that protocols for home care are followed, including cleansing of equipment and changing of invasive devices according to a schedule. Any indications of infection must be reported to the patient's physician.

Types of Infection Commonly Surveyed in Home Health Patients

Home health patients have many of the same types of infections found in both acute and long-term care facilities. Invasive devices, such as central lines, nasogastric, and tracheotomy tubes all predispose patients to opportunistic infections that may be localized or systemic. Vascular access devices are a common cause of infection especially if hygiene is not rigorous with the patient and caregivers. Urinary infections are common, especially if urinary catheters are used. Caregivers in the home often must handle and empty drainage bags and can easily spread contamination. Respiratory infections are common for a variety of reasons: patients may not follow through on deep breathing, coughing, and exercise programs. Ventilation and dialysis equipment may not be cleaned or changed as frequently as it should be. Patients often reuse equipment that is clearly indicated for single use only because of costs or inconvenience involved in getting new equipment, again leading to infection.

Intensive Care Units

Patients in intensive care units (ICUs), with serious underlying illnesses, suppressed immune systems, and dependence on invasive devices, are already at high risk for nosocomial infections. The emergence of antimicrobial resistant pathogens has made treating these infections, when they do break out, very difficult and, in some cases, impossible.

Better ICU surveillance typically puts an emphasis on paying more attention to standard hygiene measures, discarding single use gloves and gowns and disinfecting hands after each patient contact, and restricting nurse contact to assigned patients. Sectioning the ICU into four areas and restricting movement between them is also effective. The four sections are:

- An **emergency reception area** (especially for patients with multiple trauma)
- A **contamination area** for patients colonized or infected with drug resistant pathogens
- A **protected area** for non-colonized patients or patients infected with antibiotic susceptible pathogens, and
- A **quarantine area** for patients whose infection status is unknown.

High-Risk Nurseries

Babies are admitted to a high-risk nursery for a variety of reasons that include respiratory distress, infections, birth defects, circulatory problems, and a need for nutritional and temperature support. Infection rates are calculated by using as a denominator the number of patients at risk, patient-days, and days of umbilical catheter/central line use or ventilation for each of four birth-weight categories (≤1000 g, 1001-1500 g, 1501-2500 g, and >2500 g). Infection control essentially follows that for an ICU, but with a few additions. Electronic intrauterine pressure and fetal heart rate monitoring, for example, require that all fluid pathways in the pressure monitoring system be absolutely sterile, and sterile technique must be followed in placing intrauterine catheters and spiral electrodes. There is extra watchfulness for the most frequently encountered clinical perinatal infections associated with increased incidence of infectious morbidity for the newborn. These include:

- Group B streptococcal disease
- Tuberculosis
- Bacteremia
- Endometritis
- Mastitis
- Epidemic puerperal sepsis

Standardized Surveillance Definitions

In order for comparison data, internal or external, to be valid, there must be consistency in **definitions** as to what comprises a healthcare-associated infection, including onset, symptoms, and laboratory findings. Clear definitions must be in place for events, indicators, and outcomes.

- **Events** are most commonly defined according to the CDC definitions for healthcare-associated infections, but in some cases other definitions may be developed, but they must be used consistently and cannot then be compared to events using other definitions.
- **Indicators** are used as a measure of quality because they represent numerator data that is the number of events that are being targeted, such as specific types of infections, defined as narrowly as possible. The denominator data, in this case, is the population at risk for the indicator event.
- **Outcomes** are measurements of indicators, such as the number of infections per a specified denominator, such as 100 patient days, or 1000 device days. Outcomes should provide feedback.

Surveillance in Epidemiology

Surveillance in epidemiology refers to the tracking of infectious disease for incidence and prevalence, summarizing the work of public health and medical facility epidemiologists. Outbreaks of diseases cannot be adequately treated without first tracking and reporting cases of illness in order to know who is involved, where the problems are occurring, and what is causing the problems.

If outbreaks of disease can be prevented, the results can include lower expenditures for healthcare systems, lower costs of individual healthcare expenses, and less personal discomfort and pain. Detecting, preventing, and controlling both infectious and environmental disease provides enormous financial and emotional benefit to the public.

Surveillance in the hospital setting (versus the general public) is much the same except that the public being watched is well-defined as sick patients. The goal is to keep them from becoming sicker through the acquisition of a nosocomial infection.

Surveillance of Healthcare-Associated Infections

Hospital infection control programs should include permanent surveillance that will:

- Quickly detect common source outbreaks
- Identify problem areas
- Recommend priorities for infection control activity
- Meet standards that have been set

Proper surveillance of healthcare-associated infections consists of:

- Systematic, continuous observation of occurrences
- Tracking the distribution of a disease
- Responding to events that can affect infection risks

A functioning program reduces the incidence of healthcare-associated infections (HAI) and associated morbidity, mortality, and costs.

Surveillance results must be shown regularly to clinical and managerial staff to either show progress or provide evidence of the need for improvements in infection control. The National

Healthcare Safety Network has published demonstrations of how good surveillance programs yield significant reductions in nosocomial infection rates.

Use of Outcome and Process Objectives

Process objectives are the intermediate objectives that need to be carried out to achieve outcome objectives. An example of an **outcome objective** might be, say, targeting as a special population group for the goal of reducing the use of smokeless tobacco, such as Native American Indian males aged 12-24 years. From that, a task force would set and pursue **process objectives** to accomplish that mission: monitoring smokeless tobacco use, integrating smoking and smokeless tobacco control efforts, enforcing laws that restrict minors' access to tobacco, making excise taxes commensurate with those on cigarettes, etc.

Targeted Surveillance of Healthcare-Associated Infections

General surveillance of healthcare-associated infections infers a system of facility wide watchfulness to quickly detect the outbreak of an infection anywhere within a healthcare facility, to be followed up with steps to control and eradicate it. However, such widespread coverage, called blanket coverage, can be expensive. Many hospitals, therefore, perform targeted surveillance, which has been found to be more cost effective. Rather than continuously collect data on all infections, a hospital identifies specific infections to look for as well as particular procedures that hold the most risk for infection; it then targets these for surveillance, prevention, and control.

Infection surveillance data are currently used by hospitals to identify potential infection control problems and implement measures to reduce the risk of infection. There are many published reports showing how it has been used to guide performance improvement activities and reduce the rates of healthcare-associated infection.

Objective/Priority-Directed Surveillance and Limited Periodic Surveillance

Objective/Priority-directed surveillance is becoming more and more common in many hospitals. Using this system, a hospital:

- Develops a list of diseases or infections they are most likely to see in their facility
- Sets up a data base to collect and store extensive sets of information on them
- Sets priorities as to which types of infections will take precedence as targets for elimination. This determination could be based on:
  - The severity of a disease
  - The total mortality/morbidity of the disease as indicated by records
  - The frequency with which the infection appears
  - Length of stay
  - Cost of treating the infection
- Limited periodic surveillance does spot checks at regular intervals for patterns indicating possible healthcare-associated infections.

A disadvantage of objective/priority-directed surveillance is that it does not provide broad coverage of data; certain disease clusters may be missed by the surveillance team. It is instituted to keep costs down but has limited effectiveness.

SURVEILLANCE OF PNEUMONIA-RELATED NOSOCOMIAL INFECTIONS

Pneumonia-specific considerations for surveillance of nosocomial infections include the following:

- Getting more than just a single diagnosis of pneumonia by one physician for one patient
- Distinguishing between pneumonia and any other conditions the patient might have, and specify whether the pneumonia may be ventilator associated
- Taking into account that Gram-positive stain for bacteria and positive KOH (potassium hydroxide) may point toward the etiology of an infection, but such samples are frequently contaminated by airway colonizers
- Using broader criteria for pediatric patients than those criteria used to diagnose adult healthcare-associated pneumonia. It can be difficult to detect healthcare-associated infection pneumonia in the elderly, infants, and immunocompromised patients because typical signs or symptoms associated with pneumonia may be masked by the underlying condition
- Always distinguishing in reports between early and late onset healthcare-associated pneumonia
- Getting evidence that, in a single patient, the initial infection has been resolved before reporting that the patient is suffering multiple episodes.

SURVEILLANCE OF THE COVID-19 PANDEMIC

Early in the pandemic, multiple existing surveillance systems were utilized to gather data from health departments, public health, laboratories, health care providers, vital statistics offices, and academics. For example, early local testing was carried out through the Seattle Flu Study on samples that had already been collected and later through volunteer testing with the Greater Seattle Coronavirus Assessment Network Study. Health departments have voluntarily sent data throughout the pandemic to the CDC per the National Notifiable Diseases Surveillance System and National Syndromic Surveillance Program. The CDC has developed a form for standardized reporting and electronic case reporting. The CDC maintains the COVID Data Tracker Weekly Review and Cases in the United States, and monitors hospitalization rates, risk factors, and outcomes as well as mortality rates.

SYNDROMIC SURVEILLANCE

Syndromic surveillance includes collecting and analyzing data related to any indicator of increased illness or infection within the community. Indicators can include flu-like illness, flaccid paralysis, bleeding disorders with unclear etiology, rash, gastrointestinal symptoms, increased number of emergency department patients, similar chief symptoms in multiple patients, increased numbers of hospital admissions, increased need for EMS/ambulatory services, increased calls to help lines (health, emergency), increased sale of over-the-counter medications, increased use of search instruments for information about flu-like symptoms, increased animal (especially cattle and domestic animals) morbidity, mortality, and laboratory testing, school absenteeism and staff absenteeism at local businesses. The CDC runs **BioSense**, a national syndromic surveillance program to which many hospitals, pharmacies, state programs, and laboratories submit data. BioSense tracks this data and categorizes it so that spikes in syndromes, such as influenza-like illness, can be identified quickly. When a spike indicates a potential threat to a community, the CDC notifies public health authorities in that community.

Collection and Compilation of Surveillance Data

Clinical Evidence, Laboratory Evidence, and Supportive Data

Clinical evidence is derived from direct observation of the patient by infection control staff, supported by information obtained through chart review or review of other ward or unit records and the possible addition of diagnosis of infection by a surgeon or physician making direct observations during surgery.

Laboratory evidence comes from:

- Cultures
- Antigen- or antibody-detection tests
- Microscopic visualization methods
- Blood tests

Supportive data is derived from:

- X-rays
- Ultrasounds
- Computed tomography
- (CT) scans
- Magnetic resonance imaging
- Radiolabel scans
- Endoscopic procedures
- Biopsies
- Needle aspiration
- Other diagnostic studies

In cases where resolution of the problem is not immediately at hand, a thorough review of the medical literature may be called for.

Characteristics of Sufficient Data

In the question of what type of data to collect and how much, it is good to follow the lead provided by such agencies as the CDC's National Healthcare Safety Network (NHSN). It collects detailed information that includes, on each infected patient, demographic characteristics, history of infections and current infections, related risk factors, pathogens and their antimicrobial susceptibilities, and outcome. Data on risk factors in the population of patients being monitored are also collected to permit the calculation of risk-specific rates. It will use this surveillance data to develop and evaluate strategies to prevent and control healthcare-associated infections and calculate risk-specific infection rates. If a hospital collects its own similar kinds of data, it can compare its findings to evaluate the effectiveness of its infection control efforts. Guidance on data collection can also be obtained from the FDA and other agencies.

Collection of Data for Populations at Risk

Populations at risk must be defined for each institution, usually on the basis of an initial surveillance. There is no single way to define a population at risk; some procedures pose more risks than others, such as transplant surgery versus appendectomies. Some units in the hospital are associated with higher risk, for example, ICUs versus general medical floors. Targeting specific high-risk populations simplifies the collection of data by limiting surveillance and concentrating resources. Data collection should be stratified initially, if possible, so that information about populations and subpopulations is separated because this facilitates analysis and helps to identify outbreaks or deviations. For example, ICU data should not be commingled with high-risk nursery (HRN) data because the populations have completely different risk factors and expected outcomes. Electronic collection of data simplifies this process, but collecting data from questionnaires, interviews, lab reports, and medical records, while more time consuming, can suffice.

Prevalence Surveys

When resources are limited, making it difficult to indicate the extent of nosocomial infection within a hospital or region, a prevalence survey can prove useful. Since it can be performed by a small task force once or twice a year, a prevalence survey, while not an ideal replacement for incidence surveillance, tends to be more practical. It can pinpoint specific problems requiring attention and follow changes in the progress of a disease. Repeated at regular intervals, prevalence surveys yield information on both infected and uninfected patients that can be used to identify independent risk factors and to analyze the effectiveness of intervention strategies.

Repeated prevalence surveys have shown themselves to be useful for monitoring trends in HAI rates. However, prevalence rates do tend to be lower than incidence rates since prevalence studies are less effective in identifying acute or short-lived infections. Their greatest usefulness lies in looking at areas where infection is suspected or historically has been high.

Personnel Involved in Data Collection on Healthcare-Associated Infections

In the past, in the case of serious and pervasive healthcare-associated infections resistant to containment, as many healthcare professionals possible were thrown into the task of collecting and analyzing data and treating patients. Taking personnel away from their regular jobs was an expensive proposition.

Today, the microcomputer has taken over much of the work involved in surveillance to prevent runaway outbreaks. Many computer-based tracking systems use microbiologic data to detect upswings in the incidence of infection. Algorithms based on increases of detected pathogens over baseline levels apply statistical methods to determine whether and what kind of a response will be made to a possible outbreak. Now an Infection Control Officer and his or her staff can perform surveillance with the aid of records clerks and lab personnel.

Departments Involved in Surveillance Data Collection

Data from other departments or agencies can be very useful for the collection of surveillance data. The admissions department collects demographic information as part of the basic admissions questionnaire. For example, information about where a patient resides or was born can yield important risk factors, especially if diseases, such as malaria or Chagas disease, are endemic to these areas. This information is especially important if there is a large immigrant population. Additionally, data from public health departments about community-acquired infections or risks can trigger changes in surveillance in the hospital to reflect public health concerns. Some diagnoses of infections are based on clinical findings rather than laboratory results, and the pharmacy can be a valuable resource, providing information about the use of medications, primarily antibiotics, which may indicate treatment for infection. Operative reports can be used to identify high-risk populations, as not all patients will be treated in high-risk areas, such as ICUs.

Surveillance and Referral Forms Used in Data Collection

Infection control programs depend upon the accuracy of data collection and the clarity of surveillance and referral forms. Forms should be developed after determining the approach that will be used, whether prospective or retrospective, and the focus of surveillance. Collection of information should be simplified and targeted just to surveillance objectives rather than broad-based generalized requests for referral information. Thus, forms may be developed for a number of different surveillance objectives. For example, the neonatal unit would have different surveillance objectives and different reporting forms than an adult ICU. Staff involved in the use of the forms should be trained so that they understand the objectives and the type of information that is needed for data collection. Referral forms may be paper or electronic, depending upon the resources available in a facility. The duration of surveillance or points of surveillance should be clearly outlined. Forms may include questionnaires sent to particular staff or physician's office.

Data Collection for Device Utilization

Two common risk factors for healthcare-associated infections are length of stay and days of **device utilization**, including central lines, urinary catheters, and ventilators. The longer the invasive device is in place, the more likely an infection will occur, so collecting data on use and duration of invasive devices is especially important for infection control. Device records should be kept for each population or unit (such as ICU, HRN), electronically if possible. Coded information should be readily available and include the type of illness or procedure, the type of invasive device, the dates and duration of use, and indications of infection. It is important that data be kept for use of all invasive devices, not just occurrences of device-related infection, because the total number of invasive device days becomes the denominator data and it is impossible to arrive at meaningful indicator data and outcomes without this information.

Data Collection for Surgical Procedures

The collection of data for **surgical procedures** may vary according to the size and resources of the institution. Data may be collected and compiled from operative schedules, operative reports, laboratory results, medical records, and reports of antibiotic use. Data may be collected for targeted populations. If data are collected for all surgeries performed, then the results need to be stratified to account for different risk factors, such as the type of surgery, the ASO score, the wound classification, and the T point. Surgeon specific data should be provided as feedback to the individual surgeons rather than used as a basis of comparison. Some studies have indicated that providing feedback has successfully reduced rates of infection, but other studies have been inconclusive because of differences in variables. If possible, data collection should be electronically automated. Using an automated database that includes such information as the ASO score, T point, Risk Index, and codes for procedures can facilitate accurate collection of data.

Data Collection for Antibiotic Use with Surgical Site Infections

With the increase in antibiotic resistance, the use and timing of antibiotics are becoming of critical importance, and collection of data correlating **pre-, intra-, and peri-operative antibiotic use** to correlate with surgical site infections can provide valuable outcome information to be used for planning and intervention. In this case, the numerator data is defined as the type of antibiotic use. One problem encountered is gaining adequate data because some pre-surgical and peri-surgical antibiotics will be prescribed outside of the hospital so data may be dependent on questionnaires or interviews. Denominator data will be the population of those with surgical site infections. Again, some infections may not be evident until after discharge, so follow up with patients and doctors is necessary if the correlations are to have validity. Additionally, the denominator data may be stratified according to various risk factors, such as type of surgery, ASO score, generating different data according to risk factors.

Post-Discharge Data

Post-discharge surveillance (PDS) is a time-consuming procedure that is not commonly done by income conscious hospitals in the United States, unless it is part of a funded study. This is unfortunate because its importance and effectiveness has been illustrated by investigation. For example, after reviewing hospital records, German researchers found that over a given period, 45 urinary tract infections were diagnosed. When post-discharge follow-up was undertaken, however, 8 additional cases representing 15 percent of the total cases, were found. Follow-up showed that 4 percent of nosocomial pneumonia cases and 8 percent of bloodstream infections were missed without post-discharge surveillance. In all, about 12 percent of all ICU-associated healthcare-associated infections were missed when there was no PDS.

Follow-up for Exposure to Communicable Disease Within the Facility

If a communicable disease is identified as a possible source of infection, then the first step is to outline the epidemiology: the incubation period, the mode of transmission, the ease of transmission, and the symptoms. If the disease is reportable, then the local public health department must be notified immediately so that they can investigate and notify people. The physician should be notified, as well as the patient or person with the communicable disease, if they have not been informed. Next, a targeted retrospective survey must be done to identify those patients or staff who, because of time of hospitalization, bed proximity, contact, or shared use of equipment or facilities, may have contacted the disease. Physicians of patients should be notified and direct contact made with patients, preferably by telephone or in person if the disease poses a serious threat. If notification is sent by mail, follow up telephone calls should be done.

Compiling and Interpreting Surveillance Data

Steps followed in compiling and interpreting surveillance data include:

1. Recognize the need for an epidemiologic study when there is a problem needing investigation (e.g., case control, cohort studies)
2. Investigate clusters of infection appearing at a rate above expected levels
3. Generate, analyze, and validate surveillance data
4. Calculate and interpret statistical significance of computed surveillance data (e.g., mean, standard deviation) using an automated program to analyze statistical data and describe what is happening
5. Determine epidemiologically significant findings
6. Identify variances from baseline that require action
7. Determine incidence of healthcare-associated infections over a given period
8. Compare investigation results to published data or other benchmarks
9. Prepare analytical report using tables, graphs, or charts
10. Report findings to management staff

Organizing Surveillance Data

Surveillance data should be organized according to its meaningful use, taking into consideration the target audience and the purpose. Data that must be submitted in order to comply with regulations or accreditation are usually organized according to specific guidelines and may be submitted electronically. Data intended for staff members or administration should be organized for need and ease of understanding. Additionally, data should focus on what and how, rather than who. The infection control professional must determine how much data each group requires and how to present the data. For example, the administration may require raw data and narrative explanations as well as visual representations (graphs, charts) while nursing staff may require only visual representations that show percentages or rates. The infection control professional must select the best chart for the type of data and for the group for which it is intended.

Recording Surveillance Data

Systemic Approach

A systematic approach to record surveillance data requires planning and consistency. Surveillance may involve questionnaires, medical records, or electronic review.

- **Questionnaires** should be standardized and designed to obtain information that is quantifiable when possible. Questions should be clear, unambiguous, and non-threatening. Open ended questions may be appropriate for some types of information gathering, especially in relation to information that may be embarrassing.
- **Coding of data collection** should be consistent, with specific codes for units, populations, and/or individuals to facilitate analysis. Thus, the report of a patient with a cough would have the same identification code as the laboratory work for that patient.
- **Medical record review** should be systematic and targeted as much as possible. Reporting forms should be utilized that include all necessary information in one form.
- **Electronic surveillance** should involve use of threshold data reports that are generated, and should be directly integrated with the data analysis system.

Using Computerized Systems for Data Entry

The use of a computerized system for entering data can pose a number of problems because often systems in use are not integrated, so the lab reports and medical records may be on incompatible systems. There are a number of different ways to enter data:

- **Manual data entry** is probably the most common method. This can involve charting directly into the computer or copying information, such as lab reports, after the fact. The responsibility for entering data must be clearly outlined to prevent a backlog. Staff must be thoroughly trained in the correct procedures for data entry.
- **Scanners** can be programmed to read particular forms, such as those with boxes marked. Text can also be scanned so that reports from outside the system can be added.

Calculation of Rates/Ratios When Compiling Surveillance Data

A **rate** is the number of events per a given population (a rate of 3 infections per 100 patients) or per a time period (a rate of 3 infections per 1000 device days). These rates expressed in the form of **ratios** would be 3:100 and 3:1000. Rates and ratios are accessible, and much infection control data is expressed by these statistics. However, data should be stratified, taking risk factors into account, and different rates derived for different populations for validity. **Risk ratio** is the ratio of incidence of infection among those who have been exposed compared to the incidence among those who have not been exposed. A risk ratio of 1.0 suggests that there is equal risk of infection. A higher number suggests the probability that those exposed will have higher rates. Thus, a number of 1.5 shows that the exposed group is 1.5 times more likely to become infected than those not exposed. A lower number suggests exposure brings less risk of infection (immunity).

Calculating Rates of Occurrence

There are a number of ways of measuring a disease's rate of occurrence:

- **Incidence**: The rate at which new cases occur in a population during a specified period.
- **Prevalence**: The proportion of a population that has the disease at a point in time; a measure that is appropriate only for relatively stable conditions, unsuitable for acute disorders.
- **Point prevalence**: The proportion of a population that make up cases at a single point in time. This is based on a single examination, so it tends to underestimate a condition's total frequency.
- **Period prevalence:** The proportion of a population that make up cases at any time within a stated period. This is a better measure than point prevalence when repeated or continuous assessments of the same individuals are possible.
- **Mortality rate**: This, like other measures, can be combined as when, for example, each new case is put into a prevalence pool and remains there until either recovery or death.
- **Disease attack rate**: New cases of a specific disease per population at risk, expressed as percentage. It is the specific incidence rate over a limited time interval.
- **Case-fatality rate**: Ratio of deaths from a specified cause to the number of diagnosed cases of that disease.

Using Post-Discharge Surveillance when Calculating Rates

Because of the increasing trend toward outpatient/ambulatory surgery and procedures and decreased inpatient hospital stays, much follow-up after hospitalization or outpatient invasive procedures is done in the physician's office rather than the facility where treatment was provided; thus, infections or other events that occur after discharge may not be captured, resulting in errors in calculating rates. **Post-discharge surveillance** should include:

- Training physicians and office personnel to recognize and report findings that are part of surveillance parameters
- Sending surveys to physicians and patients after the patient is discharged with questions about infection specific to the operative procedure. Patients may be contacted by mail, email, or telephone, and follow-up surveys may be done during different time periods
- Providing discharge information to patients outlining possible complications and signs of infections and reporting procedures (call MD, notify clinic)
- Reviewing postoperative records in clinics
- Reviewing postoperative laboratory records

Incidence vs. Prevalence in Hospital-Wide Surveillance Programs

The purpose of surveillance of nosocomial infections is to reduce the incidence of healthcare-associated infection (HAI), thereby reducing the associated morbidity, mortality, and costs. If the incidence and distribution of a disease are known, measures can be taken to reduce the incidence.

Incidence surveillance keeps track of every patient within a hospital where there has been an outbreak of nosocomial infection; prevalence surveillance concentrates on following the etiology of the disease in patients who have contracted it. It requires that each patient be assessed, often repeatedly, by trained staff; for this reason, it is very expensive, and surveillance is often done routinely by analyzing laboratory reports and/or informal ward visits, methods that are not all that accurate.

Incidence Rates of Healthcare-Associated Infections

The incidence rate is the number of events (numerator) divided by the number of the population at risk (denominator), often expressed as the number of infections per 100 patients. Incidence may also be used to calculate **incidence density**, which is the rate at which disease occurs in relation to the size of the population without disease. Incidence density uses the number of infections (numerator) in relation to units of time (denominator), such as the number of infections that occur in 1000 patient days. Incidence may also be used to calculate **attack rate,** expressed as a percentage of an at-risk population that is infected. The attack rate is used to calculate incidence rates during outbreaks of specific populations.

Determining Prevalence of Epidemiologically Significant Findings

Prevalence is a good measure of the overall burden of infections on a facility, expressing how common infections are. Prevalence is often expressed as a percentage. In **limited-duration prevalence,** prevalence is looked at retrospectively. That is, it counts all those alive at a point in time who, during a prescribed duration of time (past 5 years, for example), had a particular disease. **Complete/lifetime prevalence,** on the other hand, counts all those alive at a particular point in time who had the disease at any time in the past or present, whether cured or in current treatment, usually expressed as a ratio of those with the disease compared to a given population.

Data Collected in Surveillance of Healthcare-Associated Infections

The following data should be collected in surveillance of healthcare-associated infections:

- Patient's name, Age, Sex
- Patient ID
- Patient's location
- Medical services already rendered
- Date of admission
- Description of infection
- Risk factors for the infection
- Infection's site
- Cultures run
- Primary diagnosis
- Severity of illness
- Physician's name
- Antimicrobial therapy

The primary numerator data, divided by the denominator to obtain an estimate of risk, consists of the number of persons with the infection or condition. The denominator is the number of persons at risk for the infection. For example, the number of nosocomial pneumonias (numerator) divided by the number of patients receiving respiratory therapy (denominator) gives the odds that a patient using a respirator will contract pneumonia. The more precise the denominator is in getting the potentially preventable risk elements the more descriptive the calculation's end result.

Numerator and Denominator Data for Healthcare-Associated Infections

Numerator data for indicator occurrences and denominator data for rate-based indicators are obtained by processing surveillance data collected during ward rounds, from patient records, pharmacy notes, microbiology and biochemistry reports, hematology results, and other sources. But before a rate-based indicator is obtained, there must first be a clear definition of the numerator and denominator.

For surgical site infections, this is a straightforward procedure, the rate being a proportion comprising the number of infections in the numerator and the number of patients undergoing the relevant operation in the denominator. However, for other infections and colonizations, the denominator should usually be occupied bed days, though this metric sometimes leaves much to be desired.

In the case of device related infections such as ventilator associated pneumonia, catheter associated urinary tract infection, and intravenous line associated bacteraemia, the denominator should be an approximation of device days of exposure.

Denominator Data for Device Related Infections

The National Healthcare Safety Network (NHSN) has established standardized numerator/denominator formulas. The **device associated** formula is as follows:

$$\frac{\text{selected device-associated infections}}{\text{patient days or device days}}$$

The population pool includes all those with infections related to specific devices, such as urinary catheters. Both the number of total patient days during the time period surveyed and the device days are recorded as a patient may be hospitalized for 6 days but have a catheter for only 4 days. Device days give more specific information. Data must be collected for sufficient time, at least 4 weeks, and in sufficient numbers to render useful data. Physician specific data can be obtained, but should not be used for comparison. One physician may order urine cultures for all those with catheters and another physician may rarely do so. Since urinary infections are common with catheters, the physician who orders lab work may have higher statistics but actually a lower rate of infection.

Calculation of Device-Related Infection Rates Using Device Days

Device-related infections are usually calculated by using the number of infection events (numerator) in relation to either the number of insertions/uses or the number of device days (denominator). For example, calculation the number of urinary infections per catheter insertions would be expressed as 1.4 per 100 insertions. Infections calculated using device days are done by adding together the total device days of the target population:

- Patient A 4 days with the device
- Patient B 6 days
- Patient C 10 days
- Patient D 7 days

Total device days = 27 days

Assuming there was one infection (numerator) during these 27 device days (denominator), the rate would be 0.037 multiplied by 1000 (the scale factor), resulting in an estimate of 37 infections per 1000 device days. Of course, a sample should involve far more than 4 patients and 27 days for the calculations to be statistically meaningful.

Denominator Data for Surgeon-Specific Surgical Procedures

Surgeon specific data can be derived by limiting the denominator data to that surgeon's patient pool. The denominator number must be adequate (usually 100-1000) and the time of the survey of sufficient length to yield meaningful data, usually at least 4 weeks. Questions about both numerator and denominator data must be resolved. Will all surgical site infections be included together? Will superficial infections be surveyed separately from deep incisional or organ/space? Will adjustments for risk factors be made? Surgeon specific data is rarely useful for comparison because of numerous variables. For example, two surgeons may do similar hip replacements, but one surgeon may specialize in sports injuries and deal with a younger, healthier population that the other surgeon whose patients are primarily elderly with chronic health problems. Infection rates may differ but, without adjusting for risk factors, the differences may be impossible to evaluate. Surgeon-specific data can be useful to help a surgeon implement changes to improve outcomes.

Interpretation of Surveillance Data

Generation, Analysis, and Validation of Surveillance Data

Most **generation of data** is from available resources, such as admissions records, questionnaires, interviews, medical records, public health reports, and laboratory reports. In some cases, creating data is part of the surveillance process. For example, urine cultures may be done routinely as part of a surveillance plan, or threshold rates may generate further testing. **Analysis** should be done in a timely manner, especially important for the detection of outbreaks. The type of analysis will depend upon the expected outcomes and the purpose of surveillance. **Validation** of data is an ongoing process. All steps in the generation and analysis of data should be reviewed regularly, especially when threshold rates have been exceeded. If, for example, there is an apparent outbreak of antibiotic resistant bacteria detected sputum cultures, then the procedures for obtaining the specimens as well as laboratory procedures need to be validated to ensure that the outbreak is not a pseudo-epidemic caused by faulty lab procedures or other deviations in infection control.

Decision Analysis in Epidemiologic Surveillance

Decision analysis, now typically a computer-assisted process, quantifies the comparative effectiveness of alternative medical interventions and sometimes also measures them against cost considerations. After variables and known probabilities for alternative medical interventions are recorded, quantitative analysis produces a decision tree that lays out the best outcomes in terms of morbidity and mortality.

In using decision analysis, there should be some uncertainty about an appropriate clinical strategy (otherwise there's no point). There are many circumstances when optimal clinical strategy has already been identified, so no analysis is needed. Also, decision analyses always require comparison of at least two clinical strategies, with at least one holding advantages and countervailing disadvantages. If one strategy clearly dominates the other, a decision analysis is not necessary.

Survival Analysis and Survival Curve

Survival models comprise various statistical methods used to evaluate time-to-event data in studies where the timing of events is important, particularly survival from illness, but also by extension other nonrecurring events that happen in a cohort over time, such as relapse or death. It involves following (usually figuratively rather than literally) the cohort, plotting the occurrence of events, and calculating their probabilities for each time interval. In most clinical situations, the chance of an outcome changes with time. The events must be distinct and the time at which they occur must be precisely known.

Survival analysis facilitates assessing the effectiveness of a given treatment and understanding the effects of various disease characteristics. When data is graphed to show the number of events occurring over time or the chance of being free of these events over time, this is what is called a **survival curve**. In most survival curves the earlier follow-up periods usually include results from more patients than the later periods and are therefore more precise.

Hazard Rate and Calendar Time vs. Study Time

The **hazard rate** is the probability that an individual will experience an event during a measured time period that the individual is at risk for that event. If the hazard rate is constant over time and is equal to 3.0, for example, this would mean that one would expect 3.0 events to occur in a time interval that is one unit long.

It is very common for subjects to enter or leave a study continuously throughout the length of the study, and allowances must be made for the non-simultaneity of results. In **calendar time**, both the entry and the exit time of subjects are staggered and can occur at any time throughout the course of the study. **Study time** deals only with the length of time that subjects as a group are studied.

Comparing Rates Over Time

In determining rates of infection, the numerator is the population at risk, and the denominator is the number of people infected. However, there can be problems in measuring either of those figures. A recent study at a long-term nursing care facility showed that monthly infection rates were calculated based on the census (number of infections per month/average monthly census) and care duration (number of infections per month/average monthly resident stay days). The average census based monthly infection rate was 16.5; average care duration based monthly infection rate was 5.4 episodes per 1000 patient care days. That is a substantial difference in rate, with the latter calculation probably being the more accurate, but the former being easier to calculate. The definition of population is not the only difficulty in obtaining comparative time-based data. In such comparisons, all other factors must also be held constant, a difficult task at best.

Use of Risk Stratification in Data Analysis

Risk stratification involves statistical adjustment to account for confounding and differences in risk factors. Confounding issues are those that confuse the data outcomes, such as trying to compare different populations, different ages, or different genders. For example, if there are two physicians and one has primarily high-risk patients, and the other has primarily low risk patients, the same rate of infection (by raw data) would suggest that the infection risks are equal for both physicians' patients. However, high-risk patients are much more prone to infection, so in this case risk stratification to account for this difference would show that the patients of the physician with low-risk patients had a much higher risk of infection, relatively-speaking. Risk stratification is also used to predict outcomes of surgery by accounting for various risk factors (including ASO score, age, and medical conditions). Risk stratification is an important element of data analysis.

Issues when Comparing Infection Rates Among Patient Groups

Infection surveillance data could be used to judge the comparative quality of care between two or more hospitals; however, this entails problems:

- It would require that all hospitals collect the same kind of data on the same types of infections
- They would have to use the same methods for identifying infections and collecting data. There is a fundamental lack of standardization in defining indicators purporting to measure similar events. Lacking standardization, indicator-rate specifications vary between entities and can yield widely different evaluations of hospital performance.
- Hospital staff recording raw data for the measurement systems are rarely provided information on exactly how the measure is to be calculated.
- Standardization between facilities is difficult because each has site specific infection rates stemming from a wide variety of factors unique to it, such as types of patients being served, underlying medical conditions, and types and complexity of treatments given and procedures performed.

Investigations of Clusters of Infection Above Expected Levels

Coordination and conduct of investigations of clusters or other adverse events should be established as part of the surveillance plan so that any adverse events trigger a chain of actions that may include the following:

- Immediate report to the infectious disease professional/committee
- Development of profile and definition of the outbreak with pertinent information, such as place, time, and/or incubation period
- Statistical analysis of data to determine the probability that adverse events occurred by chance
- Additional laboratory specimens obtained or retesting done on existing specimens. May include targeted cultures or serologic testing
- Review of medical records
- Contact staff, patients, physicians, and public health officials as appropriate
- Identification of index case
- Review of the infection control process through interviews, review of written policies and direct observation of staff procedures
- Assessment of source of infection and development of hypothesis with case control or cohort study

Monitoring Antibiotic Resistance Patterns

Data to monitor antibiotic resistance patterns may be compiled with one or two different types of data. Antibiotic resistance patterns may be surveyed for a given population through various cultures (sputum, blood, or urine) to which antibiotic sensitivities are completed. Organisms that are typically monitored include the following:

- Vancomycin resistant *Enterococci*
- Drug resistant Streptococcus pneumoniae
- Methicillin-resistant *Staphylococcus aureus*
- Drug resistant Group A *Streptococci*

Resistance patterns may also be correlated with antibiotic use. First antibiotic use must be monitored in relation to infections, whether the antibiotics were prescribed prophylactically before or during surgery/ exposure or in response to an infection. Then cultures must be taken of the target population and antibiotic sensitivity testing completed. Monitoring antibiotic resistance patterns is often part of establishing a formulary or protocols for antibiotic use. The increasing prevalence of antibiotic resistance poses a major concern for healthcare providers and is a primary concern of infection control.

Identifying Variances Through Surveillance

Initial planning can facilitate responding to variances identified through surveillance. As part of the infection control plan:

- Activities should be classified according to the risk of exposure, including the need for barrier protection.
- Standard procedures should be established for all activities that might involve exposure.
- Training and education should be provided for all staff, with a focus on standard precautions and handwashing.
- Compliance should be monitored on a regular basis, including monitoring of environmental surfaces.

Once a variance is identified, the framework that is already in place is used to help identify the organism and mode of transmission. Targeted infection control procedures, such as increased cleaning or disinfecting, may be indicated. Plans should already be in place for dealing with different types of organisms and modes of transmission, so an outbreak of *Clostridium difficile*, for example, would trigger a predetermined initial response, which may be varied according to the circumstances.

Identification of Variances from Baseline Data

Identification of variances from baseline data first requires baseline data that is representative for the target population. This involves an initial period of surveillance and review. Baseline data can be established for various periods of time, but a 1-month period is commonly used. Threshold rates should also be established. Once the baseline is established, new data is analyzed to determine if there are variances (changes), usually increases although decreases may be identified if data is collected for the purpose of charting improvements. The basis for an alert should be predetermined. For example, if infection rates increase 2 standard deviations above the monthly mean, this may trigger an alert. Alerts may be tied to time so that increases over a 3-month period trigger alerts. Once data triggers a variance alert, then statistical analysis must be completed to determine the relevancy of the variance, the probability of it having occurred by chance, in order to determine if the variance has statistical significance.

Periodic Evaluation of the Effectiveness of the Surveillance Plan

Surveillance should be done with a goal in mind, and the data collected should be used as a basis to plan strategies of intervention or to identify indicators for further study. One measure, then, of the **effectiveness of a surveillance plan** is the degree to which it has initiated changes or increased efficiency. The effectiveness of the plan should be evaluated on a regular basis, reviewing not only the type of surveillance but also the targets, as this may need to be changed, especially if there is evidence of outbreaks or changing patterns of infections that are unaccounted for. Laboratory findings are an integral part of surveillance and these findings should be reviewed as part of the overall evaluation as often the first indication of an outbreak is reflected in laboratory results. Threshold rates may require adjustment or additions in order to facilitate case finding. Questionnaires and interviews can help to evaluate effectiveness of surveillance.

Questions Asked of Studies with Results That Are Called into Question

Some questions that might be asked of any study where the results are called into question include the following:

- What kind of study was it? Meta analytical studies that gather the results of a number of small studies to make their conclusions should automatically be checked to see whether the researcher or the funding organization has an agenda.
- How was the data gathered? Was it verified? A retrospective study for which the data was not independently validated can be discarded.
- Was a survey used? If so, what questions were asked? Were they free of bias?
- What was the sample size? How was it selected?
- Were confounders taken into consideration?
- What is the reputation and experience of the researcher?
- Who funded the study? Was its outcome of benefit to them?

Evaluating Control Methods

Control methods will depend upon the hypothesis generated as to the infective agent, the source, and the mode of transmission. Control methods could include the following:

- Education of staff regarding infection control, handwashing procedures
- Isolation of patients as appropriate, according to diagnosis
- Serologic testing of contacts, including patients, visitors, and healthcare workers
- Immunization as needed
- Prophylactic antimicrobials, especially preoperatively
- Monitoring of antimicrobials
- Change in sterilization procedures
- Environmental modifications
- Reassignment of staff
- Changes in housekeeping procedures
- Establishment of new policies and procedures

Evaluation of control methods is an ongoing process that begins with the initial control methods. Surveillance should continue after all control methods have been instituted and should be of sufficient duration to track changes. If there is no decrease in the number of infections, then further investigation and control methods may be necessary.

Statistical Tools Used in the Analysis of Research Findings

Statistical tools used in the analysis of research findings include the following:

- **Analysis of Variance (ANOVA)**: Compares the means of multiple groups
- **Linear Regression**: Shows relationships between one or more independent variables and a dependent variable
- **Logistic Regression**: Determines the relationship between one or more continuous or categorical predictor variables and a binary outcome variable (is/is not, does/does not, etc.) to predict an outcome probability
- **Repeated Measures**: Special repeated analytic procedures may be required to arrive at the correct statistical conclusion when data from successive testing of the same subjects is collected over time. This is because both early and late measurements on an individual are not independent variables since they are related.
- **Chi-square test**: A non-parametric test for association in categorical data
- **Two Sample (Independent) t-test**: Determines whether the means from two independent groups are similar, within the bounds of chance variation
- **Paired (Dependent) t-test**: Determines the mean difference obtained by testing the same individuals on two different occasions (e.g., before treatment, after treatment.
- **Survival Analysis**: Compares survival curves

Measures of Averages

Measures of averages locate the center point of a group of data. They can also be referred to as measures of central tendency:

- **Mean** is the average number. However, since distribution can vary widely, the mean may not give an accurate picture. For example, if compiling data and one unit has 20 infections per 100 and the other has 1 infection per 100, the mean (21÷2) is 10.5 per 100, which has little validity.
- **Median** is the 50th percentile. For example, consider the following numbers: 1, 3, 7, 9, and 15. The number 7 is the median (middle) number. If there were an even number, the 2 middle numbers would be averaged: 1, 3, 7, 9, 14, and 15. The numbers 7 and 9 are averaged so the median is 8. If there is an even distribution, the mean and median will be the same. The wider the difference between the two, the more uneven the distribution.
- **Mode** is the number occurring with the highest frequency. There may be bi-modal or tri-modal data sets.

Measures of Distribution

Measures of distribution show the spread or dispersion of data.

- **Range** is the distance from the highest to the lowest number. The term interquartile is used in infection control to denote the range between the 25th percentile and the 75th percentile. Range is usually reported with median to provide information about both the center point and the dispersion.
- **Variance** measures the distribution spread around an average value. It is often used to calculate the effect of variables. A large variance suggests a wide distribution and a small variance indicates that the random variables are close to the mean.
- **Standard deviation** is the square root of the variance and shows the dispersion of data above and below the mean in equally measured distances. In a normal distribution, 68% of the data is within one deviation (measured distance) of the mean, 95% within 2 deviations and 99.7% within 3 deviations.

Standard Error of the Mean

The standard error of the mean (SEM) is used in inferential statistics to give an estimate of how the mean of the sample is related to the mean of the population that the sample represents.

However, a study sample, if the array is distributed normally, can be described entirely by two parameters, the mean and the standard deviation (SD). The larger the SD, the higher the variability within the sample. Samples should always be summarized by the mean and SD, but authors often incorrectly use the standard error ofthe mean (SEM) rather than the SD to describe the variability of their sample.

As the SEM is always smaller than the standard deviation, the reader may be led to expect that the variability within the sample is much smaller than it really is. The SD and the SEM are related, but they give two very different types of information. Use of the SEM is rarely justified.

UNIVARIATE ANALYSIS, CATEGORICAL VARIABLES, AND CHI-SQUARE

A univariate general linear statistical model is used to compare differences between group means to estimate the effect of covariates on a single dependent variable. For example, to test for the effects of smoking on emphysema, the researcher must be aware that there are variables other than smoking that could affect results. Including these variables in the analysis controls their influence and produces a univariate result.

A categorical variable is a qualitative variable such as patient gender in which cases are classified in one of two possible levels—in this case, male or female. With this kind of data, the researcher could conduct a Chi square test of independence to test the null hypothesis that there is no relationship between the two variables such as gender and prevalence of emphysema. That is, there should be little difference between observed and expected values.

PROBABILITY

PROBABILITY FACTORS

Relative to infection control biostatistics, there are various probability factors to consider:

- **Conditional probability** represents the chance that an event will occur in the future, given that an identical event has already occurred. Conditional probabilities for several events can be compared for examining such things as whether different treatments or exposures influence the probability of mortality.
- **Unconditional probability**, also called **total probability**, represents probabilities without any restrictions and typically is a number that lies somewhere between a set of two conditional probabilities.
- **Empirical probability**, an estimate that an event will happen based on how often the event occurs after collecting data or running an experiment in a large number of trials. It extracts probabilities from experience and observation.
- The **theoretical probability** of an event is the number of ways that the event can occur, divided by the total number of outcomes.

BAYES' LAW OF PROBABILITY

Bayes' Law of Probability, based to a large degree on subjective inference, can be used to calculate and chart predictive values when prevalence, sensitivity, and specificity are known values. Some researchers regard Bayesian inference as an application of the scientific method because updating probabilities through Bayesian inference requires one to start with initial beliefs about the hypotheses that come into play, to collect new information through research and experiment, and then to adjust the original beliefs in the light of the new information.

Results of such adjustment could mean accepting or rejecting the original hypotheses. The Bayesian interpretation of probability allows probabilities to be assigned to all propositions independent of whether the events can be interpreted as having a relative frequency in repeated trials.

Additional Concepts of Probability

Additional concepts relating to probability include the following:

- **Joint probability**: Chance of two events happening simultaneously
- **Product rule**: The conditional probability of one event multiplied by the total probability of another.
- **Independent event**: Each trial in a random study is an independent event.
- **Dependent events**: When one trial can affect the outcome of a second independent trial. This can be illustrated by pulling a card from a standard deck of cards. The chances of its being the ace of spades are 1/52. However, if that card is not the ace and is discarded, the chance of drawing the ace of spades on the next try is 1/51.
- The **addition or total probability rule**: For any two events (A & B), the total probability of the first event (A) equals the sum of the joint probability of both events, plus the joint probability of A and not B. This rule provides a method of reassembling an unconditional probability from specified conditional probabilities.

Issues of Statistical Significance

P Values

One problem with surveillance data is that sometimes there can be variations in data by chance alone, so a sudden increase in incidence of infection may not indicate an outbreak but rather a normal statistically acceptable variation. The ***p* value** calculates the probability that the results occurred by chance. *P* values are expressed in a range from >0 to 1.0.

- <0.05 is statistically significant with only a<5% probability that the event could have occurred by chance, and conversely a 95% chance that the event is significant.
- >0.05 percent is considered not statistically significant, probably occurring by chance.

It is important to realize that *p* value alone is not enough to make a determination that an event is of no significance because, for example, a limited outbreak may not generate enough data to show significance, but it can still be epidemiologically important. The *p* value is just one measurement of evidence and should be combined with other statistical analyses.

Causal Inference and Hill's Criteria

In epidemiology, a statistical association is not necessarily definitive. **Sir A. Bradford Hill (1897-1991)**, who made important contributions to research methods related to epidemiology, developed criteria to judge a causal inference. The more criteria are met, the more likely that an association is causal; that is, an exposure caused a disease.

- **Strength of association** as measured by the *p* value <0.05
- **Temporality:** Cause must precede event
- **Consistency of observations:** The same effect occurs in different populations and settings
- **Plausibility of theory:** The theory is based on sound biologic principles
- **Coherence:** The theory does not conflict with other knowledge/theories
- **Specificity:** One primary cause for an outcome strengthens causality
- **Dose relationship:** An increase in exposure should increase the risk
- **Experimental evidence:** Related experimental research may increase the causal inference
- **Analogical extension:** That which is true in one situation may apply to another

Issues Related to Hospital Reporting

There are a number of issues related to hospital reporting that can result in inaccurate data:

- **Insufficient information** may be the result of incomplete medical records or lab reports at the time of survey. There may be a failure in the reporting procedure so that some data is not reported.
- **Evaluation errors** may occur even when data is available but is overlooked or the significance is not understood so that the data is not included in a survey.
- **Insufficient laboratory testing** is a frequent finding of studies. Very often indications of infection are clinically evident but cultures that would verify infection are not ordered by the physician or are not automatically triggered by established threshold rates.
- **Negligence** may relate to reluctance to verify and report infections in order to keep infection rates low.

Because of differences in efficiency of collecting data, the facility with the lowest infection rate may be the one with the least accurate collection of data.

Issues Related to Bias

Selection bias occurs when the method of selecting subjects results in a cohort that is not representative of the target population because of inherent error in design. For example, if all patients who develop urinary infections with urinary catheters are evaluated per urine culture and sensitivities for microbial resistance, but only those patients with clinically evident infections are included, a number of patients with subclinical infections may be missed, skewing the results. Selection bias is only a concern when participants in studies are specifically chosen. Many surveillance studies do not involve selection of subjects.

Information bias occurs when there are errors in classification, so an estimate of association is incorrect.

- **Non-differential misclassification** occurs when there is similar misclassification of disease or exposure among both those who are diseased/exposed and those who are not.
- **Differential misclassification** occurs when there is a differing misclassification of disease or exposure among both those who are diseased/exposed and those who are not.

Issues Related to Time-Related Risk and Multiple Events

Most studies of healthcare-associated infections involve **time at risk** rather than patient numbers, so studies of incidence density related to invasive devices, such as intravenous lines or urinary catheters, are often based the number of infections per 1000 device days, that is days at risk. If there are 200 patients with a total of 600 device days and 6 patients develop infections, those 6 patients are no longer "at risk" because they have the infection and become part of the numerator data (number of infections), so their device days counted only up to the point where an infection is diagnosed. Additionally, frequently the same patient may have **multiple or recurring infections**, with the first infection a significant risk factor for the second. Generally, first events only are included in the data to avoid counting a subject more than once. Alternately, data may be stratified according to the number of infections to calculate risks. Longitudinal studies that account for multiple infections over time may also be completed.

Issues Related to Internal and External Validity

Many surveillance plans are most concerned with **internal validity**, adequate unbiased data properly collected and analyzed within the population studied, but studies that determine the efficacy of procedures or treatments, for example, should have **external validity** as well; that is, the results should be generalizable (true) for similar populations. Replication of the study with different subjects, researchers, and under different circumstances should produce similar results. For various reasons, some people may be excluded from a study so that instead of randomized subjects, the subjects may be highly selected so when data is compared with another population in which there is less or more selection, results may be different. The selection of subjects, in this case, would interfere with external validity. Part of the design of a study should include considerations of whether or not it should have external validity or whether there is value for the institution based solely on internal validation.

National Nosocomial Infections Surveillance (NNIS) System

In 1970, the National Centers for Infectious Diseases of the US Centers for Disease Control and Prevention (CDC) established the National Nosocomial Infections Surveillance (NNIS) system. The purpose was to help encourage hospitals to report and track healthcare-associated infections and to use standardized methods to collect and analyze data and to create a national database. About 300 hospitals, whose identity remained confidential, reported data using "surveillance components" and protocols that had been standardized and used CDC definitions. Surveillance components included:

- Adult and pediatric Intensive Care Units (ICUs)
- High-risk nurseries (HRNs)
- Surgical patients
- Antimicrobial use and resistance

All ICU and HRN patients were surveyed, but hospitals chose from a list of surgical procedures that they wanted to monitor for surgical patients as the numbers of procedures done at different hospitals can vary widely. Infection statistics were compiled and reported every 3 years. In 2004, this system was absorbed into the National Healthcare Safety Network (NHSN), now responsible for conducting and generating surveillance reports on nosocomial infections.

National Healthcare Safety Network (NHSN)

The National Healthcare Safety Network (NHSN) integrates and replaces 3 separate programs: National Nosocomial Infections Surveillance (NNIS), Dialysis Surveillance Network (DSN), and National Surveillance System for Healthcare Workers (NaSH). All healthcare facilities, such as hospitals and dialysis centers, can participate in the internet-based program that allows for reporting and sharing data. Those who apply to become members must agree to utilize CDC definitions, follow strict protocols, and submit data every 6 months. Anonymity of the institutions is protected. The program streamlines reporting of data and provides comparative data from across the United States. The system can identify sentinel or unusual events and notify appropriate participating agencies. There are 3 components to NHSN: patient safety, healthcare worker safety, and research and development. Extensive data analysis features are part of the program. Reports of healthcare-associated infection, or hospital-acquired, infections that were previously issued by NNIS are now issued by NHSN.

Biovigilance and Long-Term Care Facilities

The NHSN provides guidelines for surveillance in a number of different areas:

- **Biovigilance:** The only module currently available in the biovigilance component is hemovigilance, which includes surveillance of blood-transfusion adverse events and adverse reactions. Hemovigilance includes both active (personnel trained in surveillance) and passive (personnel only expected to report reactions) surveillance methods. The focus is patient-based as patients are individually monitored. Surveillance may be prospective or retrospective, and priority-directed (focused on specific events/patients/populations) or comprehensive (continuously monitoring all patients). Rates are generally crude with small numbers and risk-adjusted when numbers increase. The hemovigilance protocol provides the rules to healthcare providers for surveillance, and these should be studied before data is collected or reported.
- **Long-term care:** Long-term care facilities (LTCFs) can enroll in both the LTCF Component and the Healthcare Personnel Safety Component, with surveillance methods similar to those of biovigilance. The LTCF Component contains modules related to COVID-19, HAIs (urinary tract infection, catheter and non-catheter-associated), laboratory identified (LabID) events (MDRO and *Clostridium* difficile), and prevention process measures (hand hygiene and gown and glove use).

Medicare's Hospital Compare Website

The Hospital Compare website of the CMS provides information comparing more than 4000 hospitals in the United States. Complete data sets, that the infection control professional can use to generate reports, can be downloaded from data.medicare.gov. The Hospital Compare website contains general information, such as timely and effective care for specific conditions (such as heart attack and pneumonia), readmission and death rates, complications related to specific conditions, healthcare-associated infections, appropriate use of imaging for outpatients, follow-up of screening mammograms, survey of patient experiences, and the numbers of Medicare patients and Medicare payments. The healthcare-associated infection information is especially valuable for the IP because the quality measures correspond to some of those of the NHSN: central line-associated bloodstream infections (CLABSI), catheter-associated urinary tract infections (CAUTI), surgical site infections (SSI) from colon surgery or abdominal hysterectomy, MRSA bloodstream infections, and intestinal infections with *C. Difficile.* Information includes appropriate administration and use of antibiotics.

Surgical Care Improvement Project (SCIP)

The Surgical Care Improvement Project (SCIP) evolved from the National Surgical Infection Prevention (SIP) Project, which was a joint venture of the CDC and CMS intended to decrease the rates of surgical morbidity and mortality. Multiple national agencies are involved in this project. Hospitals must report rates of compliance with SCIP measures, which affects Medicare payments. These rates are subsequently published on Hospital Compare on the internet. Accrediting agencies, such as the Joint Commission, include the SCIP core measure set as part of evaluation. The SCIP core measure set includes: antibiotic prophylaxis given one hour prior to onset of surgery, appropriate antibiotic selection, antibiotic discontinuation within 24 hours postoperatively, controlled blood glucose level at 6 AM postoperatively, appropriate removal of hair, removal of urinary catheter on postoperative day one or two, perioperative temperature management, receipt of beta-blocker when appropriate during perioperative period, and thromboembolism prophylaxis as indicated.

National Electronic Disease Surveillance System (NEDSS)

The National Electronic Disease Surveillance System (NEDSS), is capable of transferring appropriate public health data, laboratory data, and clinical data efficiently and securely over the internet enabling public health authorities to gather and analyze data with greater speed and accuracy. The NEDSS Base System provides a platform upon which modules can be built to allow state health departments to build their own surveillance and analysis systems. When NEDSS began in 2001, no state had all the pieces necessary for the integrated and internet-based surveillance system, therefore the CDC allowed states to slowly integrate to the new system. With healthcare reform and the push for electronic medical records, today, all states are using NEDSS. The mission, among other things, is to implement seamless surveillance and information systems that take advantage of the best information and surveillance technology, and serve the following needs at the local, state, and national levels:

- Monitor and assess disease trends
- Guide prevention and intervention programs
- Inform public health policy and policy makers
- Identify issues needing public health research
- Provide information for community and program planning
- Protect confidentiality while providing information to those who need to know

External Benchmarking and Internal Trending

External benchmarking involves analyzing data from outside an institution, such as monitoring national rates of healthcare-associated infection and comparing it to internal rates. In order for this data to be meaningful, the same definitions must be used as well as the same populations or effective risk stratification. Using NHSN data can be informative, but each institution is different, and relying on external benchmarking to select indicators for infection control can be misleading. Additionally, benchmarking is a compilation of data that may vary considerably if analyzed individually, further compounded by anonymity that makes comparisons difficult.

Internal trending involves comparing internal infection rates of one area or population with another, such as ICU with general surgery, and this can help to pinpoint areas of concern within an institution, but making comparisons is still problematic because of inherent differences. Using a combination of external and internal data can help to identify and select indicators.

Comparison of Rates in a Periodic Report of Analyzed Data

Reports of healthcare-associated infections are often used as a basis of comparison between one facility and others or one department in a facility, such as an ICU, and another, such as a transplant unit. Even in-house comparisons must be interpreted carefully because a higher rate of infection does not always mean patients are at increased risk. Numerous factors must be accounted for if a comparison is to be meaningful:

- **Definitions** must be uniform and consistent, following CDC definitions or specific definitions that have been developed for the population at risk or facility.
- **Protocols** for data collection should be uniform so that data is collected in the same way in different units, and case finding should be consistent and accurate. There should also be consistency in obtaining supporting laboratory tests.
- **Risk factors** should be similar or results stratified to account for differences in risk factors.

Comparison of Surveillance Results to Published Data

Comparisons to **published data** are always problematic and should be utilized only for guidance in establishing priorities, as there are so many variables possible from one institution to another that comparisons may not be valid. The CDC/NHSN have developed **benchmarks** related to healthcare-associated infections based on surveillance reports of participating institutions, and these may be used for reference. Overall nosocomial infection rates should not be used for comparisons but rather risk-adjusted data for target populations because the narrower the data, the more likely that a comparison will yield valuable information. Benchmarks that were developed as part of the baseline data for an individual institution may be a more useful source for comparison for that institution than external benchmarks because of inherent differences in populations. Additionally, staff can more easily relate to data reflecting changes within their own units and variables/risk factors can be more readily identified.

Preparation of Periodic Reports of Analyzed Data

Reports should be generated by the infection disease professional on a regular basis, which may vary from monthly to quarterly or even annually, depending upon the size of the institution and the population numbers or device days. Statistics must include adequate denominator data for meaningful analysis, and this can require a longer period of time. Specific data about individual patients or healthcare workers are often protected by laws regarding privacy, so information about individuals cannot be disseminated unless anonymity can be assured. Reports to individual physicians about their own infections rates should be provided confidentially and comparison rates done without identifying physicians. Reports are usually presented to the infection control committee, but reports should also be presented to staff in areas of survey. Thus, if a study involved an ICU, the ICU staff and physicians should be aware of the study results so that they can evaluate the effectiveness of infection control procedures or institute preventive methods.

Use of Charts, Tables, and Graphs to Present Reports

Presenting data in the form of charts and graphs provides a visual representation of the data that is easy to comprehend. There are generally three types of graphs used to present reports:

- **Line graphs** have an x and y axis, so they are used to show how an independent variable affects a dependent variable. Line graphs can show a time series with time usually on the x (horizontal) axis. This graph might be used to show number of infections per week/month.
- **Bar graphs** are used to compare and show the relationship between two or more groups. The graphs can show quantifiable data as bars that extend horizontally, vertically, or stacked. Bar graphs might be used to show comparison data of different populations or to compare data from one time period to another.
- **Pie charts** are used to show what percentage an item is compared to the whole. A pie chart can show distribution of infection control resources.

Issuing a Final Report

The final report is issued to all interested parties in the facility as well as public health officials and government agencies, such as the CDC, as indicated. Preparations for the final report should begin as soon as an outbreak is identified because every step of the investigation and the findings should be outlined in the report so that it serves not only as information about this one particular outbreak but can serve as a guide for future outbreaks or a recurrence. The report should include laboratory findings, line listing, and epidemiologic curves as well as procedures and results from any case control and/or cohort studies, including selection methods for control subjects. All control methods should be outlined as well as evaluation of the goals of the control methods. Questionnaires that were used to elicit information should be included in the report in the appendix so that they can be used for reference.

Outbreak Investigation

Definition of Disease Outbreak

An outbreak can be a single instance of a rare occurrence or may consist of a sudden rise in reports of a more familiar illness. Continuing surveillance establishes a known background rate of the incidence to compare with a current situation. Should incidence exceed a certain level, it is an outbreak; ideally, this will produce a response within the health community to provide care for existing cases, prevent further spread, and bring the outbreak under control.

One feature of outbreaks is their unpredictable nature, with setbacks and surprises being common. Recent outbreaks have seen a relatively new phenomenon: sudden surges in cases or diseases spreading to another country after an outbreak was thought to have peaked. Such setbacks can arise from a single lapse in infection control or the sheer volume of international air travel. New risk groups can emerge, modes of transmission can change, and treatments can fail if drug resistance develops or variants of the original source of infection occur.

Confirming an Outbreak

Confirming an outbreak usually begins with comparing initial outbreak data with baseline data that has been established for the institution and forming a ratio of outbreak to baseline figures. The infection control professional should review laboratory findings of the past few weeks or months to look for trends or patterns and review medical records to look for other cases with similar diagnosis, laboratory reports, or symptoms that are suggestive of an outbreak. The initial report should be reviewed for completeness and accuracy. The target population should be reviewed for increases or changes in characteristics that might account for the apparent outbreak. If identification of the outbreak was triggered by laboratory findings, changes in laboratory procedures or increased testing or reporting could create the appearance of an outbreak. Molecular epidemiology may be initiated to create a DNA profile to determine if isolates originated from the same source.

Control Orders and Processes for Verification of Infective Agent

Initial control orders may be issued as sometimes confirmation is delayed because of a need for laboratory or record review of further testing, but if an outbreak is probable and any risk is posed to others, then control orders, sometimes as simple as requiring review of handwashing procedures or placing a patient in isolation according to the type of infection, may decrease the spread of an infection.

Verifying the diagnosis/infective agent should include research about the infective agent and disease to verify symptoms and determining if characteristics of the disease are consistent with the literature. A complete clinical evaluation should be completed during this phase of the outbreak investigation. Dates and sites of cultures should be verified. Laboratory testing may be completed to verify the type of organism/isolate. DNA fingerprinting may be done as well to determine if multiple infections developed from the same source.

Molecular Strain Identification Techniques

Use of Epidemiologic Markers for Bacteria

Outbreak investigations occur when a pattern of infection occurs that suggests a single causative agent. It is necessary to isolate the microorganism and to differentiate it from other strains in order to determine if there is an actual outbreak. In some cases, an outbreak may be related to an increase in resistance rather than an increase in infection rates, and this needs to be determined as well. Traditionally, **phenotyping**, which studies the appearance of the microorganism or the reactions, was done to identify epidemic strains. Phenotyping includes identification of the genus, species, biotype, serotype, and phage type. Phenotyping determines the genetic traits of the microorganism, but some microorganisms share the same or similar phenotypic markers, making it difficult to distinguish each strain of a particular species. Additionally, random mutations may occur. Newer techniques of molecular strain identification involve **genotyping**, which studies the composition of the DNA/RNA of microorganisms. Typing can differentiate strains and determine if they are indistinguishable.

Biotyping, Bacteriophage Typing, Bacteriocin Typing, and Protein Typing

Biotyping involves identifying different biochemical reactions. There are multiple methods, such as identifying the ability of a microorganism to ferment sugars. There are kits available for typing of different microbes; however, biotyping does a poor job of distinguishing among strains.

Bacteriophage typing uses bacteriophages, which are viral intracellular parasites with the ability to infect bacteria by entering, multiplying, and destroying (lysing) the cell. A series of bacteriophages with different ability to lyse a cell is used to differentiate strains of bacteria, depending upon the microorganism's susceptibility to lysis. This technique is time-consuming and not widely available because stocks of phages must be maintained. This test is most useful for identify *staphylococcus* strains. It has been replaced by DNA based genotyping methods.

Bacteriocin typing involves identifying different antibacterial toxins that are produced by an individual strain of bacteria. This method is rarely used nowadays.

Protein typing determines differences in proteins made by strains of bacteria.

Pulsed-Field Gel Electrophoresis (PFGE)

Pulsed-field gel electrophoresis (PFGE) is a method of typing that separates large DNA strands. A typical technique is to apply three pairs of electrodes to a gel plate containing DNA, produced by restriction enzymes that break the DNA into small numbers of large DNA fragments. The plate is covered with dye. A current that changes directions in a regular pattern is applied to the gel until the dye has spread across the gel. Then a solution is added that binds to DNA and causes it to fluoresce. Changing the direction of the current allows smaller DNA fragments to move more quickly than larger fragments so there is separation of long and short strands, providing the typical DNA band profile. Different organisms have different band patterns. Organisms are considered distinguishable if they have more than three bands in different positions. This typing method is very accurate, especially for *staphylococci, enterococci,* and *P. aeruginosa.*

Restriction Endonuclease Analysis

Restriction endonuclease analysis uses restriction enzymes to identify bacterial strains. Restriction enzymes are particular bacterial proteins that recognize unique chromosomal DNA and plasmids, which are circular, double strands of DNA that can replicate in a cell but are separate from chromosomal DNA. Restriction enzymes cleave (split) the DNA at specific sequences. The fragments that are cleaved can be separated by size to produce a **restriction endonuclease profile**. This method can detect small differences in bacterial strains. There are three different **types of restriction enzymes** that can be used:

- Type 1 can recognize unique chromosomal DNA but cleaves the strand at random at least 1000 base pairs (bp) from the site that they recognize.
- Type II, the most commonly used restriction enzyme in recombinant DNA methods, recognizes the unique site and cleaves at that point, producing predictable strands.
- Type III also recognizes the unique chromosomal DNA but cleave at least 25 bp away. This method is useful for bacteria, viruses, and parasites that do not have plasmids

DNA Hybridization

DNA hybridization, or genetic probing, involves a process in which DNA is denatured, which means heated to a temperature that allows the DNA to form into single strands. As the DNA is cooled, it recoils and can be joined to a complementary probe of labeled DNA (usually with radioactive phosphorous), forming a hybrid, which is measured. Essentially a DNA, or sometimes RNA, strand is marked chemically or radioactively with a substance that will bind to a particular gene, allowing this gene to be identified and isolated. This typing technique can profile similarities in sequence among various DNAs as well as the repetition of sequence in one DNA. Genetic probing is used to find specific fragments of DNA, referred to as target DNA. This form of typing does not require a viable pathogen and can identify individual strains of bacteria. It can also identify pathogens, such as rotavirus, and chlamydia, which are difficult to cultivate; however, it is a slow process and often not as sensitive as cultures.

Plasmid Profile Analysis

Plasmid profile analysis involves the development of a plasmid profile. Plasmid DNA is isolated from a microorganism, and then the plasmid DNA is separated by agarose gel electrophoresis. Plasmids can spread from one species or strain to another through process called conjugation, so in some instances, an outbreak can be traced to plasmids rather than to a bacterial strain. However, this mobility of plasmids interferes with analysis. Analysis is improved by using restriction endonuclease enzymes to digest the plasmids and create fragments that are then analyzed by electrophoresis. Plasmid profile analysis can be applied to many different bacterial strains and can be completed within one day, but epidemic strains may not contain plasmid or strains that are not part of the epidemic may contain the same plasmid profile as the epidemic strains. So, while plasmid profile analysis is a rapid and inexpensive technique for typing, it is not always accurate or sufficient.

Polymerase Chain Reaction

Polymerase chain reaction makes millions of replications of specific DNA sequences without a living microorganism. When cells divide naturally, polymerase enzymes copy the DNA found in each chromosome by separating the two strands of the DNA helix, so each strand can be copied and then replicated. This process also requires the four nucleotide bases. Additionally, a short sequence of nucleotide, primase, called a "primer" is needed to begin the replication process. This can be done within a test tube, which is heated to separate the DNA strands, then cooled so the primer can begin the process, and heated again so that the polymerase can begin to make copies using the nucleotides. This 2-hour method can be used to replicate and detect more than 22 different microorganisms that fail to grow well or at all in cultures. It can detect coding genes for toxins, virulence, and antimicrobial resistance, making this an effective tool for infection control.

Antimicrobial Susceptibility Testing

Antimicrobial susceptibility testing uses *in vitro* (test tube or agar) testing of microorganism's susceptibility to antibiotics to predict how successful antimicrobials will be in the body. The test measures how much an organism grows or multiplies when subjected to various antimicrobials in order to provide information to guide in the selection of appropriate treatment. In a typical test, bacteria are swabbed on an agar plate and then small antibiotic impregnated paper disks with different antibiotics are placed in a circle around the disk over the bacteria. The plate is incubated and then the area where growth of bacteria has been inhibited is measured to determine the "zone of susceptibility." That is if there is a large area with inhibited growth, the microorganism is considered **susceptible**. If there is no zone of inhibition or very little, the microorganism is considered **resistant**. Some microorganisms show incomplete susceptibility and are considered **intermediate**.

Ribotyping

Ribotyping is a type of DNA fingerprinting analysis that utilizes genes that provide code for ribosomal ribonucleic acids (rRNA). Various proteins along with ribosomal RNA comprise the ribosome, which is a structure within the cell in which proteins are manufactured. The ribosome uses coding from the rRNA to place the correct amino acids in proteins. The genetic coding for rRNA varies more between bacterial strains than within them, so ribotyping distinguishes between bacterial strains. Restriction enzymes are used to cleave the genes that code for the rRNA into fragments, and then electrophoresis is used to separate the fragments. Genetic probes are used to highlight fragments of different sizes so that they appear as bands in the profile. Different ribotypes have banding patterns that correspond to each type. Ribotyping has been successful in typing a variety of microorganisms, including strains of *Salmonella typhi, E. coli, Campylobacter, Pasteurella multocida,* and various forms of *staphylococcus.*

Communication During an Outbreak Investigation

Communication is a critical issue in outbreak investigation because much information needs to be collected and disseminated. Team members should be notified of the potential outbreak so that they can begin assisting with the investigation, according to their role in the team. All physicians, managers, administrators, and staff that may be involved should be notified immediately and updated frequently as well as asked to assist in reporting new incidences of infection. The laboratory should be contacted very early as further testing may be needed and laboratory staff can provide necessary information about laboratory procedures. Laboratory staff may also be alerted to save specimens for further testing. In some cases, ancillary staff, such as housekeepers or food workers, may need to be notified as well. Depending upon the type of infection, city, county, state, or federal officials may need to be notified of an outbreak.

Effective Planning for Disease Outbreaks

Outbreak investigations may vary somewhat according to the type of outbreak, the population, and the facility, so there is no one method that will suffice for every occasion. **Planning** includes establishment of an infection team, educating staff, assembling materials, maintaining telephone, email, and other contact lists, and instituting an effective surveillance system to allow early detection of outbreaks. Key components of effective planning for disease outbreaks include the following:

- Surveillance networks that collect and report data
- Well stocked laboratories for diagnosing parasitic, bacterial, and viral diseases
- Computers, relational databases, and geographical information systems (GIS)
- An early warning system to detect increases in outpatient visits, hospitalizations, and deaths from known or unknown causes
- New tools such as those of molecular epidemiology, which identifies at the molecular level potential genetic and environmental risk factors in the etiology, distribution, and prevention of disease within families and across populations
- Interaction and cooperation at local, regional, national, and international levels to control outbreaks and share information
- Trained staff sufficient to carry out a mission

Defining a Problem in an Outbreak

Defining a problem in an outbreak is done through both descriptive and analytic epidemiological practices:

- **Descriptive practices** involve determining time (when the infection takes place and the duration of symptoms as well as the incubation period), person (who gets infected in terms of age, gender, race, or other variables), and place (where the infection takes place, such as community, hospital, isolated area).
- **Analytical practices** include determining causes (contaminated environment, foodborne pathogens, airborne pathogens, unknown pathogen) and risk factors (age, gender, co-morbidities, immune status, occupation).

The infection control professional must develop specific criteria when defining a problem, and these criteria must be broad enough so that most cases are captured but narrow enough to adequately focus the investigation. The breadth of the investigation is often influenced by the pathogen (if identified). Criteria may or may not include specific symptoms or specific laboratory findings. Prior to defining the problem, the infection control professional should perform a literature review to help identify potential sources or investigative methods.

Key Terms in Outbreak Identification

Key terms in outbreak identification include the following:

Relative risk	The frequency of infection in an exposed group divided by the frequency in an unexposed group produces a percentage representing the likelihood of acquiring the disease upon exposure to it.
Endemic	An element that is a normal part of its environment.
Epidemic	The product of a sudden rapid spread, growth, or development, or the act of suddenly spreading rapidly.
Epidemic curve	The graphic depiction of the number and distribution of outbreak disease cases by their date of onset. It can yield information on the outbreak's spread pattern, strength, periods of exposure and/or incubation, time trends, and any outliers.
Epidemic period	Period over which the occurrence of outbreak cases exceeds the normal background rate
Hyperendemic	When an agent normally present in the environment expands to a high rate of incidence it is hyperendemic.
Pandemic	A worldwide epidemic that crosses many borders.
Pseudo-outbreak	Episode where the incidence of a disease increases because of factors unrelated to the disease itself, such as enhanced surveillance.

Steps of a Healthcare Outbreak Investigation

Initial Steps

The initial steps of a healthcare outbreak investigation are as follows:

1. Compare expected number of cases with the observed number before deciding the actual number is high enough to indicate an outbreak.
2. Ensure a proper diagnosis has been made, rule out lab error by reviewing clinical findings and lab results; identify and count cases; talk to affected patients; generate hypotheses about etiology and spread.
3. Establish the case definition determining which individuals should be classified with the infection.
4. Alert hospital staff to the outbreak, implement control and prevention measures. Involve staff in the investigation to get their commitment to the undertaking.
5. Analyze collected data to characterize the outbreak by time, place, and population; establish which stage the infection has reached; determine extent of problem and which population is most at risk.

STEPS OF AN EPIDEMIOLOGIC FIELD INVESTIGATION

The epidemiologic field investigation of a disease outbreak should go as follows:

1. **Do a case investigation** confirming the outbreak and making preliminary hypotheses.
2. Investigate the **cause** of the outbreak by:
    a. Reviewing known causal factors
    b. Establishing probable cause of infection through microbiology and looking at the disease's natural history
    c. Drawing inferences from the infection rate
    d. Generating testable hypotheses from case.
3. **Conduct analytic study** (if necessary) to test and refine hypotheses, controlling for chance, bias, and confounding.
4. **Test hypotheses** by reviewing data and gathering supporting (or refuting) data.
5. **Revise hypotheses** to accommodate findings.
6. Initiate control measures.
7. **Draw conclusions** (epidemiologic and causal inferences).
8. **Continue surveillance** (detection and monitoring).
9. **Communicate findings.**

DEVELOPMENT AND TESTING OF HYPOTHESES IN AN OUTBREAK INVESTIGATION

Classically, the epidemiologist's method of investigation begins with a description of how a disease is distributed within or between populations, then proceeds with analyses of the factors that determine this distribution. Along the way, hypotheses are generated by observation and tested by formal study.

Hypotheses concerning the source or route of exposure, when it is unknown, may be generated through open-ended interviews with those infected, a case control study, retrospective cohort study, or cross-sectional study. It is important to determine whether multiple sources of infection (perhaps due to cross contamination) are plausible and whether some associations are due to confounding (e.g., whether exposure to one potential source is linked to exposure to other sources) or to chance.

Other possibilities need to be considered when the study finds no association between the hypothesized exposures and risk for disease. The real exposure may not have been among those examined, the number of persons available for study may have been too small, or the accuracy of the available information concerning the exposures was inadequate.

Final Steps of an Outbreak Investigation

The final step of an outbreak investigation involves the dissemination of reports.

1. Schedule a meeting with local health authorities and people responsible for implementing control and prevention measures to communicate and review findings. Investigators will describe in the meeting what they did, what they found, and what control measures they recommend. Presenting their findings in scientifically objective fashion, they should be prepared to defend their conclusions and recommendations.
2. Follow with a written report that will serve as:
    a. A road map for action
    b. A record of performance
    c. Evidence for potential legal challenges
    d. An archival reference for the greater health community, contributing epidemiologies and public health scientific knowledge base
    e. The written report is to be formatted in the usual scientific way for publication: introduction, background, methods, results, discussion, and recommendations.

Control Measures Taken When a Possible Outbreak is Discovered

The following control measures should be taken when a possible outbreak is discovered:

- **Case finding**: Find, through the use of standard case definitions, all those individuals with signs and symptoms of the disease
- **Case management**: Refer suspected cases to healthcare facilities and, if necessary, isolate them
- **Inform**: Alert the public to the outbreak and caution those who have contacted known cases to watch out for signs and symptoms
- **Social activities**: Discourage all social gatherings, consider closing schools, and decide whether trained health staff should be put in charge of burials.
- **Food handling**: In an outbreak of foodborne disease, discourage consumption of uncooked food and food that has been exposed to dust, insects, and rodents.
- **Sanitation**: In primitive areas, exercise caution in the handling of drinking water, supervise public water sources, dispose of solid, liquid, and human waste properly, and apply pest control measures.
- **Hygiene:** Apply simple and effective personal hygiene measures such as frequent hand washing.
- **Education**: Seek community participation and quell panic.

Interpretation of Outbreak Investigation Results

In interpreting the results of investigations, it is possible that what appears to be statistically significant associations between one or more exposures and the disease may turn out to be chance and not really indicative of a true relationship.

Also, the problem of multiple comparisons often arises. Therefore, it is important to go beyond the statistical tests and examine whether a statistically significant relationship is likely to be biologically meaningful. Among the factors that should be considered are whether:

- The interval between an exposure and onset of illness matches known incubation period
- Multiple sources of infection are due to cross-contamination
- Some of the associations are due to confounding
- Some of the cases can be attributed to an exposure not found to be statistically significant
- Subjects represent background cases unrelated to the outbreak
- The outbreak involves only a small, non-statistical number of cases
- The quality of the study population and the study design are lacking
- There is agreement or disagreement with other studies

Path Models for Causation in Epidemiological Investigations

One important element of the epidemiologist's job is to take an event (say, an epidemic) and deduce its cause. But a given disease may have many causal mechanisms, and every causal mechanism has component causes in itself. Interaction is a fundamental characteristic of any causal process involving a series of probabilistic steps, making it very difficult to estimate contributions of any one factor in a chain; many paths may diverge looking backward from an outcome when tracking a cause. Such variables as genetics, environment, and an acquired susceptibility in childhood can come into play.

To handle these variables, various complex statistical and mathematical models are applied to obtain probabilities that any given path is one of causation. However, critics of causal path models say the analyses are based on hypotheses derived from observations which may have been in error or that the truly pivotal events may not have even been observed (making them "latent variables").

Environmental Factors Involved in an Outbreak Investigation

It is important to differentiate between an environmental contributing factor and an environmental antecedent to an outbreak. The contributing factor in an outbreak of *E. coli* food poisoning, for instance, might be eating spinach that has not been cooked, while the environmental antecedent would be the proximity of a field of spinach to a hog farm.

Various diseases have real or possible environmental antecedents. In the 2003 outbreak of SARS, for example, transmission appeared to be dependent on seasonal temperature changes and the multiplicative effect of hospital infection.

The use of aluminum cookware was once thought to be a risk in Alzheimer's Disease, but was never established. Zinc, on the other hand, may play a role, as the brains of Alzheimer's victims have shown either too little or too much zinc. So, although Alzheimer's has been shown to have a strong genetic component, diet and eating habits may be involved as environmental antecedents.

Investigation of the Environment

Investigation of the environment will vary according to the type of infection and the mode of transmission. An airborne infective agent would be investigated differently than one transmitted in liquids or through feces. However, the goal of the investigation is to determine what factors in the environment have contributed to the spread of the disease:

- **Equipment** should be cultured and reuse of single-use items noted. Cleaning/use procedures should be observed. Sharing of equipment, such as blood pressure cuffs or sterilized endoscopes, should be traced by staff and patients.
- **Ventilation systems** should be checked and cultured, including air vents and filters. Records of filter changes should be verified. Air conditioning and heating units should be checked as well, especially any parts that might accumulate moisture.
- **Rooms** implicated, such as operating rooms or patient areas, must be cultured and examined carefully with cleaning procedures observed and verified. Out of hospital environmental testing may be needed.

Case Finding During an Outbreak Investigation

Case finding involves active steps to identify further cases of infection. Recent surveillance data should be reviewed and the laboratory notified to review lab records for indications of infection. Further testing may be ordered to identify cases. Surveillance should be increased in the areas that are affected with requests to physicians and staff to report any suspected new cases. Contact should be made with other medical providers, hospital units, or the public health department to determine if other cases have been identified especially if the original infection may have originated outside of the hospital and then spread by contact. Medical records should be reviewed carefully for symptoms or changes in condition that may warrant concern. Interviews should be conducted with those in contact with the infected patient(s) or the identified site/source of infection, and they may be referred for serologic testing or cultures.

Creating Case Definitions

The case definition defines the characteristics of a typical case in the outbreak. It serves as a guide in identifying new cases:

- **Time**: The date of onset of symptoms, incubation times, and need for isolation should be noted.
- **Place**: Sometimes place may extend to an entire state or be limited to a particular unit or room of the hospital.
- **Person**: Characteristics about the person could include sex, age, or general condition. If all infected patients were in the neonatal unit, then the person would be characterized as an infant.
- **Clinical presentation**: Specific symptoms or parameters for the disease should be outlined, including transmission. This may include such details as fever, rash, shortness of breath, cough, or purulent discharge.
- **Epidemiology**: This might include travel history, contact with other infected patients or staff.
- **Laboratory findings**: This should specify the type of culture results or other lab findings that would verify the infection.

CDC's Case Definitions Utilized During Outbreak Investigations

The Centers for Disease Control requires state health departments to report cases to it because effective control of disease depends upon prompt communication of clear reports among healthcare organizations announcing occurrences of reportable diseases. Before 1990, the usefulness of such data was limited by the lack of uniform case definitions of infectious diseases. Then, in 1990, the CDC published Case Definitions for Public Health Surveillance that provided uniform criteria for reporting cases, making reports more specific and enabling comparison of diseases reported from different geographic areas.

The list of nationally reportable diseases changes periodically. Diseases may be added to the list as new pathogens emerge or may be deleted as their incidence declines. A great deal of information, including results of laboratory tests, must be collected before a final case classification is published for any newly emerging disease.

CDC's Breakdown of Case Classifications

The CDC's breakdown of case classifications is as follows:

- **Clinically compatible case**: A clinical syndrome is detected somewhere by healthcare personnel that is generally compatible with a CDC case definition.
- **Epidemiologically linked case**: A case in which a patient has had contact with one or more persons who:
  - Have the disease
  - Had the disease
  - Have been exposed to the same single source of infection (such as a food borne disease outbreak) to which all confirmed case patients were exposed, and the agent's transfer through the usual modes of transmission is plausible
- **Laboratory-confirmed case**: One or more of the laboratory methods listed by the CDC as necessary confirms the diagnosis
- Confirmed Case
- Probable case
- Suspected case

Active Case Findings in Healthcare-Associated Investigations

Routine case reporting consists of physicians, infection control practitioners, pharmacists, laboratory staff, or other health workers filing with a public health authority reports revealing suspected or confirmed cases of a disease. The disease in question must meet the CDC's case definition.

When a healthcare facility identifies unreported cases of disease after an active search through documents – laboratory and pharmacy audits, records of microbiology, infection control, transfusions, the clinic logs for the ER, outpatient records, or logs of dialysis treatment – reveals them, this is called an active case finding.

An additional source for case finding when a cohort study is conducted may be patient medical records, though using patient medical records may be feasible only if the investigation is limited to a single ward or a small facility.

Epidemiologic Descriptions

Epidemiologic descriptions include line listings and epidemic curves.

- **Line listing** is a two-column list with variables in one column and the number and percentage of those who match that variable in the other column. Line listings can give valuable information about possible transmission or other variables. For example, a line listing of 28 cases might begin like this:
    - Male 21 (75%)
    - Smoker 7 (25%)
    - Clinic visit 14 (50%)
    - Surgery Rm. A 28 (100%)
    - HIV positive 21 (75%)
- **Epidemic curve** is a line or bar graph that shows the characteristics of the infection over time. Line graphs show the incidence of infection compared to baseline data. Bar graphs with time on the horizontal axis and infections on the vertical are called epidemic or epi curves and are used to plot the type of outbreak and can indicate incubation periods. Source infections often show peaks with breaks between infections but person-to-person transmission is often continuous with few peaks.

Line Listings

The line listing of cases is a record containing the identity of every patient found to be involved in an outbreak along with the time and place of their contact. An essential component of every outbreak investigation, it facilitates determining which individuals are at risk and should be included in further studies.

In addition, line listing also provides a current summary of the outbreak and of ongoing case investigations, thus ensuring a complete outbreak investigation that can be maintained on a computer using database management or spreadsheet software.

For describing the time indicator for the outbreak, a graph normally referred to as an epidemic curve frequently is used to chart its progress by minutes, hours, days, etc. This can provide clues regarding the possible sources of the outbreak and methods of transmission of the disease.

Trends in Epidemic Curves During Outbreak Investigations

Graphing numbers of cases on a *y*-axis and units of time on an *x*-axis builds an epidemic curve that visually reflects the progress of an epidemic, possibly projecting its future course and providing clues about its source, pattern, the method of its spread, period of exposure, and the minimum, average, and maximum incubation periods for the disease.

A steep up-slope and a gradual down-slope indicate all cases are occurring within one incubation period. This makes it, by definition, a **single source (or "point source") epidemic**: everyone is exposed to the same source over a relatively brief period. If the duration of exposure were prolonged, it would be a **continuous common source epidemic**, and the curve would have a plateau instead of a peak. **Person-to-person spread (a "propagated" epidemic)** would have a series of progressively taller peaks one incubation period apart.

Outliers, cases that stand apart on the graph, are worth examining carefully because, if they are part of the outbreak, their unusual exposures may point directly to the source.

Case-Finding Issues Related to Surveillance Plans

Patient-Based vs. Laboratory-Based Issues

Case findings may be patient-based or laboratory-based:

- **Patient based** findings revolve around the patient, so the patient must be assessed for signs of infection, risk factors, quality of patient care, and staff compliance with infection control protocol. Patient-based plans are very time and staff intensive, requiring much time on the patient units in order to review charts, assess patient, and interview patient and staff. For large facilities, the cost of effective patient-based plans may be prohibitive.
- **Laboratory-based** findings, on the other hand, depend upon review of laboratory findings, often cultures, to determine if threshold rates have been exceeded. Laboratory findings are usually accurate, but the effectiveness of this type of plan depends on completeness of records and whether specimens are sent to the laboratory for analysis. If there are no clear protocols in place to determine when a specimen should be obtained, infections may be missed. This type of plan can utilize electronic monitoring systems, saving staff time.

Passive vs. Active Surveillance Issues

A number of different issues must be resolved as part of the plans for surveillance, including active surveillance vs. passive surveillance.

- **Passive surveillance**, on the one hand, utilizes observations of medical and laboratory staff to identify and report infections, often requiring the staff to fill out a report and submit it. Passive surveillance often results in misclassification and delays as well as failure to report infections because no one is specifically charged with reporting. Staff involved in patient care may not have or take the time to fill out reports.
- **Active surveillance**, on the other hand, is a program specifically designed for finding healthcare-associated infections and using trained/certificated staff, such as infection control personnel, whose primary purpose is infection identification, control, and prevention. Active surveillance tends to be more accurate and data more complete than passive surveillance because there is consistency and usually a more established program; however, active surveillance is also expensive because it requires dedicated staff.

Prospective vs. Retrospective

Another issue that must be dealt with when deciding upon a plan for outbreak surveillance is whether the plan should be prospective or retrospective.

- **Prospective**, or concurrent, surveillance follows patients while they are hospitalized and includes the period after discharge to evaluate for surgical site infections. Because prospective surveillance is ongoing and continually evaluated, it can identify clusters of infection as they occur as well as ensuring that the infection control personnel have ongoing working relationships with other staff. When there appears to be an outbreak or cause for concern, analysis can be done fairly quickly. This is the type of surveillance required by those participating in the NHSN system.
- **Retrospective** surveillance, however, is done after the fact by a review of charts and records with no patient contact. There is often a time delay, then, between the time a problem presents and the time it is identified. This method is less expensive.

Reporting Outbreaks

World Health Organization Disease Reporting Requirements

The World Health Organization (WHO) requires that its members report certain communicable diseases (such as AIDS or malaria) either in the form of case reports or outbreak reports. The specific diseases to be reported in case reports are determined by guidelines and legislation created by the federal government, which also determines the agency responsible for the report, the report's format, and the procedure for completing and forwarding it, and with what frequency before it is passed on to the WHO.

In the case of international reporting, the national government involved reports information to the WHO. The case report includes the diagnosis, age, sex, and date of onset for each individual diagnosed with the specific disease. Sometimes, under certain circumstances, the report also includes individual identifying data (e.g., name and address) as well as treatment and disease duration.

Elements of a Notifiable Disease Report

Epidemiologic surveillance data for nationally notifiable diseases and for some non-notifiable diseases is transmitted electronically by public health departments in the states and territories to CDC through NEDSS and NETSS each week.

Data transmitted includes date, county, age, sex, race/ethnicity, and some disease-specific information. Completeness of reporting varies by disease and state and can be influenced by:

- Type and severity of illness
- Whether treatment is sought in a healthcare setting
- Diagnosis of an illness
- Availability of diagnostic services
- Disease-control measures in effect
- Public's awareness of the disease
- Resources, priorities, and interests of state and local officials responsible for disease control and public health surveillance

These weekly reports provide a national information interchange essential to public health managers and providers to rapidly identify disease epidemics and understand patterns of disease occurrence.

Case Reports

On a local level, information about each confirmed or suspected case must be recorded to obtain a complete understanding of the outbreak as well as provide the basis for reports to higher agencies.

Usually this information includes subject name, age, sex, occupation, place of residence, recent movements, details of symptoms (including dates and time of onset) and dates of previous immunization against childhood or other diseases. Other details will vary with the differential diagnosis. If the incubation period is known, information on possible source contacts may be sought. This information is best recorded on specially prepared record forms called line lists.

History of Specific Disease Outbreaks

2003 SARS Epidemic

The appearance of one infection (unless it is a rare disease) cannot by itself immediately trigger an epidemiological investigation. There has to be additional cause such as numerous reports.

When WHO announced the outbreak of SARS in 2003, cases had already appeared in Canadian hospitals, but an investigation was not launched until the outbreak was announced in China and Vietnam. (China's early refusal, later rescinded, to admit to having a number of cases of the mysterious disease slowed down response appreciably.) Numerous cases of severe upper respiratory infections only then were discovered in a number of Canadian hospitals. Strangely, they centered on one family, even though various members had shown up in the emergency rooms of several hospitals. Their infections, all acquired from one member who had brought it back from a trip to East Asia, were spreading to hospital staff and other patients. Once the breakout had been announced in East Asia, it was detected quickly in Canada by staying alert to developments and freely exchanging information.

2014 West African Ebola Outbreak

The 2014 **Ebola epidemic** began with the death of a child in Guinea in December 2013. By March 2014, further cases were reported in Guinea and Liberia, by April in Mali, and by May in Sierra Leone. By the end of May 2014, WHO reported 383 cases and 211 deaths; by October, 13,540 cases and 4941 deaths. In September 2014, the first case of Ebola occurred in the United States. He was initially misdiagnosed and sent home before returning to the hospital, and subsequently two nurses involved in his direct care contracted the disease, while wearing the CDC approved PPE. The nurses denied knowingly ever breaching protocol while caring for the patient, but they were involved in direct care of the patient during intubation and dialysis, among other medical procedures. Initial CDC guidelines regarding PPE encompassed a range of precautions, depending on the type of care, but the guidelines were less stringent than those utilized successfully in Africa, leaving some areas of the body, such as the neck, exposed. CDC guidelines now call for applying and removing PPE involved in the care of Ebola patients under supervision, double gloving, and utilizing PPE that completely covers all parts of the body, including face shield with helmet or headpiece, and fluid-resistant or impermeable gown, shoe covers, apron. PAPR or N95 or higher respirator is recommended for aerosol-generating procedures.

2019 COVID-19 Pandemic

China first notified the WHO of an outbreak from an unknown virus in December 2019 although later studies indicated it may have been already spreading at that point. By January 2020, the first case of **COVID-19 (SARS-CoV-2)** outside of China, in Thailand, was reported, but by the end of January, the disease was reported in 21 countries because of worldwide travel with the first US case in Snohomish, Washington, on January 20. The first US death occurred on February 29 at a facility where eventually 35 deaths were linked and community spread was detected. On March 11, the WHO officially declared COVID-19 a pandemic, and by the end of March 2020, cases were occurring in all 50 states. Initially, no vaccines and few treatments were available. By May, cases were reported in almost every country in the world despite travel restrictions. By mid-2021, about 187 million people throughout the world had become infected and over 4 million had died. Of that total, over 33.7 million cases and over 600,000 deaths were in the US.

Successes and Failures of the US Response to COVID-19

The United States' response to the COVID-19 pandemic had both successes and failures:

Successes	Failures
• Data collection • Government support of vaccine development • Early effective vaccine development • Improved treatment options • Print/television/internet media providing up-to-date information. • COVID stimulus checks and unemployment benefits • Vaccination campaign leading to high vaccination rates	• Slow development of clinical trials • Inadequate testing • Inconsistency in mask mandates and quarantine regulations across states • Inadequate infection control supplies (gowns, surgical masks, N95 respirators) • Politicization of virus-response efforts • Social media misinformation • Inadequate vaccination rates and inadequate supply in the early roll out process • Increased unemployment, poverty, business closures, and mental health crises resulting from lockdowns

Recommended Precautions Prior to Vaccine Availability

Prior to the availability of vaccinations, recommended precautions for COVID-19/SARS-CoV-2 included the following:

- Avoid exposure to anyone outside of immediate family in the home or coworkers in the workplace. Outside of the home, maintain a social distance of at least 6 feet.
- Wear a mask for contact with anyone outside of the immediate family. (Mask mandates varied somewhat from one state to another, and some did not enforce mask mandates.)
- If anyone in the home is infected or has been exposed to COVID, that person should be quarantined away from other family members for 14 days after the onset of illness or 20 days with severe illness.
- Avoid social gatherings (limits varied by state regulations).
- Temperature/Health check carried out for all access to healthcare facilities.

Recommended Precautions After Vaccine Availability

Recommended precautions for COVID-19/SARS-CoV-2 varied after vaccinations were distributed. Early on, when vaccination numbers remained low, no change in recommendations occurred because infection rates remained relatively high, but as the number of vaccinations increased and the rate of infections fell, the CDC issued new guidelines stating that fully vaccinated people could resume normal activities without the need to wear a mask except where mandated (such as in healthcare facilities). Full vaccination occurs two weeks after the second dose of Pfizer and Moderna vaccines and two weeks after the single dose of Johnson & Johnson's single-dose vaccine. Those who were not fully vaccinated were advised to continue to use the same precautions: wear a mask, avoid social gatherings, and maintain social distance. However, since CDC guidelines are not, in fact, regulations, some states have established different guidelines.

Outbreaks Common in Daycare Centers

Diseases Common to Daycare Centers

Diseases common to daycare centers include the following:

- Enteric diseases.
- **Respiratory infections**: Children shed viruses prior to onset of symptoms, making respiratory infections control difficult.
- **Skin and cutaneous infections**: Lice, scabies, and exposure to herpes simplex virus (shingles) or other bacterial pathogens.

Because daycare centers gather very young children who are not yet trained in hygienic procedures and are also prone to soiling themselves, these places become large reservoirs for outbreaks for communicable diseases, particularly enterically transmitted infections, including hepatitis A, shigellosis, salmonellosis, giardiasis, and viral gastroenteritis. Transmission is facilitated because these children have a higher degree of close, physical contact with one another and with the staff of the day care center than is true for adults in group situations.

Adults who develop hepatitis A, giardia, salmonella, and Shigella and either work with children or have them in the home, may have acquired the condition from the child. Conversely, if they are in contact with children who attend day care centers, they may have spread the disease through the child. Either way, if a day care center is in the picture, it should be notified. Physicians and other healthcare providers treating for the disease should routinely question all about the presence of children in the household and provide proper notification. Daycare facilities should screen workers within one month of date of employment and annually thereafter for TB.

Risk Factors for Enteric Diseases in Daycare

Several factors increase daycare center risk for outbreaks of enteric disease. Higher risk centers are ones that:

- Accept infants less than three years of age
- Stay open for longer than 15 hours a day
- Accept enrollments larger than 50 children
- Operate for a profit
- Accept drop-ins

Compelling children to wash their hands after using the toilet has been proven effective in preventing diarrhea and enteric spread of disease in day care centers. Washing hands after changing diapers is also advisable for adult caretakers.

Key Components of Surveillance and Epidemiology

Carrier	Anyone carrying a pathogen which can be transmitted to a human being—regardless of whether that first person is infected or not or shows signs of the disease or not—is a carrier. A carrier need not be human. The disease may be carried by an animal that's unaffected by it. In the Black Plague of the Middle Ages, rats were carriers because they were infested with fleas carrying the bubonic bacillus without being affected by it. For that matter, the fleas were also carriers.
Case	In the epidemiological sense, a case is person who has been infected by the disease in question at the time in question and the place in question.
Index case	Depending upon context, an index case could be the first instance of a disease epidemic and therefore the cause of the epidemic; someone whose phenotype leads to a study of the family for that characteristic; the first case to become known in a population, or the earliest documented case of a disease that is included in an epidemiological study.
Bias	An error in the design or execution of a study will generally produce a bias that skews and distorts results because nonrandom factors have been introduced. Though bias happens in randomized controlled trials, it is more common to observational studies.
Virulence	A word with its root in the Latin word for poison, virulence indicates the ability of a microorganism to cause disease. Because the word may also be used as a measure of a pathogen's ability to do damage, it is not entirely synonymous with pathogenicity. Only a small portion of the total population of microorganisms are virulent.
Direct transmission	Disease may be spread through direct contact, such as a physical contact between a host and victim.
Indirect transmission	Disease may also be spread through indirect contact of victim with agent by way of airborne particles, vectors, or contaminated objects acting as intermediary.
Antigenicity	Also called immunogenicity, antigenicity assesses an agent's ability to stimulate antibodies to react. It is nearly synonymous with virulence except that virulence does not automatically assume an immunologic reaction.
Nosocomial	A strict definition would cover any event surrounding an individual while in a hospital, but most commonly the adjective is used to describe a disease contracted while an individual was hospitalized.
Pathogenicity rate	Essentially yet another term for virulence or antigenicity or immunogenicity, it is the relative ability of an agent to infect an organism.
Promoters	Promoters, while not the original stimulus for infection, contribute to the virulence of an infecting agent.
Biological plausibility	Even when a medical experiment points to a given conclusion, the reviewer should apply the principle of biological plausibility – given everything we know, does the conclusion make sense? – when reviewing results.
Coherence	Biological plausibility leans on several principles, one of which is coherence, which says there should be a biologically credible reason for one factor associating with another, thus implying causality.

Sampling error	In a perfect study, the characteristics of the study group and the general population would be exactly the same. Because this can never be, there is a sampling error which must be taken into consideration in tabulating results.
Chronic disease	A chronic disease has been a long-time condition for the patient and/or promises to be such in the future. Typically, chronic disease is not subject to a quick and permanent cure.
Clinical disease	If a disease exists but has not yet produced recognizable signs and symptoms, it is a subclinical illness. Once there are clinical manifestations, it is a clinical disease. Diabetes typically goes from subclinical to clinical in its course.
Clinical horizon	The point where a disease goes from subclinical to clinical.
Cluster	A cluster is a grouped number of disease events tied together as to location, time period, or pattern. A cluster can indicate epidemic or simply be random.
Cohort study	A cohort represents a subset of qualities of a population so as to isolate knowledge about a particular variable under study relative to different groups. These groups are observed over a period of time to determine prevalence of the variable.
Blinding	To avoid biasing the results of a medical study, observers and subjects must be kept unaware (blind) of purposes or many procedures regarding experimental procedures.
Statistical significance	A figure representing the chance that the evidence derived from a sample differs from what should be true for the larger population.
Statistical power	Measures the probability that the experiment has not fallen prone to the mistake of failing to observe some important difference that would affect the outcome when there really is such a difference. This power involves the relative frequency that would allow detection by the suggested experiment/test of a true difference of the defined size between populations
Risk factor	Any characteristic of a person or a person's situation that increases the potential for him or her to experience the event to which the risk factor is attached, such as contracting a communicable disease. Risk factors may be immutable or modifiable through intervention.
Utilities	A term associated with decision analysis; utilities are assigned values representing theoretical outcomes of alternative decisions.
Vital statistics	Recorded births, deaths, fetal deaths, linked birth/infant deaths, matched multiple births, marriages, and divorces are registered in the National Vital Statistics System. The information is available to those in epidemiology research.
Relational study	An investigational study of a hypothesized causal factor.
Case control study	Two groups, one with a specific disease or outcome and the other a closely matched control group (also called the comparison group) without the disease, are compared to isolate variables around the disease.
Randomized controlled trial	A study in which subjects are randomly assigned to treatment or control groups to test the efficacy of a drug, treatment, or procedure.

Validity of measurement	Assesses whether a particular measure actually represents what it purports to measure.
Validity of a study	To be valid, a study must meet conditions regarding study methods, sample representativeness, and measurement tools and the accuracy of their use.
Variable	Any part in a study that can be measured or controlled. There are several types: • Dependent variable: Effects vary with the actions of one or more other variables. • Independent variable: The thing that is being observed rather than controlled to see how it affects outcomes. • Confounding variable: A variable that is neither under study nor being controlled, and thus may be silently affecting study outcomes.
Epidemiology	The study of the spread of diseases
Descriptive epidemiology	Describes the time, place, and other pertinent data related to an event of disease dispersal
Analytical epidemiology	Develops and tests hypotheses regarding the causes of a disease
Experimental epidemiology	Studies intended to discover or demonstrate disease causality
Substantive epidemiology	The sum total of epidemiological knowledge about diseases
Induction period	Time from exposure to disease inception
Lead time	An earlier diagnosis gives medics lead time in treating disease
Lead time bias	Systematic error in a study when the follow-up studies for two separate groups do not begin at the same time
Length bias	An error made in survival time estimates because subject screening has failed to recognize a disease can be more aggressive in some people
Healthy worker effect	Studies can be skewed because too many subjects are employed. People who work statistically have better health and longevity over the general population, where the sick and disabled have been kept out of the workforce.
Present on admission	POA refers to an infection that meets the criteria for site-specific symptoms and diagnosis and is evident two days prior to admission to a healthcare facility, the day of admission (day 1) or the next day (day 2). Physician's diagnosis alone is not adequate without evidence (documented) of symptoms and/or laboratory confirmation as required for the specific type of infection.
Transfer rule	The transfer rule helps to determine responsibility for infections. If an infection meets the site-specific criteria on the day of transfer or the day after transfer from one inpatient facility/unit to another inpatient facility/unit, or the day of discharge or the day after discharge, the infection is attributed to the transferring/discharging facility/unit.
80% rule	A patient care area is designated according to the type of patients cared for in that area. If 80% of the patients are of a specific type (such as oncology patients), the CDC location code designates the area accordingly

Critical point	The point by which an intervention must take place in the course of a disease, in which anything done before the critical point will have some kind of impact on the disease, and anything done after will have no effect.
Level of measurement	In statistics, a classification scheme for determining variables; levels include interval measure (equal distances between whatever system of measurement is used), nominal or categorical measure (identifying a value by some naming convention), and ordinal measure (values in rank order).

In many studies, all of the events of interest may not be observed or, for whatever reason, the exact time-to-event was not known. This type of data is commonly called **censored data**, and it comes in three types:

Right Censored (Suspended)	The most common case of censoring, it consists of events that simply never happened. For instance, if a cohort of 15 patients exposed to rubella were observed for a survival analysis, and one never contracted the disease, the one case is referred to as right censored data or suspended data.
Interval Censored	Interval censored data reflects uncertainty as to the exact times the happened within a time interval. This type of data frequently comes from tests or situations where the objects of interest are not constantly monitored.
Left Censored	An event is only known to have happened before a certain time, but without specificity to the exact point in time that it occurred.

Preventing/Controlling the Transmission of Infectious Agents

Developing Infection Prevention Policies and Procedures

Levels of Prevention

The concept of primary, secondary, and tertiary levels of prevention offers a useful framework for specifying the actions to be taken and the order they should follow in dealing with illness. For the problem of childhood disabilities, as an example, primary prevention encompasses a reduction in risk factors like low birth weight, malnutrition, and family awareness pre-birth so that child development can be favorably influenced.

Primary Prevention

Primary prevention occurs during pre-pathogenesis and comprises a set of interventions to eliminate or reduce susceptibility that frequently require a patient to undergo behavior change. Primary prevention of coronary heart disease, for example, includes education on the risks of smoking and encouragement of smoking cessation and more direct protection measures that might include lowering cholesterol through diet, exercise, and medication and treating hypertension.

Secondary Prevention

Secondary prevention takes place early in the pathogenesis phase, applying preventive measures to stem the apparent advance toward illness before it is officially diagnosed in the patient. These measures include:

- Early detection of the disease through screening measures
- Prompt treatment
- A quick cure (if possible)

In many cases, such as coronary heart disease, secondary prevention is essentially a continuation of primary prevention, with such behavioral components as diet, exercise, and smoking cessation being more forcefully applied. In public health outbreaks, screening is a relatively common method of secondary prevention, with case investigations and selective examination being specific interventions at this level.

Tertiary Prevention

The tertiary prevention level of disease prevention begins in the pathogenesis period and carries on through the clinical diagnosis of disease. It includes such measures as:

- Slowing the progression/transmission of the disease
- Preventing complications or reducing their effects
- Limiting or preventing disability resulting from the disease
- Rehabilitating one the disease has run its course

With the tertiary level, the disease has occurred; therefore, efforts are designed to prevent it from turning into something worse and limit complications, such as disabilities.

The difference between the three prevention levels can be seen in the treatment of rickets. Primary prevention starts with informing a public about the need for vitamin D supplementation for some infants. For infants who do not receive needed supplementation, secondary and tertiary prevention is crucial. Secondary prevention includes detecting and treating subclinical rickets before it progresses to clinical rickets. Tertiary prevention involves treating children with clinical rickets to prevent such complications as hypocalcemia and seizures.

Infection Control Policies and Procedures

Review of infection control policies and procedures should be done in response to surveillance reports, as policies and procedures should be written with clear goals and outcomes in mind. A comprehensive review should include:

- **Analysis of achievement of goals**: If goals are met or exceeded, then new goals may need to be set. If goals are not met, then goals may have been unrealistic or policies and procedures or training may not be adequate.
- **Analysis of variances and/or outbreaks, assessing risk factors**: Patterns of infection or outbreaks may indicate breakdown in the system of infection control.
- Staff input:
    - Cross-sectional questionnaires regarding compliance, knowledge, and training
    - Meetings to discuss adequacy or problems with current policies and procedures
- **Training review**: Training should be ongoing and coupled with clear expectations that staff compliance with standard precautions, including hand-washing and hand sanitation, will be 100%.

Development of Policies and Procedures

Infection control policies and procedures should be developed in accordance to CDC and accreditation standards and should be a comprehensive document that outlines administrative polices, infection control measures, and employee health measures. The IP and other infection control members should be listed as well as contact information. The infection control policies and procedure manual should include policies and procedures for:

- Waste management/disposal of sharps
- Sample forms for record keeping and reporting
- Standard precautions and transmission-based precautions
- Barrier protection
- Invasive devices
- Durable medical equipment
- Sterilization and disinfection
- Laboratory specimens
- Patient transportation
- Nutritional services
- Environmental services
- Inpatient units
- Recall of contaminated equipment and supplies
- Specialized units, such as ICU, HRN, and transplant units
- Outbreak investigation
- Serologic testing and immunization
- Air and water quality

Influence of the Infection Control Officer on Hospital Strategies and Policies

Areas in which the infection control officer will influence strategies and hospital policies include the following:

- Effective practices in handwashing and antisepsis
- Effective practices in cleaning, disinfection, and sterilization
- Correcting variances from infection control norms identified through surveillance
- Scrutinizing specific inpatient care settings (e.g., nursing units, specialty units, respiratory therapy, operating room) and non-patient care departments (e.g., environmental services, nutritional services)
- Inspecting at-risk areas associated with therapeutic and diagnostic procedures and devices (e.g., intravascular devices, urinary drainage catheter, respiratory therapy, bronchoscopy, angiography)
- Overseeing or advising on medical waste disposal
- Identifying potentially contaminated equipment and supplies
- Reporting concerns about infection taking hold in outpatient healthcare settings (e.g., ambulatory care center, free standing surgery centers, dialysis center, day programs)

Role of the Infection Control Officer in Assisting the Facility to Maintain Accreditation

Joint Commission evaluates many aspects of the facility, including infection control, for accreditation. The guidelines by which hospitals are evaluated are often very specific, such as the exact time in minutes or hours after admission for pneumonia that a patient receives an antibiotic, with scores according to the elapsed time. The infection control officer must review, understand, communicate, and establish guidelines for all accreditation requirements to ensure that the various staff and departments are aware of the requirements and are documenting compliance. Because the accreditation survey utilizes tracer methodology, which evaluates the processes that are in place, extensive staff training regarding processes at all levels must be completed. Additionally, the IP can use tracer methodology as part of infection control, allowing staff to understand and practice the type of information they need to supply to the accreditation team.

Mission of CDC in Epidemiology

The mission of the CDC is to promote health and quality of life by preventing and controlling disease, injury, and disability. It seeks to accomplish its mission by working with partners throughout the nation and the world to:

- Monitor health
- Spot and investigate communicable health problems
- Conduct research to enhance disease prevention
- Build and advocate sound public health policies
- Develop and implement prevention strategies
- Promote healthy behaviors
- Encourage safe and healthful environments, and
- Provide leadership and training in the areas of disease prevention and treatment.

CDC's Study on the Efficacy of Nosocomial Infections (SENIC) Project

In 1974, the Centers for Disease Control undertook a nationwide study to evaluate approaches to infection control. The Study on the Efficacy of Nosocomial Infection (SENIC) Project had three primary objectives:

- To see whether infection surveillance and control programs lower the rate of nosocomial infection
- Describe the status of such programs and infection rates
- Observe any relationships between hospitals, patients, components of infection control programs, and changes in infection rates.

SENIC found that hospitals reduced their nosocomial infection rates by approximately 32%, if their infection surveillance and control program included four components: vigorous surveillance and control efforts, at least one full time infection control practitioner per 250 beds, a trained hospital epidemiologist, and providing practicing surgeons feedback on surgical wound infection (SWI) rates. Components needed for prevention varied for the four major types of nosocomial infection: SWI, urinary tract infection, bloodstream infection, and lower respiratory tract infection.

OSHA Standards for Preventing Healthcare-Associated Infections

Essentially following the CDC recommendation that blood and certain other body fluids from all patients be considered potentially infectious and that rigorous infection control precautions be taken to minimize the risk of exposure, OSHA has ruled that persons at substantial risk of HBV should be vaccinated if their work involves contact with blood or blood-contaminated body fluids. Such vaccination should be completed during training in schools of medicine, dentistry, nursing, laboratory technology, and other allied health professions before workers have their first contact with blood. Training records relative to bloodborne pathogens must be kept for three years.

OSHA also mandates proper training for all employees reasonably expected to come into contract with blood or other possibly infectious materials. Similarly, workers in healthcare settings must be trained on proper recognition and isolation of tuberculosis infected patients.

Designing Controls for Healthcare-Associated Infections

A healthcare center that fails to be vigilant in controlling healthcare-associated infections violates public trust. The primary elements in designing healthcare-associated infection programs are cleanliness of the facility, sterile procedures, and staff education. The physical plan of a facility should also be taken into consideration (including such things as ventilation shafts that are designed to keep microorganisms out).

An infection control program requires and officer in charge and a master plan that includes:

- Provisions for putting patients with communicable diseases into isolation
- Close observation of patients with indwelling catheters
- Effectively managing hemorrhagic patients
- Closely controlling linen management
- Frequently checking kitchen sanitation
- Maintaining care in operation of the mortuary and post mortem areas
- Making sure to include all patient, staff, and visitor areas in "clean sweeps"

Role of Epidemiology in Advising on Policies During the COVID-19 Pandemic

The role of epidemiology is to determine who has a particular disease, why they became infected, and how to treat the disease. Initially, epidemiologists went to China to try to trace the origins of the disease and conduct field investigations to help understand how the disease spread. Epidemiologists continue to monitor data provided by surveillance systems and determine rates of hospitalizations, deaths, complications, locations of clusters, distribution of COVID-19, symptoms, and demographics of those infected. They study the disease to determine factors such as incubation time, R0, risk factors, and effective treatments as well as developing guidance regarding precautions to slow the spread of the disease. Epidemiologists review the precautions in place (such as school closures and the wearing of masks) to determine how effective these measures are and to provide advice for ongoing measures.

Infections Requiring Specific Procedures and Protocols

Skin and Wound Infections

Surgical wound infections are the second most frequent nosocomial infection in most hospitals and are an important cause of morbidity and mortality. Among precautionary steps that should be included in a facilities policies and procedures are the following:

- Identify and treat existing bacterial infections preoperatively
- Enforce short preoperative stays
- Have patients bathe and shampoo with antimicrobial soap on the eve of their operation. (Hair removal is seldom practiced nowadays because razor nicks can become infected)
- Use operating room ventilation that filters incoming fresh air on a frequent basis
- Change dressings over closed wounds when saturated or when they appear infected
- Use parenteral antimicrobial prophylaxis for operations associated with high risk of infection or where infection could lead to life-threatening consequences
- Isolate patients with potentially transmissible wound or skin infections
- Record all wounds as clean, clean-contaminated, contaminated, or dirty and infected and review wound infection rates periodically

Diarrhea and Meningitis

Policies and procedures must also be in place for specific illnesses. For routine cases of clinical diarrhea, also known as Traveler's Diarrhea, antibiotics are no longer recommended due to increasing resistance, initially among *Campylobacter* species and now among other TD pathogens. In the case of severe diarrhea (and for those who are high-risk/immunocompromised), azithromycin (1 g single dose) has proven effective.

Meningitis comes in two classes, bacterial and viral, with subsets of those classes being caused by different pathogens. The four most common of the infecting bacteria are *Streptococcus pneumoniae, Neisseria meningitidis, Listeria monocytogenes*, and *Haemophilus influenzae*. Because the specific micro-organisms responsible for acute bacterial meningitis vary with time, geography, and patient age, the disease is difficult to treat and remains a major cause of nosocomial death worldwide.

Risk factors playing significant roles in post-operative nosocomial meningitis infection are CSF leak, external ventricular drainage, poor hand washing practices, and too infrequent changing of gloves.

Directly-Observed Therapy for MDR-TB and XDR-TB

The infection control plan should include provisions for referring patients and/or staff with tuberculosis for **directly-observed therapy (DOT)** when indicated. DOT requires that a healthcare worker monitor every dose of an individual's anti-tuberculosis medication, ensuring that all medications are taken and the entire course of treatment is completed. Drug protocol may be changed to 2-3 times weekly rather than daily to facilitate DOT. Regulations about DOT vary from state to state.

DOT is frequently used in these circumstances:

- Sputum cultures are positive for acid-fast bacilli
- There is concurrent treatment with antiretroviral (HIV) drugs or methadone (for addiction)
- Infection is MDR-TB or XDR-TB
- Co-morbidity with psychiatric disease or cognitive impairment exists
- Patient is homeless and lacks adequate facilities
- Patient has demonstrated lack of reliability in treatment

When patients are discharged from the hospital, plans must include continuation of DOT through the use of home health agencies or having the patient return to a clinic for administration of drugs.

Infection Prevention and Control Strategies

Hand Hygiene

Strategies for Handwashing

All patients are considered potentially infectious, so **handwashing** must be done before and after every direct contact with a patient or when removing gloves. Contamination of the hands is one of the most common causes of person-to-person transmission of infection and all medical personnel must be trained in handwashing techniques and observed regularly for compliance:

- Routine handwashing is done under running water with plain soap rather than antimicrobial soap because of issues related to resistance.
- Hands must be lathered thoroughly, covering all areas of the hands and wrists with soap, and then rinsed.
- After handwashing, care should be taken to avoid contact with surfaces that might serve as vectors, such as faucet handles and doorknobs.
- The faucet should be turned off by using the elbow or upper forearm or holding a piece of paper towel as a barrier.
- Hands should be dried using disposable towels.

CDC Precautions Regarding Handwashing and Gloves

The CDC's precautions regarding handwashing and the use of gloves are as follows:

- Gloves, not necessarily sterile but clean, are to be worn when touching blood, body fluids, secretions, excretions, and contaminated items.
- Gloves should be donned before touching mucous membranes and non-intact skin.
- After contact with material that may contain a high concentration of microorganisms on one part of a patient's body, healthcare personnel should change gloves before performing any task or procedure on another part of the same patient's body. This ensures against the possibility of cross-contamination between infection sites.
- Remove gloves promptly after use, before touching non-contaminated items and environmental surfaces, and before leaving the room or tending to another patient.

Hand Disinfection with Alcohol-Based Rub

While soap and water handwashing has been the standard for many years, in fact studies have proven that **alcohol-based rubs** kill twice as much bacteria in the same amount of time. They are waterless and act quickly to kill bacteria and are less irritating to the hands than repeated washing. The procedure for application is as follows:

- Hand disinfection is done for at least 15 seconds by using an alcohol-based rub, such as Purell, and should be done before and after contact with a patient or after removal of gloves.
- All hand surfaces should be thoroughly coated with the alcohol-rub, including between the fingers, the wrists, and under the nails, and then the hands rubbed together until the solution evaporates.
- The hands do not need to be rinsed after using alcohol-based rubs.
- Alcohol-based rubs disinfect but do not mechanically clean hands, so hands that are dirty or contaminated should be washed first with soap and water.
- Certain bacteria are not sufficiently eliminated with alcohol-based rubs, requiring the mechanical hand washing with soap (e.g., *Clostridium difficile*).

USES AND AVAILABLE SOLUTIONS

Hygienic hand rubs are used before and after the following:

- Performing invasive procedures or patient care
- Touching wounds, urethral catheters, or other indwelling devices
- Donning gloves (and after doffing gloves)
- Having contact with blood secretions or sites where microbial contamination is likely to have occurred
- Having contact with a person known to be colonized with a significant nosocomial pathogen (such as MRSA or MDR *Klebsiella*).

An aqueous solution of 4% chlorhexidine gluconate/detergent or Povidone, an iodine/detergent solution containing 0.75% available iodine, may be used to disinfect. An alcoholic hand rub, ideally from a dispenser at the patient's bedside, is the most efficient and least time-consuming procedure for hand decontamination. The solution may be 0.5% chlorhexidine, povidone-iodine in 70% isopropanol or ethanol, or either 60% isopropanol or 70% ethanol without antiseptic. Apply not less than 3mL of the preparation to the hands and rub to dryness (approximately 15-30 seconds).

SURGICAL HAND DISINFECTION

Surgical hand washing aims to remove and kill transient flora and decrease resident flora toward reducing the risk of wound contamination should surgical gloves undergo damage. Agents are the same as those used for hygienic hand washes, the primary difference between the surgical scrub and the hygienic hand wash being that, for the former, more time is spent in scrubbing (an extra 2 to 3 minutes) and it includes both wrists and forearms.

Sterile disposable or autoclave-able nailbrushes may be used to clean the fingernails only, but not to scrub the hands. A brush should only be used for the first scrub of the day.

After hand washing with soap and water, a hand rub with an alcohol base formulation (70%) should be used if possible. This enhances the destruction or inhibition of resident skin flora. If an alcohol preparation is used, two applications of 5 mL each is suggested, both rubbed to dryness. Sterile towels should be used to dry the hands thoroughly after washing and before alcohol is applied.

SURGICAL HAND RUBS VS. SURGICAL HAND WASHES

In a recently issued guideline on hand hygiene, the CDC recommends the use of hand rubs over surgical hand washes, indicating that the efficacy of alcohols as disinfectants in controlling all types of hand flora – infectious, transient, and resident – is superior to antimicrobial soaps.

This is backed up by studies which have shown that a solution of 80% ethanol was superior to using a combination of 61% ethanol with 1% chlorhexidine. Other studies have shown its superiority, too, to surgical hand washing. The use of a well formulated alcohol-based hand rub can also decrease skin dryness and produce significantly less skin irritation than an antimicrobial soap.

Alcohol-based hand rubs have been in common use for surgical hand disinfection for several years in Europe, where their *in vivo* efficacy is usually tested under practical conditions against a reference treatment. To pass this test, a commercial hand rub product cannot be significantly less effective after three hours compared to a reference alcohol. This type of testing is not currently conducted in the United States.

Chlorhexidine

The biguanide, chlorhexidine, is one the more widely used disinfectants, in part because of its low cost and the fact it is relatively non-irritating to skin. Though considered a bactericidal, virucidal, and fungicidal, chlorhexidine is less effective against these agents than many other disinfectants. It is fairly effective as a sporicidal agent, but to be effective chlorhexidine must remain in contact with a surface to be disinfected for not less than five minutes.

While it remains effective in the presence of some organic materials, cleaning before application is recommended. Its primary effectiveness is at low concentrations for disinfecting clean, small objects; its ineffectiveness against some important microorganisms is balanced off by its broad germicidal activity. It is not as effective as alcohol is as a sanitizing antiseptic for hands. Care must be taken around hard or alkaline water, as it will cause precipitation of the active ingredients necessary for disinfection. Chlorhexidine disinfectants include Chlorhex and Hibiclens Phisohex.

Iodophors

Iodine and iodophors, known for their rapid action and relative freedom from toxicity and irritancy, are well established chemical disinfectants despite the fact that Gram-negative bacteria have been found to survive or grow in the substances, just as they do in phenolics. The disinfective ability of iodine, like chlorine, is neutralized in the presence of organic material; hence, frequent applications are needed for thorough disinfection.

Without modification, iodine tinctures can be irritating to tissues, can stain fabric, and be corrosive. However, when these compounds are incorporated in a "tamed" form such as in surgical scrubs, they have proven to be bactericidal, sporicidal, virucidal, and fungicidal without irritating tissues, but they do require prolonged exposures to be effective.

Phenol Derivatives

Commonly found in mouth washes, scrub soaps, and surface disinfectants, phenols make up the most common type of agents found in household disinfectants. Household antiseptic brands like Lysol and Pine-sol are effective against bacteria (especially Gram-positive bacteria) and enveloped viruses (which include BRS, BVD, Coronavirus, IBR, PI3, Pox, Rabies, and Stomatitis). They are not effective against non-enveloped viruses and spores such as Bluetongue, Papilloma, Parvo, and Rota virus. Common spore forming bacteria include those which cause tetanus and anthrax.

Hexachlorophene, a type of phenolic antiseptic that binds strongly to the skin, had been used widely in surgical soaps like pHisoHex. However, it was determined that absorption of the substance through the skin can cause damage to the central nervous system, particularly in infants, so the use of hexachlorophene is now severely restricted. Phenol no longer plays a significant role as an antibacterial agent for hand washing either. Phenol derivatives are still used as antimicrobial agents in germicidal soaps and lotions.

Triclosan

In the United States, 79% of liquid soaps and 29% of bar soaps contain the antibacterial agent triclosan, an antibiotic designed to kill a wide variety of germs. The germicide has been put into soaps and toothpastes for the last 30 years, a prominent brand containing it being Procter & Gamble's Dial.

According to a recent study, this may be contributing to the rise of drug-resistant microorganisms. The triclosan used by hospital personnel in soaps to prevent the spread of infection comes in much higher doses, about 10 times as much as is found in soap used in the home. The irony is that the doses found in supermarket soaps are too small to prevent infection but large enough to make microorganisms resistant to the ingredient over time. Germs that can resist triclosan have already been observed in laboratories. Right now, *Escherichia coli*, a major offender in cases of food poisoning, has the ability to fight off triclosan if it mutates only a single gene.

Quaternary Ammonium

Regrowth of bacteria on the skin occurs slowly after use of alcohol-based hand antiseptics, presumably because of the sublethal effect alcohols have on some skin bacteria. Adding chlorhexidine, quaternary ammonium compounds, octenidine, or triclosan to alcohol-based solutions can result in persistent activity, which is why many types of quaternary ammonium compounds are used as mixtures and often in combination with other germicides, including alcohols. These compounds, properly diluted, have low odor, are not irritating, and have good activity against some vegetative bacteria and lipid containing viruses.

QA disinfectants, while effective against Gram-positive and Gram-negative bacteria and enveloped viruses, are not effective against nonenveloped viruses, fungi, and bacterial spores. They have limited effectiveness in soaps, detergents, and hard water salts.

Hand Hygiene in Countries with Limited Resources

Over 2 million children die each year from diarrheal diseases, largely the result of poor hygiene, sanitation, and water supply in underdeveloped nations. Improving the quality of water supplies cuts the risk of diarrhea by about 16%, and making clean water more available reduces the risk by 20%. Installing adequate facilities to dispose of bodily waste and promoting hygiene, however, are far more effective than either of those measures – washing hands with soap alone cuts the risk of diarrhea by 47%, almost three times as effective as improving water quality.

A strategy to increase hand washing being tested in six countries has public private partnerships marketing hand washing as if they were consumer products like cars or shampoo. Consumers begin to see a toilet as a home improvement, not as a health intervention. They use soap to make hands look, feel, and smell good, not to prevent sickness.

Personal Protective Equipment

Devices and wearable items such as surgical gowns, gloves, masks, and respirators act as barriers between infectious materials and the skin, mouth, nose, eyes, and other mucous membranes. FDA evaluates the performance of personal protective equipment (PPE) such as this before it is cleared for marketing.

Proper use of PPE by workers involved in patient care helps prevent the spread of infection because:

- It helps protect wearers from infection or contamination from blood, body fluids, or respiratory secretions
- It reduces the chance that healthcare workers will infect or contaminate others
- It reduces the chance of transmitting infections from one person to another

The use of PPE alone does not fully protect against acquiring an infection, however. Hand-washing, isolation of patients, and proper coughing or sneezing etiquette are also important to minimize risk of infection. Protective clothing should be changed whenever torn or ripped.

Gloves

Barrier precautions are used to prevent infection in accordance with mode of transmission and likelihood of contamination with blood or other body fluids or wastes:

- Gloves are worn when hands may make contact with body fluids, including mucous membranes, or instruments that have made contact with body fluids, or any skin that is not intact, such as cuts, scrapes, or chapped.
- Gloves should be worn to protect the patient from any cuts or other breaks in the skin of the caregiver.
- Sterile gloves are used for sterile procedures.
- Gloves are used not only to prevent the spread of pathogenic agents from one patient to another but also to protect the healthcare worker. There are limitations to the degree to which gloves can control infections because transmission is complex. For example, gloves offer no protection to infections caused by endogenous flora.

Types of Gloves

There are a number of different **types of gloves** available. Traditionally nurses and surgeons have relied on latex gloves, which pose a danger to those who are allergic to latex. Now healthcare workers in almost all departments use gloves, so they must be widely available in all patient rooms and departments, so strength and versatility are important.

- **Latex** is strong, flexible and has some reseal ability, but contains proteins that cause allergic reactions.
- **Chloroprene/Neoprene** similar to latex in strength and flexibility, resists puncture, but tears more easily. It contains chemical accelerators.
- **Nitrile** is strong and resistance to tears and punctures. Less flexible than latex, it contains chemical accelerators.
- **Vinyl** is weak, inflexible, tears and breaks easily and contains chemical accelerants.
- **Polyurethane** is durable, resistant to tears and punctures and superior to latex. It contains no proteins or chemical accelerants.
- **Copolymer** punctures easily but is resistant to tears, and is stronger than vinyl but less flexible than latex. It contains chemical accelerants.

Goggles and Face Shields

The face is particularly vulnerable to splashing and splattering of blood and body fluids because staff are often leaning over the patients during procedures. The mucous membranes of the eyes, nose, and mouth can become contaminated, so **protective eyewear and face shields** should be worn when contamination of the face is possible:

- **Goggles** should be non-vented or indirectly vented with an anti-fog coating and should allow for direct and peripheral vision. They should be large enough to cover eyeglasses if necessary and still fit snugly to provide protection.
- **Face shields** provide protection to the eyes and face. The shields should have both crown and chin protection and should extend around the face to the ears. Small, thin disposable shields that attach to surgical masks provide more limited protection.

Both goggles and face shields should be washed with soap and water after each use and disinfected with 70% alcohol if contaminated.

Gowns

The CDC guidelines for barrier precautions call for the use of a **clean non-sterile gown**. Sterile gowns are reserved primarily for surgical procedures. There are a variety of different types of aprons and gowns that are available, primarily for the protection of the healthcare worker, but gowns also reduce contamination of uniforms and thus protect patients:

- Gowns should be moisture-resistant and easily cover clothing.
- Gowns are worn to prevent contamination from blood or body fluids during activities or procedures that may result in splashing or splattering.
- Gowns should be changed after caring for the patient or procedures that may have resulted in contamination.
- Gowns should be handled as little as possible, sliding down raised arms and fastening at the neck, with gloves pulled over sleeves.
- Gowns should be removed before gloves to reduce hand contamination, and the hands should be washed immediately after gloves are removed.

Masks and Respirators

Masks can provide protection from droplets, but they do not provide protection from smaller airborne microorganisms. Respirators that contain filters must be used for airborne precautions.

- **Masks** are used primarily to protect patients from droplets during sterile procedures, but are used when working within 3 feet of a patient on droplet precautions. They provide protection of the mucous membranes of the nose and mouth from spraying or splattering of blood or body fluids.
- **Respirators** must be used for protection against airborne transmission. The National Institute for Occupational Safety and Health (NIOSH) establishes requirements for respirators, which must filter 95% of 0.3 μm-sized particles in order to protect against *Mycobacterium tuberculosis.* These are referred to as N95 respirators.
    - The disposable N95 can be reused if not visibly damaged or dirty with TB patients but must be disposed of after use if patients are also on contact precautions (smallpox, SARS).

Fit Testing for Respirators

Respirators that are not properly fitting will not provide adequate protection against airborne particles. **Fitting** must be done prior to use for anyone who will use a respirator. OSHA has established guidelines for fitting and use of respirators. The staff must be tested with the same make, model, and size of respirator they will use.

- Numerous factors can affect seal, including facial hair, makeup, bone structure, scars, and dentures.
- Sensitivity testing involves placing the subject's head into a hood and then squeezing a test solution of saccharine or denatonium benzoate into the hood in increments to determine when the subject can taste the solution.
- The qualitative fit test involves wearing the respirator for 5 minutes; then, the hood is placed over it and the test solution is squeezed into the hood to determine if the respirator fits tightly enough to prevent the subject from tasting the solution.
- Exercise, such as talking, moving, bending, and jogging must be done to check security of seal.

Healthcare Worker's Responsibilities in Infection Control

Healthcare workers have a primary role in preventing and controlling infections, especially those whose work puts them in direct contact with patients, such as nursing staff in the operating room and nursing units or laboratory technicians. Healthcare workers must be knowledgeable about diseases and disease processes as well as infection control, including signs and symptoms of infections, risk factors, and preventive methods. Specific responsibilities for healthcare workers include:

- Using proper hand hygiene at all times, including handwashing and use of antiseptic hand cleaner both before and after patient contact.
- Using barrier precautions, including personal protective equipment such as gloves, gowns, and masks or respirators as needed.
- Using aseptic technique and proper procedures for urinary catheters, central venous lines, and other invasive procedures.
- Reporting any indications of infection to the physician and to the infection control committee as per protocol.

Nail Care

The subungual (beneath the nails) area of the fingers harbors high levels of microbes, especially *Staphylococcus*, Corynebacteria, Gram-negative rods such as *Pseudomonas* spp. as well as yeast. Both long nails and artificial nails have been implicated in transmission of infections. Because of this, the CDC recommends that healthcare workers who have contact with patients, supplies, medicine, food, or equipment not wear artificial nails or nail tips and keep nails trimmed to about 1/4 inch. Fingernail polish that is freshly applied does not increase bacterial count, but chipped polish can harbor bacteria, so most infection control policies allow either no nail polish or unchipped nail polish. Sequin, rhinestones, or other nail decorations also have the potential to harbor bacteria. While bacteria in the subungual area are most concentrated in the 1 mm closest to the skin, there are other problems associated with long nails:

- Scratching patients
- Puncturing gloves
- Interfering with palpation

Antisepsis

Modern surgical techniques for avoiding infection are based on asepsis, the absence of pathogenic organisms, and sterilization is the chief means of achieving it. Sterilization of surgical instruments can be pursued through steam cleaning in autoclaves but, of course, this will not work on human skin which, as Louis Pasteur determined in the mid-19th Century, is a major transporter of infection.

There is great variation in the ability of antiseptics to destroy microorganisms ranked against their effect on living tissue. Silver nitrate, with low potency but mild enough be used on the delicate tissues of the eyes and throat, is routinely put into the eyes of newborns to prevent infections that could lead to blindness. In contrast, mercuric chloride is a powerful antiseptic that irritates delicate tissue (and is now avoided because of its mercury content).

Antiseptics also differ in the time they take to work and the time they remain effective. Iodine kills bacteria within 30 seconds. Other antiseptics have slower, more residual action. Since so much variability exists, phenol is used as a standard (the phenol coefficient) in comparing the bacteriostatic action of antiseptics.

Antisepsis vs. Asepsis

A distinction should be made between antisepsis and asepsis.

Antisepsis	Asepsis
• Removes transient microorganisms from the skin and reduces resident flora • Patients undergoing surgery are subject to antisepsis procedures • Antisepsis techniques in the operating theater involve the use of sterile instruments, a gloved, no-touch technique, and proper preoperative skin preparation that includes flooding the field with antiseptic.	• Any procedure used to reduce the risk of bacterial contamination. • All the furniture and fixtures in the room of the patient who has gone off to surgery will undergo asepsis to reduce risk of infection upon their return.

Antiseptic Solutions

Background of Antiseptic Solutions

Lister, in 1865, introduced the practice of using carbolic acid for antisepsis in the operating theater. Today, skin may be washed with a variety of solutions such as those listed below to sterilize hands and instruments and produce a sterile field for surgery; it also maintains microorganism-free environments for laboratory work and on hospital wards. No evidence indicates any one of these solutions being superior to another:

- **Alcohols**: Most commonly used is ethanol (60-90%), 1-propanol (60-70%) and 2-propanol/isopropanol (70-80%) or mixtures of the two. Short-acting bactericidals effective against Gram-positive and Gram-negative organisms, they are also a fungicidal and virucidal.
- **0.5% Chlorhexidine**: Used to treat gingivitis, as a bactericidal it is persistent and has a long duration of action. It is effective against Gram-positive organisms but does not kill spore forming organisms, instead disrupting the bacterial cell wall.

Because of concerns about its mercury content, mercurochrome (an organomercury antiseptic) is now obsolete, no longer being recognized as safe and effective by the FDA. Occlusive adhesive drapes are sometimes used during surgery, but there is no evidence that they reduce infection rate and they may actually increase skin bacterial count during surgery.

Octenidine Dihydrochloride and Sodium Chloride

Octenidine dihydrochloride:

- A cationic surfactant and bis-(dihydropyridinyl)-decane derivative
- Similar in action to the QAs, but is of a somewhat broader spectrum of activity
- Currently used in continental Europe to an increasing extent because of concerns about the carcinogenic impurity of 4-chloroaniline

Sodium chloride

- Also known as table salt, has only a weak antiseptic effect, and is used as a general cleanser and antiseptic mouthwash.

Sodium hypochlorite

- Still used as a disinfectant, sodium hypochlorite was formerly used in diluted form with potassium permanganate in Dakin's solution.

Reducing Infections Associated with Intravascular Devices

Short-Term Intravascular Devices

Strategies for reducing infection risks associated with intravascular devices include:

- **Site selection** away from the internal jugular or femoral veins, using a PICC if possible.
- **Tunneled catheter or ports** should be used, if possible, because of lower infection rates than non-tunneled catheters.
- **TPN catheters** used only for TPN and no other procedures/infusions.
- Experienced **trained staff** should insert intravascular devices, using **maximum aseptic technique** for insertion.
- **Dressings** may be transparent or gauze, but the insertion site should be examined frequently by palpation and the dressing removed for inspection in the case of any tenderness. Change dressings at least 1 time weekly.
- **Catheter material** of Teflon or polyurethane should be used, which demonstrates lower rates of infection than polyvinyl chloride or polyethylene. Catheters that are impregnated with antimicrobials have demonstrated reduction in infections.
- **Catheter sites should be rotated** every 72-96 hours (for adults) for short peripheral venous catheters but only as needed for others.
- **Avoid antibiotic ointments** at insertion site because of danger of fungal infections or resistance.

Types of Infections Common in Short-Term Intravascular Devices

Short duration central lines are inserted <21-30 days for the purpose of administration of medicine, blood, fluids, and nutrition. Because they are invasive devices, they pose a risk of infection. Studies have shown that infection in short duration devices is often caused by bacteria on the skin invading along the outside of the catheter. Different types of infections are common:

- **Colonization** of bacteria either on the outside or inside of the catheter may occur.
- **Localized infection** at the insertion site involves swelling, erythema, and discharge.
- **Exit infection** can occur where tunneled catheters exit the skin.
- **Tunnel infection** occurs along the portion of the catheter that is tunneled under the skin before entering a vessel.
- **Bloodstream infections** may be related to a catheter infection, with the same microbe, but they may occur as primary infections without evidence of local inflammation.

Long-Term Central Line Devices

Long term central lines are in place for >30 days and can cause a variety of infections, usually from microbes entering the catheter and moving down the inside to the bloodstream. There are three types of long-term central lines in common use.

- **Non-tunneled catheters** consist of subclavian silicone or peripherally-inserted central catheters (PICC).
- **Tunneled catheters** usually are inserted between the nipple and the sternum and have a Dacron cuff about 5 cm from the exit point. This cuff anchors the catheter to fibrous tissue.
- **Implantable ports** include a catheter and metal port, all inserted under the skin in a subcutaneous pocket, usually in the upper chest but sometimes in the arm.

While infections may be similar to short term central lines with the addition of port pocket infection, of added concern is the development of biofilms that adhere to the catheters, leading to bloodstream infections and antibiotic resistance. The implantable port has a lower rate of infection than other types of lines.

Categorization of Central Line-Associated Bloodstream Infections (CLABSI)

Surveillance for central line-associated bloodstream infections (CLABSI) is both active and prospective. Surveillance should continue in any healthcare facility and is not required after discharge but must be reported if discovered:

- **Bloodstream infection (BSI):** The major category for these types of infections.
- Laboratory-confirmed bloodstream infection (LCBI): Requires a positive blood culture.
- **CLABSI:** LCBI occurring after central line or umbilical catheter has been in place for more than two days at the time of the infection and was in place the prior day. If the central line or umbilical catheter had been in place for more than two days and was removed, the LCBI criteria must be met on the day of removal or the next day.
- **Mucosal barrier injury laboratory-confirmed bloodstream infection (MBI-LCBI):** Must now be reported and applies to patients with hematopoietic stem cell transplant within a year or who are neutropenic for 2 out of 7 days that include date of a positive blood culture and up to 3 days after positive blood culture.

Reducing Infections Associated With Procedures

Angiography, Angioplasty, and Percutaneous Transcatheter Embolization

Strategies for reducing infection risks associated with angiography, angioplasty, and percutaneous trans-catheter embolization include:

- Using standard precautions with barrier protection, such as gloves, gowns, and goggles, as well as strict aseptic technique with surgical drapes that are liquid resistant
- Avoiding shaving when possible or using electric shaver
- Using antiseptic on insertion site
- Antibiotic prophylaxis in selected individual, such as the immunocompromised, or selected procedures, such as embolization
- Avoiding cutdown procedures, which have higher rates of infection
- Removing catheters as soon as possible
- Avoiding non-permeable plastic dressings in favor of gauze or semi-permeable transparent dressings
- Avoiding disposing of contaminated fluids or flushing of catheter into an open container
- Limiting reuse of equipment to those allowed by federal regulations
- Cleaning and disinfecting any non-disposable equipment following manufacturers' directions
- Environmental precautions as per operating room

Bronchoscopy

Bronchoscopy poses risks of spreading infection distally from the upper respiratory tract, transmitting infection to other patients from contaminated equipment, and transmitting infection to staff. Of primary concern are pathogens that survive and multiply in water, such as *Pseudomonas* or mycobacteria. Pseudo-epidemics may occur if scopes are environmentally contaminated as colonization may be from the scope rather than related to infection in the patient. **Control strategies** include the following:

- Thorough mechanical cleaning immediately after use to prevent drying of secretions.
- Sterilization or high-level disinfection with EPA-approved agents as directed, manually or with automated endoscopic reprocessor, with dismantling of all components of the scope to ensure proper disinfection and sufficient duration. Sterile rinses and sterile transport cases must be used to ensure that environmental contamination does not take place.
- Monitoring of automated endoscopic reprocessor for contamination.
- Use of disposable devices for parts that are difficult to adequately clean.

Reducing Infections Associated with Urinary Catheters

Strategies for reducing infection risks associated with urinary catheters include:

- Using aseptic technique for both straight and indwelling catheter insertion
- Limiting catheter use by establishing protocols for use, duration, and removal, training staff, issuing reminders to physicians, using straight catheterizations rather than indwelling, using ultrasound to scan the bladder, and using condom catheters
- Utilizing closed-drainage systems for indwelling catheters
- Avoiding irrigation unless required for diagnosis or treatment
- Using sampling port for specimens rather than disconnecting catheter and tubing
- Maintaining proper urinary flow by proper positioning, securing of tubing and drainage bag, and keeping drainage bag below the level of the bladder
- Changing catheters only when medically-needed
- Cleansing external meatal area gently each day, manipulating the catheter as little as possible
- Avoid placing catheterized patients adjacent to those infected or colonized with antibiotic-resistant bacteria to reduce cross-contamination

Issues Associated with Urinary Catheters

Urinary infections are the most common healthcare-associated infection in both acute and long-term care facilities, almost always caused by invasive devices, such as **catheters** and cystoscopes. Most people with continuous catheter drainage are chronically infected within 30 days. Catheters are frequently over used and left in for too long, increasing risk of infection. Infections have occurred both in endemically and epidemically and may involve local inflammation, abscess formation, and, in males, infection can spread to the testes, prostate, and other reproductive organs. Because urinary tract infections are routinely treated with antibiotics, they have a role in increasing resistance of microorganisms to treatment. Fungal infections have increased markedly as a result. The urinary drainage bag serves as a reservoir for microorganisms, which can be transmitted on the hands of staff handling the bags. Contaminated bags can be implicated in pseudo infections, where only the urine in the bag is infected.

Reducing Infections Associated with Hemodialysis

Strategies for reducing infection risks associated with hemodialysis include the following CDC precautions:

- Use standard precautions and gloves. Wash/sanitize hands between each patient.
- Items taken into dialysis area should be disposed of, used on only one patient, or cleaned and disinfected prior to returning to central area for use on another patient.
- Use single-dose medications or multi-dose vials for one patient and do not return to central area; conversely, prepare medications from a multi-dose vial in central area and deliver separately.
- Do not use a common medication cart for multiple patients.
- Maintain separate clean and contaminated areas that are non-adjacent.
- Use external venous and arterial pressure transducer filters/protectors for individual patients, change between patients, and do not reuse.
- Clean and disinfect entire dialysis station, including all furniture and equipment (with control panels), between patients.
- Use leak proof containers to transport dialyzers and tubing for reprocessing according to industry standards.

Dialysis Events

Facilities providing hemodialysis must report the number of patients receiving dialysis service on the first two working days of the months. All patients must be monitored throughout the month for three NHSN **dialysis events**:

- **IV antimicrobial starts:** Includes all starts of antibiotics or antifungals (but not antivirals) even if patients are transfers and administration began elsewhere. To be considered separate events, more than 21 days must separate IV antimicrobial starts.
- **Positive blood cultures:** Suspected source must be indicated—vascular access other than vascular access for dialysis (infection from other site), contamination, or uncertain. There must be more than 21 days between positive blood cultures to be reported as separate events even if the organisms are different.
- Evidence of infection at local access site: Pus must always be reported.

Measure definitions include blood stream infections (BSI), access-related bloodstream infection (ARBI), local access site infection (LASI) and vascular access infection (VAI). Vascular access types include non-tunneled central line, tunneled central line, graft, fistula, and other access device. Numerator data are reported monthly.

Reducing Infections Associated with Ventilators

Issues Associated with Ventilators

Mechanical **ventilation** carries a risk of respiratory infection and pneumonia; usually from the patient's own microbes. Some infections are related to trauma and swelling that compromises tissue, resulting in aspiration of normal flora of the oropharyngeal area, and/or inhalation of microbes in aerosol form. Contaminated equipment may provide a reservoir for microbes, especially in moisture containing tubes, nebulizers, or other equipment. Additionally, the ventilator essentially inoculates the respiratory tract with microbes. Nebulizers have been related to significant numbers of infection because the moist environment encourages colonization, especially if the nebulizers are reused for more than 48 hours. Humidifiers are often added to ventilators, but these tend to cause condensation in tubes, again providing fertile ground for microorganisms, unless heat moisture exchangers, which recycle exhaled heat and moisture, are used. Manual ventilator bags have been implicated in spread of infection because the inside of the bag was not sufficiently sterilized.

Ventilator-Associated Events (VAE) and Ventilator-Associated Pneumonia (VAP)

According to the NSHN, ventilator associated events (VAE), which refer to those that are associated with mechanical ventilation in adults, comprise three different tiers. VAE criteria include sustained increase in the daily minimum PEEP value (≥3 cm H_2O, for at least an hour) and sustained increase (≥20%) in FiO_2 after a period of stability. Eligibility requires two full days of mechanical ventilation with the earliest day of event (worsening of oxygenation) on day three and fulfillment of criteria on day four for all three tiers:

- **Ventilator-associated condition (VAC):** Criteria include increased temperature (>38 °C) and change in WBC count (≥12,000 or ≤4,000) and a new microbial agent.
- **Infection-related ventilator associated complication (IVAC):** Criteria include purulent respiratory secretions and/or positive culture (leading to possible VAP) OR purulent respiratory secretions and positive culture or positive culture/positive diagnostic test for a number of different agents without purulent respiratory secretions (leading to probable VAP).
- **Ventilator-associated pneumonia (VAP), possible or probable:** Both possible and probable VAP must meet criteria for VAC and IVAC.

Patients on extracorporeal life support or high frequency ventilation are not included in VAE surveillance.

Review Video: Medical Ventilators
Visit mometrix.com/academy and enter code: 679637

Reducing Infections Associated with Durable Medical Equipment

Oxygen Equipment

Oxygen equipment can easily become contaminated and implicated in healthcare-associated infections. Control includes the following:

- Use standard precautions, including washing hands and wearing gloves when working with oxygen equipment to avoid spreading contamination.
- Avoid humidification when possible. Flow rates of 1-4 L/min per mask or nasal cannula allow for adequate humidification from the respiratory tract, but higher flow rates or flow directly to a trachea requires humidification. In-line fine particle nebulizers have become contaminated when oxygen is mixed with ambient air from an oxygen wall outlet.
- Decondensate any tubing as needed.
- Use only sterile solutions for humidification or inhalation.
- Use disposable equipment (regulators, masks, tubing, humidifiers) and replace according to manufacturer's directions. Equipment should never be shared among patients. Nasal cannulas and facemasks should be cleaned regularly as replaced scheduled intervals.
- Store oxygen cylinders (green tanks) properly in upright position and only in areas that are designated as clean.

Wheelchairs and Walkers

Wheelchairs are ubiquitous in the healthcare facility and often are used to transport many different patients between various units in the hospital without intervening cleaning or disinfection. However, they may become contaminated with urine, feces, and food. Organisms on the hands can be easily transmitted to the arms of the chairs or walkers and then to the next occupant. **Walkers**, while often dedicated to one patient, pose a similar danger if used for multiple patients. Control of transmission should include:

- Barriers for transportation, such as a clean sheet between the patient and the wheelchair with waterproof disposable pads if necessary to protect against urine, feces, blood, or other discharge.
- Inspection after use should be done each time and if soiled, it should be immediately removed from service, washed, and disinfected with an approved EPA disinfectant.
- Scheduled cleaning should be done on a regular basis for all wheelchairs and walkers in use, including either manual cleaning and disinfecting or use of automated cleaning and infection control systems.

Handling Medical Equipment of Patients in Isolation with a Communicable Disease

Medical equipment may be cleaned to remove contaminants (dust, soil, large numbers of microorganisms and organic matter [e.g., blood, vomit]) as a necessary prelude to disinfecting and sterilizing it. Whilst disinfecting reduces the number of smaller microorganisms so that they are not immediately harmful to health, bacterial spores will still remain. Sterilization removes them. Each medical instrument that has come into contact with a patient is a potential source of infection. It should be considered a high-risk item when it has made close contact with broken skin or mucous membranes or has been introduced into a body, which requires sterilizing. Intermediate risk items (mainly non-invasive respiratory equipment) need only to be disinfected. Stethoscopes, blood pressure cuffs, and such make only slight skin contact and therefore need only cleaning and drying. Boiling equipment in water for 10 minutes disinfects, killing all organisms except for a few bacterial spores. Autoclaving sterilizes by using steam under pressure at a temperature of 134 °C for 3 minutes or 121 °C for 15 minutes.

NHSN Patient Safety Components

The CDC's National Healthcare Safety Network is a surveillance system that focuses on 5 components: Patient Safety, Long-Term Care Facility, Outpatient Dialysis, Healthcare Personnel Safety, and Biovigilance. Within the **Patient Safety component**, there are five modules of surveillance:

- **Device-Associated Module:** Covers bloodstream infections, central line insertion protocols, urinary tract infections, ventilator associated events, and ventilator associated pneumonia.
- **Procedure-Associated Module:** Covers surgical site infections.
- **Antimicrobial Use and Resistance Module**
- **Multi-Drug Resistance and *Clostridium Difficile* Infection (MDRO/CDI) Module**
- **Coronavirus Infectious Disease 2019 (COVID-19) Module**: This is a new module described as off plan, meaning that this data is not included in annual reports and facilities have to manually upload their data.

Data is collected through a variety of surveillance methods. One key method is through "patient-based, prospective surveillance" conducted by a trained infection preventionist (IP). The IP screens various sources (laboratory data, patient records, pharmacy, physician/nurse notes, etc.) for infections acquired during a patient's stay. The IP is assisted by others trained to collect "denominator data" such as hand hygiene or central line insertion practices. Additional information is collected specific to each module, for instance, the number of antimicrobials used for patient care, positive MRSA, and/or VRE culture.

Device-Associated Module

Almost all patients admitted to a healthcare facility have exposure to some type of invasive medical device during their stay in the facility, and this exposure increases the risk of infection. **The Device-Associated Module** of the NHSN Patient Safety Component defines the type of devices associated with increased risk of specific infections. These include but are not limited to:

- Central line-associated bloodstream infection (CLABSI): Laboratory-confirmed BSI with central line or umbilical catheter in place for >2 days on the day of the event
- Central line insertion practices adherence (CLIP)
- Catheter-associated urinary tract infection (CAUTI): Infection occurring >2 days after insertion of catheter with symptoms and positive urine culture
- Ventilator-associated events (adults) (VAE): Include ventilator-associated condition (VAC), infection-related ventilator-associated complication (IVAC), and possible or probable ventilator-associated pneumonia (VAP)
- Ventilator-associated pneumonia (pediatrics, NICU, and adults) (VAP)

NHSN provides guidance for surveillance activities to monitor infections and processes (such as central line insertion) associated with these devices, for data collection, and for reporting data.

Procedure-Associated Module

The Procedure-Associated Module of the NHSN Patient Safety component includes:

- **Surgical site infections:** Includes deep incisional (primary or secondary) (DIP/DIS) occurring within 30-90 days of operative procedure, organ space occurring within 30-90 days, and superficial incisional (primary or secondary) (SIP, SIS) occurring within 30 days.
- **Post-procedural pneumonia:** Procedural-associated infections are attributed to the procedure that resulted in the infection, not the location where the infection occurred. Post-procedural pneumonia can occur with or without exposure to mechanical ventilation (ventilator-associated pneumonia). Post-procedural pneumonia may include postoperative pneumonia (especially with thoracic-abdominal surgery) and healthcare-associated pneumonia. Risk factors include surgery, hemodialysis, infusions, and wound care, especially in patients who are immunocompromised, colonized by bacteria (such as MR*SA)* or have co-morbidities. Preventive measures include early ambulation, deep breathing, and routine use of incentive spirometry.

Operative Procedure Guidelines

The NHSN and the CDC provide a list of codes (ICDM-9 CM/CPT) for **operative procedures** and define operative procedures for purposes of surveillance as any surgical procedure contained in the list and in which at least one incision is made through the skin or mucous membrane. A reoperation through an incision that was left open is also considered an operative procedure. Operative procedures must take place in an operating room or other room that meets guidelines for an operating room, such as a cardiac cath lab or an interventional radiology lab. Data collection must include the type of wound closure (primary vs non-primary). Data collection for surgical site infections must now also include diabetic status, height, and weight. The NHSN provides lists of procedures that must be monitored for 30 days and for 90 days, depending on risk factors associated with the type of surgery:

- Superficial incisional SSI: 30 days
- Deep incisional and organ space SSIs: 30-90 days

ANTIMICROBIAL USE AND RESISTANCE MODULE

The Antimicrobial Use and Resistance (AUR) Module of the NHSN Patient Safety Component requires electronic medical administration record (eMAR) or a bar coding system to report and analyze antimicrobial use. Participating facilities include acute care hospitals, LTC facilities, IRF, oncology hospitals and critical access hospitals. AUR comprises two approaches:

- **Antimicrobial use:** Collected data each month includes summary level data as well as numerator (antimicrobial days) and denominator (admission and patient days) data. Reports show antimicrobial use by location and class of antimicrobial.
- **Antimicrobial resistance:** Collected data includes numerator (patient level susceptibility results for 19 specific microorganisms) data, such as birth date, gender, admission date, type and source of specimen, and susceptibility data. Denominator date includes patient days and admissions. Results may be presented as line list or facility-wide antibiogram. Reporting rules require the same organism from invasive specimen source (blood, CSF) once per patient every 14 days and from non-invasive sources (urine, feces, sputum) once per patient every month.

CDC/NHSN GUIDELINES TO PREVENT SURGICAL SITE INFECTIONS (SSIS)

CATEGORY 1: SUPERFICIAL INCISIONAL SSIS

Comparison of data requires that precise and standardized definitions be utilized for the descriptions of surgical site infections. The CDC/NHSN developed the *CDC Definitions of Nosocomial Infections* to be used in reporting. The type of wound is classified according to these definitions, and then the Risk Index is applied to determine the severity of infection as well as rates of infection. Surgical site infections are identified by degree of infection among other criteria. The first category comprises:

- **Superficial incisional infection** occurs within 30 days of surgery and involves only skin and subcutaneous tissue of the incision, and patient has one of the following:
  - Purulent drainage
  - Organisms isolated from culture of wound fluid or tissue
  - Localized signs of infection, and wound is deliberately opened by physician, resulting in positive wound culture
  - Diagnosis of superficial infection by surgeon or attending physician

Category 2: Deep Incisional

The second category of the CDC/NHSN surgical site infection may include those wounds that have both superficial and deep incisional characteristics. The definition for the second category comprises:

- **Deep incisional infection** occurs within 30 or 90 days of surgery (according to the type of surgery which is accessible in the NHSN manual), infection appears related to the surgery and involves deep soft tissues (fascial and muscle layers) of the incision, and patient has one of following:
  - Purulent drainage from incision but not organ/space component of surgical site
  - Spontaneous dehiscence of wound or deliberately opened by surgeon when patient has one of these symptoms: fever (38C), localized pain or tenderness, unless wound culture is negative
  - Abscess or other evidence of deep incision infection found on direct examination, histopathology, or radiology
  - Diagnosis of a deep incisional infection by surgeon or attending physician

Category 3: Organ/Space

The third category of the CDC/NHSN surgical site infection definitions comprises the following:

- **Organ/space infection** occurs within 30 or 90 days of surgery (depending on type of surgery performed), appears related to surgery, and involves any part of the body, excluding the skin incision, fascia, or muscle layers, that is opened or manipulated during the operative procedure. Specific sites are assigned to organ/space SSI to further identify the location of the infection. Patient has one of the following:
  - Purulent drainage from a drain that is placed through a stab wound into the organ/space
  - Organisms isolated from an aseptically obtained culture of fluid or tissue in the organ/space
  - An abscess or other evidence of infection involving the organ/space that is found on direct examination, during reoperation, or by histopathology or radiology
  - Diagnosis of an organ/space infection by a surgeon or attending physician

Interventions to Decrease Risk of SSIs

Interventions to decrease risk of surgical site infections (SSIs) include:

- **Preoperative**: These measures include antibiotic prophylaxis, proper surgical hand preparation, screening for MR*SA* and nasal colonization of *Staphylococcus aureus,* avoiding hair removal or clipping hair instead of shaving, delaying elective procedures if remote infection is present, and using a presurgical checklist. Patients should quit smoking or refrain from smoking for at least a month prior to surgery when possible. Patients should shower the evening before surgery.
- **Intraoperative**: These measures include avoiding hypoglycemia and hypothermia, providing supplemental oxygen, and maintaining aseptic technique. Environmental controls include at least 15 air exchanges per hour with ≥3 fresh air (with air incoming at ceiling and outgoing at floor), maintenance of closed door into operating room as much as possible, adequate cleaning and disinfecting of environment, and sterilization of instruments.
- **Postoperative**: These measures include hand hygiene, aseptic wound care, covering wound with sterile dressing for 24-48 hours, and educating patient and family about wound care.

Key Terms Defined by the CDC's NHSN System

The following concepts are utilized by the CDC's NHSN System to characterize whether infections were acquired prior to, or during, a hospital stay:

7-day Infection Window Period (IWP)	The period of time, starting 3 days before and ending 3 days after the collection date of the first positive test (laboratory, imaging, or exam) for infection
Date of Event (DOE)	The date when the first element is utilized that meet criteria of a NHSN site-specific infection for the first time within the identified 7-day IWP
Present on Admission (POA)	If the DOE falls within the period of 2 days before admission date, to 1 calendar day after admission date, the infection is deemed present on admission
Healthcare-Associated Infection (HAI)	If the DOE falls one or after the 3rd day of admission (including the admission day), the infection is considered healthcare-associated
14-day Repeat Infection Timeframe (RIT)	This time frame is a 14-day period within which no new infections of the same type are reported. This is applied to both POA and HAI instances.
Secondary BSI Attribution Period (SBAP)	A 14- to 17-day period (depending on the DOE) in which a bloodstream specimen must be collected in order for a secondary infection to be attributed to a primary infection.
Location of Attribution (LOA)	The location of attribution signifies the inpatient location when the date of event is marked. If the patient is in the operating room or in interventional radiology, these cannot be considered LOA's. In these instances, the LOA must be where the patient's data is being collected.
Device-Associated Infection	Diagnosed because a patient has used a medical device such as a ventilator within the 48-hour period prior to onset of infection. For catheter-associated UTIs, an indwelling urinary catheter must have been in place within the 7 days before positive laboratory results or signs and symptoms meeting criteria for a UTI have presented.
Secondary Bloodstream Infection	Must yield a culture of the same organism displaying the same antibiogram as the primary nosocomial infection site. Should a blood culture positive for nosocomial UTI and organisms and antibiograms of both blood and urine specimens be identical, infection is reported as UTI (as the primary disease) with secondary BSI.

Patient Placement, Transfer, and Discharge

Placement and Transport of Patients with Communicable Diseases

Containing communicable diseases means keeping the infected and those who may be infected separated from the general public. Isolation of infected persons accomplishes this while allowing for the focused delivery of specialized healthcare to them in their homes, hospitals, or designated healthcare facilities. This is standard for patients with tuberculosis (TB) and certain other infectious diseases. In most cases, isolation is voluntary; however, many levels of government have the authority to compel isolation and to declare and enforce quarantine. But, because it is difficult to enforce, problems have arisen when there has been resistance to this authority: what options are open for dealing with people who choose not to obey?

As for transportation, care should be taken that ambulance staff and receiving staff are notified of the patient's communicable status. Both patient and transporting staff should wear protective clothing and face masks when warranted.

Patient Placement Issues

The use of standard precautions obviates the requirement for most patient placement in private rooms, but private room placement is necessary under some conditions:

- **Airborne transmission**: Airborne precautions must be used. Room should have negative pressure if possible.
- **Droplet transmission**: Droplet precautions must be used. Patient may share a room with another patient infected with the same microorganism if there are no other contraindications.
- **Microorganism transmitted by contact**: Contact precautions must be used. Patient may share a room with a patient colonized or infected by the same microorganism.
- **Contaminated environment**: Patients producing large amounts of body fluids or waste, such as blood or stool that cannot be contained should be placed in a private room.
- **Poor hygiene**: Patients not willing or are too confused or unable to properly maintain hygiene should be placed in private rooms.
- **Private rooms** should be assigned, when possible, by admissions utilizing a list of specific diagnoses.

Transfer/Discharge Planning

Infection control and transfer/discharge planning must be a joint effort so that the transfer and discharge documents provide the information that the individual or staff at transfer facilities need. Information should include:

- Contact telephone numbers/email addresses/street addresses for IPC to contact patient for discharge surveillance and patient or transfer facility staff to contact IPC if problems arise
- An outline of risk factors for infection incurred during hospital stay, including stay in ICU or specialized units and use of invasive devices, such as central venous lines, ventilators, and/or urinary catheters
- Information sheets outlining signs of infection for all risk factors, especially if patient is discharged home without nursing care
- Public Health notification if indicated by local or state regulations
- Follow-up appointment dates, with physicians or infection control
- Specific directions for medication or treatments, especially important for antibiotics or wound treatment

Specific Infection Control Strategies in Obstetrics

Infection control strategies for obstetrics comprise the following efforts to identify and prevent infections:

- Temperature monitoring will identify most infections for inpatients.
- Post-discharge questionnaires or telephone surveys of patients and physicians can identify potential problems.
- Preoperative shaving should be replaced with clipping and depilatories or done immediately prior to procedures.
- Glucose/blood sugar control increases resistance to infection.
- Antibiotic prophylaxis should be with 60 minutes of incision and discontinued within 24 hours to provide protection and prevent resistance.
- Central venous lines using internal jugular of femoral sites should be avoided if possible or used for short periods of time. PICCs have lower infection rates. Coated catheters and use of heparin flushes may also lower chances of infection.
- Alcohol-based hand sanitizers should be used properly before and after all patient contact.
- Nursing/breast care instruction should be provided to all maternal patients.

Common Types of Infections of Concern

Most infections in the obstetric units are caused by migration and multiplication of the normal vaginal and cervical flora although exogenous sources are sometimes implicated. Common types of infections include the following:

- Post-partum endometriosis most-often related to Caesareans or prolonged difficult vaginal deliveries with rupture of membranes. The infection may spread and can develop into sepsis.
- Surgical site infections for Caesarean and episiotomy, resulting in serious infection if not promptly identified and treated. While most infective agents are endogenous, exogenous organisms, such as *Staphylococcus aureus* may be causal.
- Urinary infections usually related to catheterization. They are common after delivery.
- Mastitis, usually occurring after discharge. It is usually related to poor maternal nursing practices, such as improper care of nipples, poor feeding technique, pumping-related issues, and not emptying breasts.
- Blood-stream infection is uncommon and usually relates to *E. coli*. It is also associated with central venous lines.
- Intra-amniotic infection, most often related to rupture of membranes and prolonged labor, resulting in polymicrobial infection from normal flora.

Infection Control in Labor and Delivery Units during the COVID-19 Pandemic

Infection control in labor and delivery units for those with high risk for COVID-19 (SARS-CoV-2) must protect the patient, a support person, the neonate, and the staff. Patients with existing or suspected COVID-19 infection should be tested and others at the discretion of the facility. All infection control procedures, including appropriate use of PPE, must be followed. Facilities may limit visitors to one essential support person, but any visitors to the unit should be screened for COVID-19 and for fever before allowed access and must wear face masks and appropriate PPE as determined by the facility. The visitors are restricted to only the patient's room and no other areas in the facility, such as the nursery. Infected patients and their infants should be isolated from other patients. Neonates of an infected mother are considered infected as well. Isolating neonates in the NICU should be avoided, if possible, because of risk to other neonates. Mothers with infection may usually decide if they want the child isolated with them or away from them although if the mother or the neonate is seriously ill, separation is necessary.

Specific Infection Prevention Strategies For Neurological/Spinal Cord Injuries

Common Types of Infections of Concern

The most common infections in **neurology/spinal cord injuries** are the following:

- **Urinary tract infections** are very common and related to clean or sterile intermittent or continuous catheterization as well as urinary stasis and/or anatomic abnormalities. Infection is most often related to intestinal flora. Infections about the urethra and perineal skin are often related to condom catheter use. Bacteremia can result from severe infections.
- **Decubiti** occur in about 1/3 of patients with spinal cord injuries and are a frequent cause of infection that can invade underlying bone. Ulcers are related to pressure and contamination. Decubiti often are colonized by multiple organisms, both aerobic and anaerobic. While skin openings may be small, underlying subcutaneous and muscle tissue may be extensively compromised.
- **Respiratory tract infections**, usually pneumonia, affects about 1/3 of patients with high cervical injuries, related to invasive devices for ventilation or weakness of muscles that decreases cough reflex.

Infection Prevention Strategies

Infection control strategies for the common infections in **neurological/ spinal cord injuries** include:

- **Urinary tract infection:** Patients should be monitored for fever and/or changes in spasms or voiding habits that may indicate infection. When possible, intermittent catheterization (sterile rather than clean in the hospital) should be used rather than continuous. Antibiotic prophylaxis has not proven to be effective but bacterial interference, colonizing of the urinary tract with nonpathogenic *E. coli 83972,* has shown promising results.
- **Decubiti:** Procedures for regular monitoring of skin condition, turning patients, and avoiding friction to prevent pressure from developing are critical. Both staff and patients must be educated about prevention and skin care and cleanliness. Nutrition and hydration must be adequate to maintain integrity of the skin.
- **Respiratory infections**: Proper use of ventilation equipment must be monitored. Assisted coughing, such as through respiratory therapy and postural drainage, can reduce infections. Prophylactic antibiotics are not recommended, but patients should receive immunizations for pneumonia.

Specific Infection Prevention Strategies in Oncology

Infection control strategies for oncology patients are aimed first at preventing infections due to these individuals' immunocompromised state:

- Transmission-based precautions are appropriate for some patients, especially those immunocompromised.
- Handwashing and aseptic techniques are especially important for person-to-person transmission.
- Central venous line precautions include using antimicrobial/antiseptic-coated catheters, using clear dressings that do not obscure site, and observing carefully for signs of infection.
- Protective isolation with use of glove and gown barriers has proven to be effective in reducing the spread of infection but is costly and not recommended for all patients.
- Total protected environments can be difficult to provide and expensive but may be used in selected case.
- Air filtration using HEPA filtered air can be used to maintain ultra-clean air in a patient's room. The use of particulate respirators, such as the HEPA and N95 mask, by either the patient or the staff, can help to reduce inhaled pathogens.

Common Types of Infections of Concern

Oncology patients are often especially at risk for both healthcare-associated and community-acquired infections because of decreased immunity, surgeries, invasive devices, and extended hospitalizations. Most infections are related to normal flora so cultures do not always identify the causative agent. Bacterial infections are the most common, followed by fungus infections and viral infections. Common infections include:

- **Respiratory tract infections** may range from rhinitis to pneumonia, occurring most commonly in patients with leukemia, lymphoma, or solid tumors involving the head, neck, or lungs.
- **Bloodstream infections** pose special risks for hematologic malignancies, but can be related to the use of tunneled central venous lines, antibiotic resistance causing an increase in Gram-positive organisms, and surgical procedures.
- **Urinary tract infections** are common and often related to catheterization.
- **Surgical site infections** are more common with extensive surgical procedures.
- **Gastrointestinal infections** may be hard to differentiate from diarrhea caused by chemotherapy, but surgery and antibiotics are risk factors.

Infection Control in Oncology Units during the COVID-19 Pandemic

Infection control in oncology units for those with high risk for COVID-19 (SARS-CoV-2) include measures to protect the patient and healthcare providers. Patients should be screened before appointments or hospitalization to determine if they have symptoms of COVID-19 or have had recent exposure. When possible, appointments may be conducted via telemedicine rather than in person. Visitors should be limited, typically with only video or telephone calls permitted although pediatric patients are usually allowed one parent or guardian to be present. Strict isolation procedures must be followed. Masks and the use of hand sanitizer are required for all outpatients and visitors, and social distancing must be maintained. Any patient suspected of having COVID-19 must be tested. All high touch surfaces must be frequently cleaned with disinfectant.

Specific Infection Prevention Strategies for Transplant Patients

Potential Sources of Infection

Infections pose a serious threat to transplant patients, especially during the first year. While opportunistic infections have decreased, healthcare-associated infections have increased, with the most being related to bacterial infections. Transplant patients consistently show higher rates of infection than other patients. There are numerous potential sources:

- Donor-infected organs can transmit HBV, HBC, Herpesvirus, HIV, Human-T-cell leukemia virus, type I. Additionally, donors who are immunocompromised prior to harvesting of the organs may have nosocomial bacterial or fungal infections that can be transmitted. Organs can also become infected during harvesting.
- Healthcare workers may transmit pathogens through droplets, airborne particles, or contact, frequently transmitting pathogens on their hands or clothing.
- Blood and blood products can transmit CMV, but transmission is rare. HCV transmission has been reduced to <1%.
- Environmental reservoirs/sources can include the water system, demolition activities, equipment, and surfaces. Some pathogens, such as MRSA and VRE, may be endemic to the hospital environment.

Kidney Transplant Patients

Kidney transplant patients are at risk for rejection (as are all transplant recipients) and infection.

- Urinary catheterization results in infection in about 50% of patients and poses a danger to the kidney if the infection spreads or becomes systemic; however, most infections, especially after three months, are asymptomatic and self-limiting.
- Diabetes mellitus that develops shortly after transplant poses a higher risk of infection than chronic diabetes that existed prior to transplant.
- CMV-positive donor kidneys in young patients increase the risk of serious viral infections.
- Delayed graft function may increase risk of bacterial infection.
- History of chronic pyelonephritis increases postoperative risk of infection.
- Cadaver donor organs are related to post-operative infection, possibly because of contamination or trauma to the organ during harvesting.
- Preoperative hemodialysis increases risk of bacteremia.
- Acute rejection episodes increase risk of bacteremia.

Liver Transplant Patients

Immunosuppression as well as the type of surgery and host responses can all be implicated as risk factors for different types of transplant patients. Liver transplant patients face a host of risk factors because long-term liver disease has often resulted in general debilitation and malnutrition.

- Endogenous infection of invasive candidiasis is common.
- Infections may arise from vascular and anastomotic complications.
- Hepatic artery thrombosis can result in gangrene and abscess formation.
- Biliary changes may cause blockage and stone formation, leading to infection.
- T-tubes inserted during surgery to maintain patency of anastomoses are prone to infections.
- Portal vein thrombosis may lead to infection.
- HCV in the host may recur, compromising the new liver and often leading to fungal infections.
- Gastrointestinal colonization of VRE is increasingly common in liver transplant patients, causing minor clinical difference in the host but serving as a reservoir of infection in the facility.

Heart and/or Lung Transplant Patients

Heart and/or lung transplant patients are especially susceptible to bacterial pulmonary infections, with infections occurring in 35-48% of hosts. Some risk factors place patients at increased risk:

- CMV positive donor places sero-negative heart and/or lung and transplant patients at increased risk for postoperative CMV pneumonia, invasive aspergillosis, and pulmonary bacterial infections.
- Preoperative colonization of *Aspergillus fumigatus* in cystic fibrosis patients poses the risk of postoperative tracheobronchial aspergillosis.
- Colonization of resistant Pseudomonas strains in the damaged lungs, especially in cystic fibrosis patients, can result in residual infection in other parts of the respiratory tract, providing a source of infection for the donor organs.
- Invasive devices such as central venous lines, circulatory assist devices, and ventilators may result in colonization and infection, especially pneumonia and sternal surgical site infections.
- Decreased ability to cough and clear mucous because of loss of cough reflex, pain, or weakness can contribute to pneumonia.

Small Bowel Transplant Patients

Small bowel transplants use primarily cadaveric donors to treat intestinal failure requiring parenteral nutrition to provide adequate nutrition and hydration. Small bowel transplants may be done alone or with liver or other organ transplants. About two-thirds of the patients are pediatric. However, there is significant morbidity and mortality related to the small bowel transplants with 5-

year survival rates <50%. Virtually all recipients develop infection to some degree, sometimes with multiple recurrences. About 55% of deaths are caused by sepsis.

- Intensive immunosuppression may result in adenoviral infections of the small intestine as well as bacterial and fungal infections.
- Cytomegalovirus or Epstein-Barr infections caused by sero-positive donors to sero-negative recipients can lead to severe complications as large viral loads may be transmitted with the transplantation.
- Multivisceral grafts increase the chances of infection.
- Bacterial translocation may result in intra-abdominal infections and abscess formation.

Pancreas Transplant Patients

Pancreas transplants have the highest rate of complications compared to other transplants, resulting in infection rates that range from 7-50%. Pancreas transplants may be done with (>90%) or after kidney transplants or alone for those who have type I diabetes but functioning kidneys. There are a number of factors that increase risk:

- Underlying disease, such as uremia and diabetes, with immunosuppression impairs healing and increases the susceptibility to infection.
- Enteric drainage of pancreatic enzymes into the bowel predisposes to infections by enteric bacteria.
- Peritoneal cavity drainage of enzymes provides a medium for pathogenic agents and increases the risk of infection and has a high rate of mortality.
- Anastomosis of pancreas to an internal organ may result in leakage that increases chance of infection.
- Graft necrosis associated with vessel thrombosis or rejection provides another medium for pathogenic agents and can result in infection.

Time of Onset for Infections in Transplant Patients

Days 1-30: Infections that arise in the early postoperative period are often surgical site infections or other healthcare-associated infections.

- Bacterial infections are most common.
- Fungal infections, especially *Candidiasis* and *Aspergillus* usually occur early.
- Viral infections are less common but usually involve HSV or the herpesvirus, HHV-6.

Days 31-180: Most infections during this time period are opportunistic infections rather than nosocomial because of continued immunosuppression that increases susceptibility.

- CMV is the most common pathogen for all types of transplants.
- HBV and HCV may reactivate about 90 days after surgery.
- Various pathogens may cause infections, including *Mycobacterium tuberculosis* and *Nocardia.*

Days 181 and onward: Infections acquired after 6 months are usually community-acquired rather than healthcare-associated although the risk of opportunistic infections remains as well. Varicella zoster virus and dematiaceous fungi infections are late infections, usually after 6 months.

Common Viral Pathogens of Transplant Patients

Cytomegalovirus (CMV)

Cytomegalovirus (CMV) is the most common pathogen related to transplant infections affecting 40-90% of recipients. There are three types:

- **Primary infection**: The seropositive organ is transplanted into a seronegative recipient, posing the most risk of rejection and other complications.
- **Reactivation infection**: A latent viral infection reactivates in response to immunosuppression.
- **Superinfection**: A new strain of the virus infects a seropositive recipient.

Infection control strategies may vary:

- Serologic matching of donor and recipients can prevent transmission; however, the limited number of seronegative transplant organs may preclude transplant surgery for many patients.
- Early diagnosis with the CMV antigenemia assay can yield information about the degree of infection and likelihood of CMV disease.
- Targeting patients at the highest risk for disease through surveillance methods, such as monitoring with CVM antigenemia assay and instituting prophylaxis to prevent asymptomatic disease from activating, is the most practical infection control.

Human Herpesvirus-6 (HHV-6)

Human herpesvirus-6 is the newest identified viral pathogen of transplant patients, infecting 31-55% of solid organ transplants with the usual onset of symptoms (bone marrow suppression, encephalopathy, fever, and pneumonia) about 2-4 weeks after transplant. HHV-6 is a DNA virus distinct from other herpesviruses but most like CMV. There are two variants of the disease HHV-6A and HHV-6B. HHV-6A is more virulent than HHV-6B, but at the current time HHV-6B is the most common infection. HHV-7 is a closely related virus that often co-infects, but its significance is not yet established. Most infection with HHV-6 is endogenous from reactivation of latent virus acquired in early childhood, but primary donor transmission can also occur.

Infection control strategies include:

- Early diagnosis with culture assay.
- Antiviral medications ganciclovir and foscarnet are effective against HHV-6 infection.
- Antiviral prophylaxis with ganciclovir has been given BID for a week prior pre-stem cell transplant and 120 posts. Studies demonstrated a significant reduction in infection for those receiving prophylaxis.

Herpes Simplex Virus (HSV) and Varicella-Zoster

Herpes simplex virus infection may occur from reactivation or primary transmission from the donor. Infection may become disseminated, most frequently affecting the liver with a high mortality rate.

Infection control strategies include:

- Serologic matching can prevent primary transmission but the limited supply of organs may make this impractical.
- Antiviral prophylaxis with low dose Acyclovir (200-400 mg TID) for 1-3 months has proven very effective in preventing HSV infections.

Varicella-zoster virus infection may result in primary infection over two years from the time of transplant, resulting in visceral dissemination and sometimes death. This delay time may cause the symptoms to be misdiagnosed.

Infection control strategies include:

- Immunization has proven to be safe and highly effective, reducing the incidence of infection and the severity.
- VZ immunoglobulin is given to susceptible transplant patients exposed to VZV, but is not completely protective.
- High-dose acyclovir during the 2-3 week incubation period may reduce incidence and severity of infection.

Hepatitis B (HBV)

Hepatitis B virus is a concern for both liver and kidney transplant patients because infection markedly increases mortality rates. HBV is transmitted in blood, semen, and vaginal fluids. Recurrence of HBV is most common in those already seropositive (about 83%) compared to those seronegative (about 58%) at the time of transplant, but both figures are high. Mutant varieties of HBV (precore mutants) pose an even greater threat of graft loss. HBV progresses more slowly in kidney transplant patients than in liver transplant patients, with cirrhosis and death occurring in 6-8 years compared to 2-2.5 years for liver transplant patients.

Infection control strategies include:

- Standard precautions should prevent bloodborne transmission.
- Antiviral prophylaxis with Hepatitis B Immune Globulin (HBIG) has markedly reduced recurrence rates.
- Combination therapy with HBIG and lamivudine prevents recurrence disease in >90% of liver transplant patients infected with HBV.
- Hepatitis B vaccine should be provided to adults at risk, especially staff working with patients with HBV. Children are now routinely immunized.

Hepatitis C (HCV)

Hepatitis C virus causes end-stage liver disease in about half of the liver transplant patients, and 95% remain with viremia after transplant, resulting in recurrence in 30-70% of patients within a year. HCV is also common in hemodialysis patients as it is a bloodborne pathogen, and 10-60% of rental transplant patients develop chronic liver disease. Co-infection with HGV occurs in about 25% without clinical impact. Most infections are reactivation, but primary transmission can occur.

Infection control strategies include:

- Standard precautions prevent bloodborne transmission. Up to 10% of those with needle stick injuries develop HCV.
- Antiviral prophylaxis using HBIG developed for hepatitis B has been shown to reduce incidence of HCV viremia because it also contains some antibodies to HCV. An investigational Hepatitis C Immune Globulin, Civacir, is currently in trials to evaluate its prevention of recurrence of HCV infection in liver transplant patients. Civacir is made from pooled blood and serum of individuals with antibodies to HCV.

Adenoviruses (AdV)

Adenoviruses (AdV) comprise at least 49 serotypes and cause infections in up to 10% of pediatric transplant pediatric patients and 15% of adult, especially affecting those receiving bone marrow transplants. AdV can cause disseminated disease resulting in hemorrhagic cystitis (kidney transplants), hepatitis (liver transplants), conjunctivitis, and pneumonitis (lung transplants). AdV 11, 34, 35 are implicated in hemorrhagic cystitis while 2, 5, 7, and 9 are implicated in pulmonary infection, especially in children. Infection may be from seropositive donors or reactivation. Nosocomial outbreaks have occurred. A recent military study demonstrated serotypes 4 and 7 were transmitted through asymptomatic shedders via the respiratory tract.

Infection control strategies include:

- Ribavirin, ganciclovir, and IgG have been tried with varying reports as to effectiveness.
- Vaccine (serotypes 4 and 7) was available to the military from the 1970s to 1990s and was successful, but the vaccine was lost. A new version of vaccine for serotypes 4 and 7 was introduced in 2011 and is approved for use in military personnel ages 17 to 50.
- Droplet precautions should be considered, especially with respiratory infection.

BK Virus (BKV)

BK virus (BKV) has recently emerged as a cause of renal dysfunction after transplant, resulting in loss of graft. BKV is a DNA polyomavirus, and is ubiquitous, with about 80% of the population seropositive. The transmission mode is not yet established. JC virus (JCV) often coinfects and may be a cause of nephropathy as well. About 5% of kidney transplant patients develop BKV infection (hemorrhagic and nonhemorrhagic urinary infection, nephritis, increase in creatinine, and replication of decoy cells of the urinary epithelium), usually reactivation, within 3-24 months after surgery. Diagnosis is by PCR assay.

Infection control strategies include:

- Reduction in immunosuppressive medications with the addition of cidofovir (10-20% of the recommended dose of cidofovir) has been the treatment of choice with varying degrees of effectiveness.
- Leflunomide at immunosuppressive doses was shown in one study to eradicate BK virus. Other studies are ongoing or in progress.

Common Bacterial Infections of Transplant Patients

Mycobacterium Tuberculosis

Mycobacterium tuberculosis in transplant patients occurs in 0.35-5% of patients, a relatively low number, but the mortality rate for those infected is 30%. About a third of those infected develop disseminated disease involving extrapulmonary sites that include the gastrointestinal tract, the urinary tract, and the central nervous system. While most *M. tuberculosis* infection is reactivation of latent disease, nosocomial transmission of infection has occurred, especially if patients are undiagnosed so that airborne precautions are not used. Transmission has also occurred from living and cadaveric donor organs. Infection control strategies include:

- Airborne precautions for diagnosed or suspected infections.
- Identifying infected patients/staff includes tuberculin skin testing followed by confirming radiography.
- Prophylaxis with Isoniazid:
    - Tuberculin reactivity ≥ 5mm
    - Newly-converted positive tuberculin
    - Chest-x-ray showing old active TB with no prior treatment or inadequate treatment
    - Close contact with infected individual
    - Seropositive TB donor organ

Staphylococcus Aureus and Enterococci

Staphylococcus aureus is the most common cause of bacterial infection in liver, heart, kidney, and pancreas transplant patients with >50% of infections occurring in the ICU. Intravascular cannulas cause about 54% of MRSA infections, but nosocomial transmission occurs. While nasal colonization has been implicated in infection in liver transplant patients, using mupirocin to eradicate nasal colonization has not affected infection rates, probably because of nosocomial transmission with exogenous colonization. Isolate studies have demonstrated nosocomial cross-transmission.

Enterococci are a primary concern for liver transplant patients. Vancomycin-resistant *Enterococcus faecium* (VREF) cause 10-15% of liver failures, according to recent studies. Nosocomial transmission occurs frequently, especially with prolonged hospitalization and ICU stay. Intra-abdominal infections occur about 40 days after surgery with mortality rates of 23-50%. VREF colonization puts patients at continued risk for infection and poses a reservoir for healthcare-associated infections. Antibiotics have been ineffective in reducing mortality rates.

Nocardia

Nocardia infections occur in about 2-4% of organ transplant recipients with onset from 2-8 months after surgery with pulmonary infection common but 17-38% of those infected have central nervous system involvement which often includes brain abscesses. Lung, heart, and intestinal transplants have the highest rates of infection. Mortality rates are high for those who are infected. *Nocardia* is found in the soil and decaying vegetation, and transmission is through inhalation. Some species are more virulent than others. Healthcare-associated infections have occurred in clusters in transplant units related to environmental dust. Risk factors include high dose cortisone, high levels of calcineurin inhibitors (cyclosporine and tacrolimus), and CMV infection within 6 months. Calcineurin inhibitors are commonly used for immunosuppression for kidney transplants.

Infection control strategies include:

- Environmental monitoring
- Antibiotic prophylaxis with trimethoprim-sulfamethoxazole is effective.
- Airborne precautions of those infected have been recommended by some.

Legionella

Legionella pneumonia occurs in 2-9% of solid organ recipients with *Legionella pneumophila* and *Legionella micdadei* the most common forms. Some studies have reported incidence as high as 17% in heart transplant patients. Inhalation of aerosols may transmit the disease but aspiration of the bacteria occurs more frequently. *Legionella* has been traced to potable water systems providing hospital drinking water, ice machines, and ultrasonic nebulizers. Patients may develop pneumonia with or without characteristic dense nodular areas and cavitation, pericarditis, necrotizing cellulitis, and graft rejection.

Infection control strategies include:

- Routine annual culturing of water supply to check for Legionella, especially important if there are large numbers of transplant patients.
- Positive water culture should result in the laboratory having diagnostic tests, such as urinary antigen, available.
- Early diagnosis of high-risk patients should be done by routine urinary antigen testing up to two times weekly.
- Water disinfecting methods:
  - Superheating water to 70° C and flushing distal outlets.
  - Installing copper-silver ionization units.

Common Fungal Infections of Transplant Patients

Candidiasis

Candidiasis is the most common fungal infection in transplant patients, with the exception of heart transplants. While some infections are mild, thrush and cystitis, others are invasive and life threatening, especially with the immunocompromised patient. Infection of all organs is about 5%, but liver and pancreas transplant patients have infection rates of 15-30%. Infection may occur in the surgical site or be disseminated, posing a serious threat to the site of anastomosis. Almost all transmission of Candida is nosocomial. Endogenous transmission is common in liver transplants, but heart and lung transplants are often infected from the donor organs. Some cases have been traced to contaminated medical equipment.

Infection control strategies include:

- Antiviral prophylaxis with 1-2 months of fluconazole post-transplant is used at some centers, but azole-resistant strains are appearing, and there is an associated increase in *aspergillus*, so prophylaxis may be considered for only high-risk patients.
- Monitoring of invasive devices to ensure that they are not contaminated with *candida.*

Aspergillus

Aspergillus infections primarily involve pneumonia and sinusitis, but 25-35% disseminate systemically, and *Aspergillus* pneumonia infections have mortality rates to 85%. *Aspergillus* is a serious fungal infection in immunocompromised transplant patients, especially lung transplant patients with 8% infection rates within 9 months of surgery. Liver transplant patients have infection rates of 1-4% but disease occurs earlier, within 2-4 weeks. Heart transplant infection rates are 1-6% with disease within 1-2 months. Aspergillus affects renal transplants the least with <1% infection rates. Prophylaxis with antifungals has not proven to be effective.

Infection control strategies include:

- Monitoring environment and improving air filtration with HEPA filtration or use of laminar air flow rooms for patients at high risk.
- Construction precautions to prevent dust and debris from circulating in patient care areas.
- Standard precautions
- High resolution CT scans should be used for early diagnosis rather than chest x-rays so treatment with voriconazole (drug of choice) can begin.

Pneumocystis Jirovecii

Pneumocystis jirovecii (formerly *carinii)* was classified for many years as a Protozoan, but DNA analysis has caused it to be reclassified as a fungus, though it does not respond to antifungal treatment. The variety that causes *Pneumocystis* pneumonia, commonly referred to as PCP, has been renamed as *Pneumocystis jirovecii.* While most infection is thought to be endogenous, there is sufficient evidence that person-to-person transmission has occurred in nosocomial outbreaks affecting transplant patients in contact with PCP infected HIV patients. While renal, heart, and liver transplant patients are vulnerable to *Pneumocystis,* without prophylaxis 80% of lung transplants become infected, with infection usually occurring 4 months after surgery although the length of time varies depending upon the degree of immunosuppression.

Infection control strategies include:

- Transmission precautions to separate PCP-infected patients from contact with transplant patients.
- Prophylaxis with trimethoprim-sulfamethoxazole should be given to all transplant patients. There is no consensus on the length of prophylaxis, with durations varying from 6-12 months to indefinite.

Specific Infection Prevention Strategies for Burn Patients

Burn Wound Cellulitis

Burn patients are at exceptional risk for infection because the barrier of protective skin is breached, eschar provides a medium for microorganisms, and immunosuppression occurs. Classifying burn infections can be done in different ways. The CDC has guidelines for classification of unexcised burns.

Burn wound cellulitis is characterized by erythema of uninjured tissue around burns that is more than the usual irritation and includes one of the following:

- Pain, tenderness, and edema
- Systemic signs of infection
- Progressive erythema and edema
- Lymphangitis/lymphadenitis

This type of infection usually suggests a need for different antimicrobial treatment. When the erythema spreads beyond 1-2 cm from the burn, it may be indicative of infection with β-hemolytic *Streptococcus.*

Burn Wound Impetigo

Burn wound impetigo is an infection of previously healing and re-epithelialized partial-thickness burns, skin grafts, or donor sites. One important criterion for burn wound impetigo is that the deterioration is not caused by mechanical disruption of the tissue or by a failure to completely excise the wound but by an invading organism. Burn wound impetigo can occur with or without indications of systemic infection, such as temperature >38.4 °C, leukocytosis, and/or thrombocytopenia, may be present as well. The wound may develop multiple small superficial abscesses that infect and erode the tissue. The most common cause of burn wound impetigo is *Staphylococcus aureus.* Prompt debridement of the abscesses, cleansing of the area, and application of topical antimicrobials, such as Bactroban, must be done in order to stop the spread of the infection. A change in antimicrobial treatment may be necessary as well.

Invasive Infection in Unexcised Burns

Invasive infection in unexcised burns occurs when microorganisms invade partial or full thickness burns, causing a change in the appearance of the burn as well as separation and/or dark discoloration of the eschar. Other evidence of infection may include:

- Inflammation of surrounding tissue
- Biopsy indicating invasion of microorganisms into adjacent uninjured tissue
- Blood culture isolating organisms.
- Signs of systemic infection, such as hypotension, leukocytosis, hypothermia, or hyperthermia.

The systemic response to a severe burn can be similar to that of an invasive infection, so careful observation of the wound and biopsy should be done because mortality rates increase markedly when the organism invades the blood stream.

Staphylococcus aureus, Pseudomonas aeruginosa, Enterococci, *Enterobacter* spp. and *Escherichia coli* are the most frequent causes of infection. Since the frequent use of antimicrobials with burn patients, there has been a subsequent increase in the number of *Aspergillus* fungal infections.

Open Burn-Related Surgical Wound Infection

Open burn-related surgical wound infection usually involves an invasive infection of the excised burn site, grafts, or donor sites, and the invasive organisms are similar to those of unexcised wounds, with *Staphylococcus aureus* and *Aspergillus* frequent causative agents. The wound presents with culture-positive purulent exudate and includes at least one of the following:

- Loss of graft, synthetic or biologic
- Change in wound appearance
- Erythema around the periphery of the burn wound in adjacent tissue
- Systemic signs of infections, such as temperature 38.4 °C, leukocytosis, and/or thrombocytopenia

Surface colonization by organisms in the wound may not be the same as the invading agent, so wound biopsy may be necessary. For example, *Candida albicans* frequently colonizes but rarely invades unless the immune system is severely depressed, often an impending sign of death. Changes of antimicrobial treatment as well as topical treatments are usually indicated for open burn related surgical wound infections.

COMMON RESERVOIRS FOR ORGANISMS THAT INFECT BURNS

There are a number of reservoirs for organisms that infect burns. Many of these reservoirs can serve as sources for transmission on the hands of healthcare workers:

- **Burn wounds** are colonized within the first few hours by Gram-positive organisms from sweat glands and hair follicles and within days by Gram-negative organisms, so collectively the burn wounds of all patients on the unit may harbor organisms that can spread from one patient to another.
- **Gastrointestinal tract flora** can contaminate burn wounds directly if wounds are in proximity to fecal material or indirectly through cross contamination.
- **Normal flora**, especially Gram-positive cocci, on the skin are the cause of early burn infections and an increasingly important reservoir, with nasal colonization often implicated in burn infections.
- **Environment** can harbor organisms on many inanimate surfaces. Hydrotherapy equipment has been a frequent cause of wound infection as contaminated equipment spreads the infection to subsequent patients being treated.

INFECTION PREVENTION STRATEGIES IN BURN UNITS

Strategies for preventing and controlling transmission of infection in burn units include the following:

- Handwashing and sanitizing before and after every patient contact.
- Barriers such as gloves and water-impermeable aprons or gowns to reduce contact transmission.
- Environmental controls include providing patients with individual equipment, such as stethoscopes and blood pressure cuffs, and thorough cleaning and disinfecting of all surfaces. Mattress covers should be checked. Gloves should be worn to use computers and keyboard covers cleaned daily.
- Raw fruits and vegetables should not be fed to patients or allowed to contaminate kitchen utensils.
- Surveillance of all burn patients that might serve as reservoirs of infection, including convalescent patients no longer in acute care.
- Use of topical antimicrobials, such as silver sulfadiazine, to control infection, but with testing of outbreak strains for resistance.
- Protocol for systemic antimicrobial to treat active infection but avoid development of resistance.
- Early wound excision and closure to reduce wound infection.

USE OF HYDROTHERAPY

Hydrotherapy has been used in burn treatment but implicated in a number of nosocomial outbreaks, primarily of *Pseudomonas aeruginosa.* In some cases, rigorous cleaning protocols have reduced infection; in others, suspension of hydrotherapy treatments was needed. Because of problems with infection, there has been decrease in the use of hydrotherapy. Methods to control transmission of infection include:

- Protocol for draining tub after use and cleaning and disinfecting all parts of the hydrotherapy tub and agitators, with a chlorine germicidal agent circulated through agitators. Tank to be rinsed and dried thoroughly.
- Environmental cleaning and disinfecting of complete area and transportation equipment.
- Disinfectant may be added to filled tank.
- Disposable plastic liners, shown to reduce but not eliminate infection.
- Barriers such as long gloves and aprons or gowns impervious to fluid to prevent contact with water or patient.
- Faucets without stream diverters or aerators, which might harbor organisms, flushed with hot and cold water before use.

Infection Control Issues in Patients with Cystic Fibrosis

Cystic fibrosis (mucoviscidosis) is a progressive congenital disease that particularly affects the pancreas and lungs causing digestive and respiratory problems. It is caused by a genetic defect that affects sodium chloride movement in cells, including mucosal cells that line the lungs, causing the production of thick mucus that clogs the lungs and provides a rich medium for bacteria. Cystic fibrosis patients usually suffer from recurrent respiratory infections of the lower respiratory tract. The most common infective agents are *Pseudomonas aeruginosa* and *Burkholderia cepacia* complex. Patients with chronic infections serve as reservoirs for patient-to-patient transmission of infection, with proximity and duration of contact as precipitating factors. Cystic fibrosis patients should be maintained on universal and droplet precautions and placed in private rooms or cohorted with someone with the same pathogen.

Infection Prevention Strategies for Healthcare-Associated Pneumonia

CDC recommendations for traditional preventive measures for healthcare-associated pneumonia include:

- Decreasing aspiration by the patient
- Preventing cross-contamination or colonization via hands of healthcare workers
- Appropriate disinfection or sterilization of respiratory-therapy devices
- Use of available vaccines to protect against particular infections
- Educating hospital staff and patients.

Research is looking to new measures for reducing oropharyngeal and gastric colonization by pathogenic microorganisms.

Infection Prevention Strategies in Respiratory Therapy

Respiratory equipment has been implicated as the cause of many healthcare-associated infections, so preventing and controlling transmission of infection during respiratory therapy is imperative. Control measures include:

- Specific procedures for different types of respiratory equipment/procedures
- Standard precautions at all times
- Cleaning all equipment prior to disinfecting/sterilizing
- Disinfecting/sterilizing all equipment as directed by manufacturer, with steam sterilization or high-level disinfection
- Disposable equipment used by only one patient and changed as directed by manufacturer
- Scheduled draining of condensate in ventilator/other tubing
- Using closed-continuous feed humidification system/ heat-moisture exchange (HME)
- HME changed daily
- Single-dose sterile medications used at all times
- Sterile/pasteurized nebulizer fluid administered aseptically
- Avoiding intubation when possible
- Avoid high-volume humidifiers unless sterilized daily and used with sterile water
- Nursing practices aimed at reducing pneumonia (turning, kinetic beds, Elevating the head of the bed, deep breathing, and coughing exercises)

Infection Prevention Strategies in the Operating Room

Strategies for preventing and controlling transmission of infection in operating rooms includes:

- Preoperative surgical scrubs for 3-5 minutes and aseptic techniques at all times
- Positive-pressure ventilation with respect to corridors and adjacent areas
- ≥15 air exchanges per hour (ACH) with at least three fresh air exchanges
- Filtering of all recirculated and fresh air though filters with 90% efficiency
- Horizontal laminar airflow or introduction of air at ceiling and exhaust near the floor level
- Operating room closed except to allow passage of essential equipment and staff
- Clean visible soiling with approved disinfectants between patients
- Wet-vacuum operating room at end of each day
- Sterilize surgical equipment and avoid use of flash sterilization
- Perform environmental sampling of surfaces or air as part of epidemiological investigation
- Establish protocols for patients with airborne precautions, such as tuberculosis

Infection Prevention Strategies in Hospital Nurseries

Because newborns, even those with communicable diseases acquired in utero, are not disease transmitters, isolation of these children is seldom an issue. On the other hand, neonates are quite susceptible to communicable disease organisms, so sterile precautions are necessary along with restrictions on contact.

Family visitation, beneficial to any child, carries potential risks of transmitting pathogens to neonates. While many hospitals allow unlimited visitation for immediate family – and this includes siblings because studies indicate bacterial colonization among neonates does not increase after sibling visits – all visitation needs to be screened to restrict those, regardless of age, who have been exposed to communicable diseases like chicken pox or tuberculosis or have symptoms of infectious diseases such as fever, diarrhea, or a droplet-producing cough.

Cohorting of Well Newborns

The nosocomial infection rate of *Serratia marcescens* in a pediatric cardiac ICU recently studied was correlated to patient census and nurse staffing indicating that, when neonate nurseries become overcrowded and/or the number of nurses is inadequate, transmission of healthcare-associated infections between infants either by airborne spread or by decreased distance between infants, can lead to inadvertent cross-contamination of equipment and exposure to transmitted pathogens.

Inadequate cohorting of infected infants can then also become a factor. **Cohorting** infants (separating newborns who have acquired the same type of infections and keeping them apart from well babies) has two advantages: it puts barriers before the spread of the infection and it assigns responsibility for the cohorted children to a specifically selected set of nursing and medical personnel.

Infection Prevention Strategies in Ambulatory Care Centers

Ambulatory care centers comprise a wide range of facilities, from those that are within the hospital to freestanding, prison-based, or physician's office surgical centers. They pose a particular challenge for the IP, who must work with personnel and computer systems in order to collect data. Numerator and denominator data may be difficult to establish, and patient populations may vary widely. Because stay is short-term, many infections or problems may present only after discharge. Control strategies include:

- Definitions that allow for comparison
- Procedures for surveillance and identifying staff to assist/train
- Targeting particular types of infections or populations
- Reporting procedures for results of surveillance
- Strict adherence to standards of asepsis and care
- Post-discharge surveillance: Letters, telephone calls to patients and physicians
- Institution of outcomes and changes based on results
- Standard infection control procedures as per hospital operating rooms
- Identify sentinel events such as death or impairment resulting from nosocomial infection

Infection Control Strategies Related to Nutritional Services

Nutritional services staff should be trained to safely deliver food to patients. Disposable dishes and silverware are not necessary for infection control, but the following strategies are important:

- Nutritional services staff deliver food trays to all patients except for those on airborne precautions.
- Medical personnel deliver trays to those on airborne precautions.
- Trays must not be delivered if the overhead table is contaminated with equipment, such as a bedpan, or body fluids, such as blood. Medical staff must be notified so that they can remove the material, disinfect the table, and deliver the tray.
- Nutritional services staff pick up all trays except those on airborne precautions.
- Trays must not be picked up if they contain medical equipment (such as syringes) or are contaminated with body fluids or wastes. Medical staff must be notified so that they can resolve the issue. Nondisposable dishes or utensils contaminated with body fluids must be placed in a decontamination bag or container and taken to central supply services for reprocessing.

Disease-Specific Infection Control and Prevention

Tuberculosis

One of the world's deadliest diseases, TB infects about a third of the world's population; nearly 9 million each year come down with active cases. Two million die each year. Estimates of infection in the US are approximately 9 million. About 10% of those infected will develop active TB, which can be treated with antibiotics (as can infections, which are more easily treated). Recently, multi-drug resistant strains of *Mycobacterium tuberculosis* have appeared that are difficult to treat. Even more recently, extensively multi-drug resistant strains are being encountered that are virtually impossible to treat with existing drugs.

Tubercular patients can infect other patients and healthcare workers, with the level of risk varying by setting, occupation, patient population, and effectiveness of TB infection control measures – higher in facilities that manage large numbers of smear-positive TB patients who do not receive rapid diagnosis, isolation, and treatment, particularly in the absence of other infection control measures. Ideally, TB patients are isolated in rooms specially engineered to reduce risk of transmission. Healthcare workers having contact with them should wear respirators.

CDC Guidelines

The primary emphasis of the TB infection control plan should be on achieving these three goals: early identification, isolation, and effective treatment of persons who have active TB. An effective control program should first use measures for identifying, isolating, and treating TB cases; training staff on TB and such practices as wearing respiratory protection and keeping doors to isolation rooms closed, and, third screening HCWs for TB infection and disease.

Buildings should be engineered to prevent the spread and reduce the concentration of infectious droplet nuclei through local exhaust ventilation, controlling direction of airflow to prevent contamination of air in areas adjacent to the infectious source, diluting and removing contaminated air via general ventilation, building rooms with reduced air pressure, and cleaning the air via air filtration or ultraviolet germicidal irradiation (UVGI).

Provide prompt triage for patients coming in for treatment who may have infectious TB, moving them quickly into isolation. Personal respiratory protective equipment should be used wherever the risk for infection with M. *tuberculosis* may be relatively higher.

Facility Ventilation Management

Crowded living conditions and poor ventilation are conducive to the transmission of *M. tuberculosis.* Epidemics of tuberculosis were quite common in American big city slums of the early 20th Century, and there are still troubling incidences of the disease in such overcrowded conditions as those found in many prisons.

Improvements in housing conditions help prevent outbreaks. In hospitals, ventilation systems may be supplemented with high efficiency particulate air (HEPA) filtration (which will also remove droplet nuclei from the air) and ultraviolet germicidal irradiation (UVGI) in high-risk areas. UVGI lamps can be used in ceiling or wall fixtures or within air ducts of ventilation systems. Such systems may be used along with negative pressure systems in rooms used for isolation of TV patients.

COVID-19

Infection control measures for COVID-19 (SARS-CoV-2) in the healthcare environment are as follows:

- **Daily environmental cleaning of patient rooms:** PPE (N95, gown, gloves, shield, or goggles) must be worn during cleaning. Disinfectants should be EPA-approved for emerging viral pathogens, including SARS-CoV-2. All surfaces and dedicated equipment in the room and bathroom must be wiped clean and disinfectants left in place or wet for required time. Cleaning should be done from dirty to clean, sides to center, high to low, left to right, or clockwise. Trash must be double bagged. Floors must be cleaned from farthest corner toward door. Any surfaces that are contaminated with body fluids must be disinfected immediately with bleach.
- **Terminal cleaning of patient rooms:** The door to the room must remain closed for 35 minutes for negative pressure rooms or those with a HEPA units and for 1 hour for non-negative pressure rooms. PPE, disinfectants, and cleaning procedures for floors and surfaces are similar to those used for daily cleaning, and all surfaces should be considered contaminated. Rooms should not have curtains, but all other linen should be double bagged. Ceilings and ceiling fixtures should be dry dusted and walls washed (top to bottom) with disposable pads. All wall fixtures, cabinets, counters, furnishings, and equipment must be disinfected. Trash must also be double bagged.
- **Patient transport**: Staff must wear full PPE and prepare the patient prior to transport. A patient who is not intubated should wear a mask and have the entire body below the neck covered with a sheet. If the patient is intubated, transport should wait long enough for aerosols to settle after intubation (45 minutes in negative pressure room and 3.5 hours in standard room). One staff member should open doors and ensure no surfaces are touched during transport, and staff moving the patient should touch only the equipment and no other surfaces.
- **Visitor policies:** Video visits only are allowed although exceptions may be made at the end of life to allow one family member to be present and one parent may usually stay with a child.
- **Nurse ratios**: Nurse-to-patient ratios have varied during the pandemic from the ideal of 1:1 or 1:2 for those in critical care. California, the only state with specific ratios required by law, waived those ratios in response to increased patient loads and inadequate staffing and this has been true throughout the United States.

Disinfection of COVID-19 Exposed Medical Equipment

Disinfection of used medical equipment associated with infection with COVID-19 (SARS-CoV-2) is consistent with standard high-level disinfection used for other highly infectious organisms. EPA-approved products will indicate that they are effective for SARS-CoV-2/COVID-19 and will have a registration number. Bleach (1:1000) readily kills the coronavirus. The EPA provides a list of disinfectants to use for COVID-19 (SARS-CoV-2)—List N. Non-invasive medical equipment, such as blood pressure cuffs and air hoses, have a low potential for spread of disease but should be cleaned according to manufacturer's recommendations, such as by wiping with EPA-approved isopropyl alcohol or sodium hypochlorite. This type of equipment should not be immersed. Semicritical and critical equipment that is contaminated with body fluids must be cleaned with water or soap and water before disinfection and/or sterilization.

Pertussis

Pertussis (also known as whooping cough) is primarily a disease whose greatest danger is to young children. In the United States, of the total reported 9 deaths from pertussis reported to the National

Center for Immunization and Respiratory Diseases, children 3 months of age or younger accounted for 100% of these deaths. Incidence has dropped more than 80% since the 1940's when an effective vaccine was introduced. Worldwide, however, there are nearly 161,000 deaths per year.

Pertussis is passed through expelled droplets. The first stage of the disease appears to be a head cold, but this is quickly followed by the second, paroxysmal stage, in which the patient has bursts, or paroxysms, of numerous, rapid coughs and may, in extreme case, turn blue. Complete recovery can take months. Prevention is by inoculation. Azithromycin and clarithromycin have some effectiveness in treatment (as erythromycin is no longer recommended). States provide information about cases of pertussis to the CDC, including demographic information, through the National Electronic Disease Surveillance System.

Herpes Simplex Virus

Signs of **genital herpes**, a sexually transmitted disease caused by the herpes simplex virus type 2 (HSV-2), are generally minimal, one or more blisters (if any) on or around the genitals or rectum that may never be noticed. Some do suffer recurrent painful genital sores.

Outbreaks are recurrent, decreasing over the years, and almost always being less severe and shorter than the first outbreak. More common in women, at least 45 million people ages 12 and older, or one out of six adolescents and adults, have had genital HSV infection in the US. Generally, the virus is passed only during sexual contact with someone who has a genital HSV-2 infection. Persons with herpes should abstain from sexual activity with uninfected partners when lesions or other symptoms of herpes are present. Since a condom may not cover all infected areas, even correct and consistent use of latex condoms cannot guarantee protection from genital herpes.

There is no treatment that can cure herpes, but antiviral medications can shorten and prevent outbreaks.

Meningitis

Meningitis (also called spinal meningitis) is an infection of the spinal cord and the fluid that surrounds the brain. The severity of illness and the treatment differ depending upon whether a case has been caused by a virus or bacterium, viral meningitis generally being less severe. Viral meningitis resolves without treatment, and bacterial meningitis can be treated with a number of effective antibiotics if treatment is started early.

Bacterial meningitis, while not highly contagious, is spread through the exchange of respiratory and throat secretions. However, anyone who has been in contact with meningococcal meningitis (HiB) is at increased risk of acquiring the infection. There are vaccines against Hib, against some serogroups of *N. meningitides,* and many types of *Streptococcus pneumoniae*. Inoculation is recommended at high school entry and for collegians in dormitories, microbiologists, military recruits, immune deficiency, and anyone traveling to areas of outbreak.

Vaccination to prevent meningitis due to *S. pneumoniae* (also called pneumococcal meningitis) is recommended for all persons over 65.

Dermatitis

It is the water in the chronic hand washing necessary in clinical settings that is the cause of irritant hand dermatitis (dry, fissured, inflamed and sometimes very painful skin), not so much the soap. Repeated wetting and drying removes protective oils, making the skin less pliable and more prone to cracking. Cleansing agents serve only as secondary agents that also remove protective lipids from the skin and change pH. Temperature of the water is also a factor, the warmer the water, the more protective oils that are removed.

Low humidity and cold weather aggravate the condition, and healthcare workers may be more prone to the condition if they have a history of eczema.

Hand dermatitis is a problem because it affects the hand's barriers to microorganisms, making them more prone to passing pathogens on. The best treatment is to ease up on hand washing and, therefore, reduce contact with patients until the condition clears up.

Ectoparasites

Ectoparasites, parasites that that live on the outside of a host, include such "bugs" as lice, fleas, ticks, mites, and scabies. Their potential danger is illustrated by a recent paper recounting several typhus deaths that occurred in the United States after contact with flying squirrels, which were presumably carrying lice.

Common sources are household pets whose vermin can be controlled with pesticides known to be safe to animals and humans. Precautions can be taken against encounters with ectoparasites such as ticks which carry Lyme Disease; they can be kept at bay by protectively covering the body from the waist down when walking in wooded areas. Infestations of head lice, body lice, scabies, and chiggers are common causes of rash and pruritus in children. Head lice are an annoyance, but body lice are a vector of human diseases, including typhus, relapsing fever, and trench fever. They are transmitted through infested clothing; the best way to control outbreaks is by changing and laundering clothes and linens.

Measles

After a long, successful campaign of encouraging measles vaccinations, measles has nearly been eradicated as a threat in the USA. However, the contagious virus causing it is frequently imported into the United States by persons from other countries, where measles continues to be a major killer: 207,500 deaths worldwide in 2019, most of them in Africa. Each imported measles case could start an outbreak, especially if under-vaccinated groups are exposed. Measles remains, worldwide, the leading cause of vaccine-preventable child mortality, with the remaining global disease rate primarily attributable to underutilization of measles vaccine in developing nations.

Mumps

Mumps is a viral infection whose symptoms are fever, headache, muscle aches, tiredness, and loss of appetite followed by swelling of salivary glands. It is spread through direct contact with respiratory secretions or saliva or through fomites anywhere between 3 days prior to appearing to about 9 days after. There is no treatment for the disease, which is self-resolving, but it can be prevented through use of the MMR (measles, mumps, and rubella) vaccine. Complications, which are very rare, can include encephalitis/meningitis, orchitis, oophoritis, mastitis, spontaneous abortion, and deafness, which is usually permanent.

Rubella

Since the introduction of the rubella vaccine in 1969, the number of cases of the disease, also known as German measles, in the United States has decreased 99%, from 57,686 cases in 1969 to 271 cases in 1999. There has been a recent increase due to an influx of adults who have not been immunized, most of them illegal immigrants from Mexico and Central America. Outbreaks have been identified in poultry and meat processing plants that employ large numbers of foreign-born workers. Though there are rare outcomes like thrombocytopenic purpura, encephalitis, neuritis, and orchitis, its greatest danger is to the unborn children of susceptible pregnant females; possible outcomes of intrauterine rubella infection include miscarriage, stillbirth, abortion, and combinations of birth defects. Rubella is transmitted through expelled droplets. It is prevented through vaccination with the MMR (measles, mumps, and rubella) vaccine.

Infection Prevention Strategies for the Use of Medical Maggots

Medical use of maggots is slowly regaining acceptance since FDA approval in 2004 as a medical device for wound debridement. Used extensively before the introduction of antibiotics, they fell out of favor, but maggots eat infected or necrotic tissue, cleaning the wound effectively and stimulating new tissue. The eggs are sterilized so the maggots do not transmit infection unless they become contaminated so careful handling is critical. They arrive in a sterile container, which should be examined to be sure it is intact. The maggots should be used right away, following prescribed procedures. Maggots excrete enzymes that can be very irritating to healthy tissue if too many are applied or if they are left in place for too long. Maggots are left in the wound for 48 hours and then must be carefully collected and disposed of in a red plastic biohazard bag tied and placed inside another bag to ensure that none escape and exposed of as hazardous waste.

Infection Control Strategies for the Use of Medical Leaches

In 2004, the FDA approved medical leeches as a medical device to relieve venous congestion, especially in skin grafts and reattachment/reimplantation.

Hirudo medicinalis is about 1-2 inches long before feeding. It has three jaws and bites into the tissue with teeth, which are surrounded by an oral sucker that aids attachment along with the rear ventral sucker. The teeth leave a bite mark. Leeches must be maintained in non-chlorinated water before use. While feeding, they will swell with about 15 mL of blood and then drop off after feeding. The wound will continue to bleed slowly, forming new venules. The leech should be retrieved with tweezers and immediately placed in a container of 70% alcohol and disposed of as medical waste. *Aeromonas hydrophila* lives in the gut of the leech and is necessary for the leeching function, but approximately 20% of patients develop infection, so prophylactic antibiotics are often given with treatment, especially for the immunocompromised.

Immunization Guidelines

Active and Passive Immunization

Active immunization utilizes antigens from parts of the infectious pathogen (acellular vaccines), attenuated (weakened) live organisms from disease-causing pathogens, or bacterial toxins treated with chemicals to cause the body to develop antibodies or T lymphocytes against the disease. Some vaccinations provide lifetime immunity but others lessen the severity of disease. Other vaccinations, such as tetanus, require boosters at particular intervals. Because active immunization contains antigens, they may put people who are immunosuppressed, such as those with AIDS or who are on immunosuppressive drugs or chemotherapy, at risk for contracting the disease.

Passive immunization utilizes antibodies, immune globulin, from another person or animal that was actively immunized against a disease. These antibodies survive for about 14-21 days, conferring temporary resistance to a disease. One advantage to passive immunization is that it provides protection right away. Immune globulin derived from animals, such as horses, poses more of a potential for adverse allergic reactions than human-derived immune globulin.

Review Video: Immunomodulators and Immunosuppressive Agents
Visit mometrix.com/academy and enter code: 666131

Issues Related to Immunization Status of Patients

The patient's immunization status is often neglected and not questioned during the admission procedure, so this information is frequently not in the patient's record. While most individuals who went to school in the United States were required to have childhood vaccinations, many adults do not take influenza, mumps, measles, chicken pox, hepatitis B or tetanus booster. Many others are not tested for tuberculosis, so immunization of patients is an area of concern for IPs. The IP should work with admissions to ensure that all patients are queried about their immunization status, including the last influenza shot and last tetanus booster. When appropriate, patients should be offered immunizations during hospitalization, especially if there is a possibility of exposure to infective agents as occurs with outbreaks. Ideally, immunizations would be given prior to hospitalization, but this involves consistently educating physicians of the need through an ongoing infection control education program.

Immunization Procedures for Patients Exposed to Influenza

Influenza, a viral respiratory disease, is transmitted by person-to-person contact through droplets generated when people sneeze or cough as well as by direct contact with sputum. Those exposed may be infectious the day before symptoms and five days after, and outbreaks often affect both staff and patients. The CDC provides guidelines for immunization and treatment of patients exposed to influenza:

- Rapid influenza virus testing done for those with recent onset of symptoms and viral cultures from a subset of patients to identify the virus type and confirm testing results
- Droplet precautions for all those suspected or confirmed wit influenza, with those suspected separated from those confirmed
- Current season's vaccination administered to those not immunized
- Providing influenza antiviral prophylaxis and treatment according to most current recommendations
- Limiting visitors or posting notices to advise people with symptoms not to visit

Immunization for Tuberculosis Prevention

The single vaccination available for tuberculosis is the **Bacille Calmette Guerin (BCG) vaccine** developed in the 1930's. Though it is the most widely used vaccination in the world, it has not been used for many years in the US, partially because tuberculosis has not been a major threat in the past half-century, but also because there are questions about its effectiveness. The question is asked, if the vaccine is effective, why is a third of the world's population infected and annually 2 million people die of it?

Its effectiveness in reducing childhood incidence of tuberculosis is generally accepted; however, immunity does not seem to stay through adulthood. It is not used with children in the US because there is such a slim chance that infants and young children will be exposed.

Immigrants from other parts of the world are assumed to have been vaccinated with the BCG vaccine to prevent tuberculosis. The TB skin test is the best available test for TB infection, and one characteristic of the BCG is that it gives false positives on the skin test. Thus, there is no way of knowing whether the immigrant has had the vaccine or is actually tubercular. The safest course is to presume he or she is tubercular. Repeated vaccination even increases the likelihood of causing a positive skin test even though it probably does not increase protection against TB.

COVID-19 Vaccination

Emergency Use Authorization for the COVID-19 Vaccine

Current COVID-19 (SARS-CoV-2) vaccines are approved by the FDA under Emergency Use Authorization (EUA), which allows the use of unapproved medical products for emergency situations. For the vaccines, the FDA requires that phase 1 (small number of participants), phase 2 (hundreds of participants), and phase 3 (thousands of participants) clinical trials be completed. The EUA request is made after analysis of phase 3 data from which at least 50% of participants have had at least 2 months of follow-up. The EUA request must include a safety database of over 3000 participants who have been followed for at least a month after the last injection to assess for adverse events/effects. All data submitted to the FDA regarding vaccines are assessed by scientists and physicians and reviewed by an advisory committee. Manufacturers are required to include a plan for follow-up regarding safety, mortality rates, hospitalizations, and other adverse events/effects as well as to continue clinical trials.

Adverse Reactions, Contraindications, and Recommendations for the COVID-19 Vaccine

Adverse reactions to the COVID-19 vaccine are rare, but have occurred. Most reactions are limited to local erythema, edema, and pain, which usually subsides within a day or two. Some people develop flu-like symptoms with fatigue, fever, chills, myopathy, headache, and nausea. A few people develop "COVID arm," an itching painful rash at the injection site. People with the preceding symptoms should still get the second injection if receiving Pfizer or Moderna vaccines. Some may experience a severe allergic and anaphylactic reaction requiring medical attention, and these individuals should not receive a second dose. The Johnson & Johnson vaccine has been implicated in the development of Guillain-Barré syndrome. The Pfizer and Moderna vaccines have been implicated in mild cases of myocarditis in adolescents and young adults. The only absolute **contraindications** are immediate or severe allergic reactions. While vaccination is recommended for those with underlying health conditions, those who are immunocompromised may have reduced immune response.

The CDC recommends that all healthcare workers be fully vaccinated; however, this is not a mandate. Healthcare facilities can require all workers to be vaccinated, but not all choose to do so. As of mid-2021 the vaccination had been approved for children ages 12 and older, with studies for younger children in process.

Rabies Vaccination

Unless there is some likelihood a person will come into contact with rabid creatures, there is insufficient reason to obtain rabies vaccination. People who might consider it are animal control officers, zoo workers, kennel operators, and laboratory technicians who work where experiments are conducted on live animals.

Pre-exposure prophylaxis provides protection to persons who run the risk of being bitten by rabid animals or might have a delay in obtaining post-exposure therapy after a possible exposure. Rather than eliminating the need for additional therapy after a rabies exposure, it decreases the number of doses of vaccine that need to be given after a bite and eliminates the need for rabies immune globulin. This is of particular benefit to those who could be exposed in places distant from any effective treatment available.

Risk Categories for Exposure to Rabies

The risk categories for exposure to rabies include the following:

- **Continuous**: The rabies virus is always present, possibly in high concentrations. Bites are possible, but so are exposures from aerosol sources affecting the mucous membrane and one can become exposed without knowing it. In this category are workers in rabies biologics plants and rabies lab researchers. PPE immunization is advised, with blood tests every six months and boosters when antibodies fall below a cutoff point.
- **Frequent:** There may be aerosol exposure to mucous membranes or other non-bite exposures as well as bite exposure, so that there may be no recognition of exposure. But the danger is more infrequent than continuous. PPE and boosters or blood workups every two years are recommended for veterinarians, spelunkers (for the danger from rabid bats), rabies diagnostic lab workers, and wildlife and animal control officers in rabies epizootic areas.
- **Infrequent:** Episodic exposure to a source that is always recognized. This applies to veterinary students as well as vets, animal control people, and wildlife workers in areas where rabies is not terribly endemic.
- **Rare:** The population at large, for which rabies vaccine is not recommended.

Issues in Countries with Limited Resources for Injections

Every year, unsafe injections worldwide account for cases of hepatitis B, hepatitis C, liver cancer, cirrhosis and HIV infections and leading to as many as 500,000 deaths. A high proportion of these are in developing nations.

The first thing to keep in mind is that many hospitals in these areas do not have access to disposable needles or autoclaves, and the sterility of their reusable hypodermic needles can be seriously questioned. In fact, one theory about the rapid spread of AIDS in Africa is that dirty needles are a major factor.

Though poverty is the prime cause this situation, lack of policies on and education in the use of needles puts not just injection recipients but also healthcare workers at risk for acquiring diseases through contaminated needles and syringes. Also put at risk, through exposure to contaminated sharps not properly disposed of, is the community at large.

Transmission Based Precautions

History of CDC Isolation Guidelines

CDC Isolation Guidelines, 1970

In 1970, CDC began recommending that hospitals use seven isolation categories (Strict Isolation, Respiratory Isolation, Protective Isolation, Enteric Precautions, Wound and Skin Precautions, Discharge Precautions, and Blood Precautions) to more easily decide which precautions to take based almost entirely on the epidemiologic features (primarily their routes of transmission) of the diseases grouped in each category.

Specific isolation techniques were indicated for each isolation category. But because some diseases in a category could require fewer precautions than others, more precautions were suggested for some than were necessary. This disadvantage was offset by the convenience of having a small number of categories; the simple system required personnel to learn only a few established routines for applying isolation precautions. To make the system even more user friendly, instructions on isolation precautions for each category were printed on color coded cards and placed on the doors, beds, or charts of patients.

CDC Isolation Guidelines and Universal Precautions, 1980's

In 1985, driven largely by the growing HIV epidemic, the CDC altered isolation practices dramatically by introducing a new strategy which became known as **universal precautions (UP)**. For the first time, emphasis was put on applying to everyone universally the already existing Blood and Body Fluid Precautions regardless of presumed infection status. UP expanded precautions to using masks and eye coverings to prevent exposure of mucous membrane exposures and taking greater precautions against needle-stick infections. Reports in 1987 and 1988 emphasized blood as the single most important source of HIV and that infection control must focus on preventing exposures to it. A new system, Body Substance Isolation (BSI), focused on isolating all moist and therefore potentially infectious body substances (blood, sputum, feces, urine, wound drainage, saliva, etc.) from all patients, regardless of their presumed infection status, primarily through the use of gloves.

CDC Changes to Categories of Isolation Guidelines, 1980-1990

By 1980, the primary need for isolation precautions was becoming nosocomial in nature rather than the previous concern with the spread of infectious diseases brought into the hospital from the community.

The CDC's 1983 guideline changed the categories of isolation to Strict Isolation, Contact Isolation, Respiratory Isolation, Tuberculosis Isolation, Enteric Precautions, Drainage/Secretion Precautions, and Blood and Body Fluid Precautions. As with its previous categorical approach, the CDC tended to over-isolate some patients. But an alternative approach, attacking each disease individually, was also recommended to correct for this. A CDC issued chart listed all diseases posing the threat of in-hospital transmission, and the epidemiology of each infectious disease was considered individually by advocating only those precautions (e.g., private room, mask, gown, and gloves) needed to interrupt transmission of the infection.

Recommendations for Tuberculosis (AFB) Isolation were updated in 1990 after heightened concern about nosocomial transmission of drug-resistant TB, particularly around persons with human immunodeficiency virus (HIV).

CDC Revision to Isolation Guidelines, 1996

By the early 1990s, there was considerable confusion about which body fluids or substances required precautions under UP and BSI. The CDC released a 1996 guideline containing three important changes to eliminate confusion. It did the following:

- Melded into a single set of precautions the major features of UP and BSI, calling them Standard Precautions, to cover all patients regardless of their presumed infection status.
- Collapsed the old categories of isolation precautions (Strict Isolation, Contact Isolation, Respiratory Isolation, Tuberculosis Isolation, Enteric Precautions, and Drainage/Secretion Precautions) along with the old disease-specific precautions into three sets of precautions based on routes of transmission and called Transmission-Based Precautions; these were intended to be used additional to Standard Precautions.
- Listed specific syndromes highly suspicious for infection and identified appropriate Transmission-Based Precautions to be used on an empirical, temporary basis until a diagnosis could be made.

Indications for Use of Isolation Guidelines

In 1996, the CDC revised its *Guideline for Isolation Precautions in Hospitals* that identifies appropriate precautions to use on an empiric, temporary basis until a diagnosis can be made. It also lists specific clinical syndromes or conditions that should be regarded as highly suspicious for infection.

The **first tier** of precautions is the Standard Precautions, to be practiced with all patients regardless of their diagnosis or presumed infection status, including patients with whom transmission-based precautions should also be followed.

In the **second tier** of the guidelines are listed precautions intended only for the care of specified patients known to be or suspected of being infected or colonized with pathogens transmittable through any or all of three routes: airborne, droplets, or contact that is either direct with another person or indirect through the medium of contaminated surfaces.

Tier I: Standard Precautions

Through the years, the CDC has issued a number of different guidelines for isolation precautions. The 1996 CDC isolation guidelines were an update from the universal precautions (UP) guidelines that dealt with blood and some body fluids but did not directly address other types of transmission. There are now two tiers of isolation precautions. Tier I deals with standard precautions that should be in place for all patients.

Standard precautions include protection from all blood and body fluids and include the use of gloves, face barriers, and gowns as needed to avoid being splashed with fluids. Hand washing remains central to infection control and should be with plain (not antimicrobial) soap or instant antiseptic.

Standard Precautions for Bloodborne Pathogens and Patient Placement

The Standard Precautions regarding bloodborne pathogens basically boil down to avoiding cuts from sharp, contaminated instruments. Used, disposable hypodermic syringes, for instance, are never to be recapped but immediately placed in the closest puncture-resistant container for transport to a reprocessing area. Healthcare workers are directed to never point a needle toward any part of their body or manipulate them using both hands.

Should mouth-to-mouth resuscitation become necessary, it must be performed only with the use of mouthpieces, resuscitation bags, or other ventilation devices.

A patient who contaminates the environment and will not (or cannot) follow rules of proper hygiene and environmental control, must be placed in a private room. If none is available, the problem must be taken up with infection control professionals. Patients with the same type of infection, same colonizing organism, may share a room.

Standard Precautions for Protective Clothing, Patient Care Equipment, Surfaces, and Linens

According to the CDC's Standard Precautions, there must be a hospital-wide program for the routine care, cleaning, and disinfection of environmental surfaces, beds, bedrails, bedside equipment, and other frequently touched surfaces.

Masks, eye protection, and face shields protect mucous membranes of the eyes, nose, and mouth during procedures and patient-care activities that are likely to generate splashes or sprays of blood, body fluids, secretions, and excretions. Likewise, gowns protect skin and prevent clothing from getting soiled during the same kinds of activities. Remove and dispose of a soiled gown as promptly as is possible, and wash hands to avoid transfer of microorganisms to other patients or environments. Assume that any used patient-care equipment is contaminated and wear protective clothing when handling it. Ensure that single use items are discarded properly and reusable equipment is not used for the care of another patient until it has been cleaned and reprocessed appropriately.

Soiled linen must be handled, transported, and processed in a manner that prevents skin and mucous membrane exposures and clothing contamination.

Tier II: Airborne Transmission-Based Precautions

Tier II of the CDC isolation guidelines protects from three types of transmission. The first type provides protection from diseases spread by small airborne droplets (<5 mm), including measles, tuberculosis, varicella, and COVID-19.

Airborne precautions include placing patient in a private room with monitored negative airflow and the door closed. People who are susceptible to the disease, such as those not immune against measles, should not enter the room. Respiratory precautions (a mask) should be worn if the patient has suspected or confirmed tuberculosis. Patient should wear mask outside of room.

Tier II: Droplet Transmission-Based Precautions

Unlike the pathogens transmitted by airborne mechanisms, microorganisms transmitted through droplets consist of particles larger than 5 μm in size. They infect by making contact with the mucous membranes of the nose or mouth of a target. They are contained in droplets generated from a carrier's cough or sneeze, or even talking. They may also be producing in the performance of suctioning or bronchoscopy.

Droplet precautions in isolating a patient are exactly the same as for the patient whose disease is transported through means other than large droplets, except for one thing: Because large droplets do not remain suspended in the air and generally travel only short distances, usually 3 ft or less, special air handling and ventilation is not necessary, and the room's door may remain open.

While some hospitals may prefer staff to wear a mask upon entering the room, at the very least, a mask should be worn when working within 3 ft of the patient.

Transport advisories are exactly the same as those for patients with airborne pathogens.

Tier II: Contact Transmission-Based Precautions

Tier II of the CDC Isolation guidelines includes the third type, contact, which provides protection from diseases spread by direct hand-to-hand or skin-to-skin contact, such as those with significant infection or colonization and those who have suspected or confirmed multi-drug resistance, which may include vancomycin-resistant *Enterococci* and *Staphylococcus aureus.*

Contact precautions include placing the patient in a private room or room with someone with the same infection. Gloves should be used as for standard precautions but should immediately be removed and hands sanitized after contact with infective material. A clean protective gown should be worn inside the room for close contact with patient, including caring for a patient who is incontinent or has uncontained drainage. The patient should not leave the room if possible and equipment should be dedicated for patient use or disinfected before use by other patients.

Some diseases may require some combination of airborne, droplet, and contact precautions: Lassa fever, Marburg virus, and smallpox.

Precaution Considerations for Patients with Tuberculosis

Respiratory Protection and Duration of Isolation

Admit patients into negative pressure isolation rooms when:

- Coughing and chest x-ray suggest there may be tuberculosis
- There is a positive acid-fast smear
- Multi-drug resistant tuberculosis is known when admitted or re-admitted
- There is a known HIV infection
- There is an undiagnosed cough or pulmonary condition
- Medical conditions, with cough and an undiagnosed pulmonary infiltrate, predispose to tuberculosis.

Isolation should be maintained until there is evidence of response to therapy. Such evidence consists of:

- Three consecutive negative AFB smears with no organisms on smear
- Decreased cough
- Decrease in maximum daily temperature
- Resolution of night sweats
- Improved appetite

Possible Staff Exposure

It is estimated that *Mycobacterium tuberculosis* causes the greatest number of deaths of any infectious pathogen: three million deaths annually worldwide. Hospital staff should therefore use extra precaution against infection when treating tubercular patients by wearing gowns and gloves and using HEPA filtration masks.

Should a staff member suspect he or she has had any possible exposure, it has got to be reported immediately to a supervisor for referral to a screening exam. While a Mantoux skin test helps identify those infected with *M. tuberculosis* but not yet showing symptoms, sputum or other bodily secretions can be cultured for growth of mycobacteria to confirm the diagnosis. It may take 1-3 weeks to detect growth and 8-12 weeks to be certain. With a positive test result, a daily dose of isoniazid (also called INH) may be prescribed. It will be taken for up to a year, with periodic checkups.

Isolation Guidelines for COVID-19

CDC-recommended isolation guidelines for COVID-19/SARS-CoV-2 are as follows:

- For most adults, isolation and standard and transmission-based precautions should continue for 10 days after onset of symptoms and for at least 24 hours after non-medicated resolution of temperature. Patients who are critically ill may need to be on isolation and precautions for 20 days.
- Patients should be in negative pressure rooms if at all possible.
- PPE: Staff should use standard and transmission-based precautions, including N95 respirator or higher (or facemask if N95 unavailable), gown, gloves, and face shield or goggle.
- Transport and movements of patients must be limited.
- Screening for all visitors, patients, and staff for COVID must occur at points of entry.
- Supplies for hand hygiene and cough etiquette must be readily available at healthcare facility entrances, waiting areas, and patient check-in.

Identifying Patients That Require Isolation

Identifying patients with communicable diseases involves four different types of surveillance:

- Admitting history/admission physical can help to identify high-risk behaviors or symptoms that may not be current but can indicate a communicable disease. Questioning answers to elicit more information is also helpful.
- Admitting diagnosis serves as a key element to determine if further evaluation should be done, especially if the diagnosis is a common opportunistic infection involving particular infectious diseases. For example, cytomegalovirus is often related to HIV infection.
- Symptoms, such as chronic or severe cough or diarrhea, should trigger further investigation to determine if there is a contagious cause.
- Laboratory review should be ongoing after threshold rates are established for different lab tests. Any abnormality that is suggestive of an infectious disease process should be evaluated to determine if further follow-up or isolation is needed.

Initiating and Discontinuing Isolation Precautions

While isolation is usually intended to protect others from an infected patient, **protective environments (PE)** are usually used to protect a severely immunocompromised patient. Most often, protective environments are provided in specialized hospital units, such as those for stem-cell transplant. Patients who are identified by diagnosis should be placed immediately in the protective environment and maintained in the environment until immune or clinical status improves. Protective environments include:

- Placing patient in a private room (or room shared by cohort) with positive airflow from the room to the outside so that contamination from the hallway or other rooms is avoided. ACH is ≥12 and HEPA filtration is used to prevent contamination.
- Gown and gloves are used to reduce transmission of pathogens, but mask is not needed unless the patient is also on droplet precautions.
- One to one nursing should be utilized.
- Patient should leave room only if medically necessary and in clean linens with face mask if necessary and 2-person transport.

Initiating and Discontinuing Airborne Isolation Precautions

Airborne infection isolation should be initiated with suspicion or confirmation of a diagnosis of disease that has airborne transmission, such as varicella-zoster virus (VZV), measles, variola (smallpox), and tuberculosis, with droplet size <5 µm, or patients with multiple drug-resistant strains of organisms. Isolation should be continued until confirmation that patient is not infective. Isolation procedures include:

- Placing patient in a private room with ≥ 12 air exchanges per hour (ACH) under negative pressure with air from the outside in and exhaust, preferably, to the outdoors, or recirculation provided through high-efficiency particulate air (HEPA) filters.
- Door to the room should remain closed and sign or color/coding should be used at door to alert medical staff to isolation.
- Mandatory respirator use for personnel entering the room when indicated because of disease transmission (TB and smallpox) or lack of immunity (measles, VZV).
- The patient should be transported in clean linens and wearing a facemask.
- Procedures should be conducted in the room whenever possible.

Emergency Preparedness and Management

Epidemiologist's Role in Disaster Planning

Of the five most common causes of death in emergencies and disasters—diarrhea, acute respiratory infection, measles, malnutrition, and, in endemic zones, malaria—all of these causes except malnutrition are communicable diseases directly related to environmental health conditions. Acute respiratory infections and diarrhea are the chief killers, hitting children particularly hard. Even malnutrition is greatly exacerbated by communicable disease.

People caught in natural or man-made mega disasters are markedly vulnerable to communicable diseases, for disasters have ways of reducing resistance to disease through malnutrition, stress, fatigue, and unsanitary post disaster living conditions. To prevent disease, epidemiologists promote preparations for disaster such as keeping adequate quantities of safe water, providing community sanitation facilities and appropriate shelter, and encouraging immunization. Outbreaks of such diseases as measles are a common hazard in emergencies, often with a high fatality rate, making periodic community vaccination campaigns vital.

Steps To Take in Preventing the Spread of Infection and During an Outbreak

To prevent spread of infection, the IP should:

- Identify best infection control strategies, policies, and procedures
- Periodically review with all personnel the infection control policies and procedures
- Apply the infection control policies and procedures
- Initiate or discontinue isolation/barrier precautions for infected patients when warranted
- Advise on appropriate patient placement
- Inspect and evaluate infection control measures as put into practice in patient environments/check for any existing hazards
- Review medical equipment and supplies for their suitability in infection control
- Advise on the patient transfer/discharge planning process
- Collaborate on immunization programs for patients and staff
- Assist engineering personnel in the development of infection control plans for air and water quality

During an outbreak, the IP should:

- Verify outbreak's existence
- Establish case definition, period of investigation, and case-finding methods
- Define the problem in terms of time-to-event, place, persons, and risk factors
- Formulate hypothesis on source and mode of transmission
- Institute and evaluate control measures

Public Health Considerations in Disaster Planning

A vulnerability analysis should be carried out in preparation for a disaster. Estimates need to be made of potential demands on healthcare facilities and the need for healthcare workers as well as the disease implications of damage to reservoirs and water mains, power failures, material and manpower shortages due to injury or lack of transport, and communication difficulties.

When designating and laying out disaster relocation centers, keep in mind, for hygienic reasons, that people sleeping on beds or mats should have a minimum of 3.5 square meters of floor area or 10 cubic meters of air space. Beds or mats should be separated by a minimum distance of 0.75 meters. In planning for adequate ventilation, the amount of fresh air needed will be approximately 20–30 cubic meters per person per hour.

To facilitate the management and control of communicable diseases, relocation camps should hold no more than 10,000-12,000 people, preferably subdivided into independent units of no more than 1,000 people.

SULLAGE AND PUBLIC DEFECATION

Sullage, wastewater from kitchens, bathrooms, and laundries, can contain harmful microorganisms, particularly from soiled clothing during an outbreak. When it collects in poorly drained places and causes pools of organically polluted water, its danger is that it may then serve as breeding places for mosquitoes that transmit some viruses as well as the parasitic disease lymphatic filariasis.

Defecation in rivers and streams should be discouraged but, if absolutely necessary, confined to an area downstream of other human use. Dumping raw sewage into the sea should also be discouraged in areas of high population density or when there is fishing in the area. Open defecation should be discouraged along public highways, in the vicinity of hospitals, feeding centers, food storage and preparation areas, and in fields containing crops for human consumption. When more hygienic alternatives are unavailable, limit open defecation to specific, well-defined areas, which should be closed as soon as alternative sites for defecation are available.

HUMAN FECES

Microorganisms contained within **human feces** can enter the human body by way of contaminated food, water, utensils (eating and cooking), and by contact with contaminated objects. This spreads the major causes of sickness and death in disasters and emergencies like diarrhea, cholera, and typhoid.

Intestinal worm infections like hookworm which contribute to anemia and malnutrition are transmitted through contact with feces contaminated soil and render people more susceptible to other diseases. The intestinal form of schistosomiasis (also known as bilharzia), caused by parasitic worm species living in the veins of the intestinal tract and liver, is transmitted through feces.

Though some fly species (and cockroaches) are attracted to or breed in feces and carry fecal material on their bodies, there is no evidence that this contributes significantly to the spread of disease. However, high fly densities will increase the risk of transmission of trachoma and *Shigella* dysentery.

Food Safety During Disasters

Public health problems surrounding food safety during disasters include the following:

- Flood waters often pick up large quantities of wastes and pathogenic bacteria from farms, sewer systems, and septic tanks, so food may become contaminated by surface water polluted by this sewage and wastewaters
- Aggravating the situation, particularly if sanitary conditions are poor, will be the overcrowding of survivors forced out of their homes
- With electric power knocked out, cold storage will not be available; at all stages of the food chain, from production to consumption, foods may be subject to bacterial growth
- Lack of safe drinking-water and sanitation will also hamper the hygienic preparation of food and increases the risk of food contamination
- Food is especially susceptible to contamination when it is stored and prepared out of doors or in damaged homes where windows and possibly even walls are missing
- Environmental contamination combined with improper handling of food increases the risk of epidemics of cholera and shigellosis

Supplying Potable Water During a Disaster

Among public health considerations in supplying potable water in a disaster:

- Maintain stocks of water supplies at hospitals, nutrition centers, and elsewhere so that water does not have to be diverted from the general water supply when disaster strikes; Otherwise, should the general water supply be polluted, impaired, or insufficient, hospitals would soon be swamped with patients suffering from water related disease.
- Inform the public that tap water may be contaminated and should not be consumed without treatment
- Information about simple household methods of filtration, sedimentation, storage, and disinfection should be provided
- Distribute a stock solution of bleach or water chlorination tablets (e.g., sodium hypochlorite) at central pick-up points in each neighborhood for home water disinfection
- Provide clear instructions on the proper use of chlorine solutions and tablets
- Have a supply of buckets stored for collecting water from a safe supply and containers with lids for storing it

Returning the Water Supply to Normal After a Disaster

Public health considerations when the water supply has been turned back on include:

- During any disaster in which water may be contaminated, increase the chlorine level in the public water supply to as high as 1 mg/L to prevent polluted water that may enter the distribution system from contaminating the water; discontinue as soon as the risk is reduced.
- After making repairs to damaged intake pipes, new sections of pipe should be disinfected by filling them with a strong chlorine solution and then flushing them out with treated water before being put back into service.
- Where a dam or reservoir wall has been badly damaged and is dangerous, the reservoir should be partly or completely drained.

Symptoms and Precautions for Emerging Infectious Diseases

Severe Acute Respiratory Syndrome (SARS)

Severe Acute Respiratory Syndrome (SARS) is caused by a coronavirus (Co-V) and presents as a respiratory illness with fever, cough, dyspnea, and general malaise is extremely virulent, spreading easily from person to person through close contact by way of contaminated droplets produced by coughing or sneezing. SARS has a high mortality rate. Some possibility exists that SARS may also have airborne transmission in some cases with aerosol-producing procedures. High rates of infection have occurred in healthcare workers and others in contact with infected patients, so prompt diagnosis and proper isolation are essential. Precautions include:

- Contact and droplet precautions, including eye protection and appropriate personal protection equipment.
- Airborne precautions (recommended by the CDC), especially with aerosol-producing procedures (ventilators, nebulizers, intubation).
- Immediate notification of public health authorities and institution of contact tracing.
- Activity restrictions of exposed healthcare workers planned in coordination with public health officials.

Emergency Preparedness for COVID-19

Emergency preparedness efforts faltered even before the initial outbreak of COVID-19/SARS-CoV-2, but these unfortunately failures were not uncovered until the COVID-19 pandemic exposed them. Emergency preparedness plans were outdated and focused on response to natural disasters (hurricanes, floods, tornados) and mass casualty events (train wrecks, airplane accidents) more than on pandemics. When caseloads began to rise and people quarantined, many businesses shut down, including some critical to providing necessary equipment, such as PPE. Because many healthcare facilities utilized just-in-time ordering, inventories of supplies were often very low and some equipment outdated, leaving healthcare workers without the PPE that was critical to their safety. Many facilities had not identified alternate supply chains and costs escalated, leaving facilities and even states bidding against each other. The Strategic National Stockpile was low on supplies and equipment and much was outdated or in need of repair. As people were laid off from their jobs and businesses closed, applying for unemployment was chaotic in many areas and funds inadequate.

Quarantine Guidelines for COVID-19

The following quarantine guidelines were issued for confirmed or suspected exposure to COVID-19/SARS-CoV-2 during the COVID-19 pandemic:

- **Healthcare workers**: Contact tracing and work restriction for healthcare personnel are no longer recommended for asymptomatic individuals in favor of universal symptom screening; however, if community transmission increases, these procedures may be reconsidered, especially with prolonged exposure (uncovered eyes, mouth, nose) ≥15 minutes in 24 hours or during aerosol generating procedures. Work restrictions may include exclusion for 14 days following last exposure. Restrictions may be relaxed during staff shortages. Fully vaccinated staff do not need to be restricted from work after an exposure.

- **People with COVID-19 symptoms or suspected exposure** should stay home for 14 days after last exposure and maintain 6-foot social distance.
- **All others**: Practice social distancing, wear masks when appropriate, and monitor for symptoms.
- **Mask guidelines**: Fully vaccinated individuals do not need to wear a mask or maintain social distancing for activities unless required by federal, state, local, tribal, territorial laws, rules, and regulations (including business and workplace restrictions).

Pandemic Influenza

Pandemic influenza is a worldwide epidemic of influenza that causes serious respiratory illness or death in large populations of people. Pandemics can occur when a virus mutates, creating a new subtype that infects humans and spreads easily from person to person. The influenza of most concern recently has been avian flu, which primarily affects birds, but has infected other animals, including humans, primarily those in contact with infected flocks. There are a number of subtypes of avian flu and symptoms may range from typical influenza-like respiratory infections to severe pneumonia. Should a further mutation occur and a pandemic occur, the implications for healthcare are profound because of the potential number of infected patients overwhelming the medical system. Precautions include:

- Standard precautions with careful hand hygiene
- Contact precautions with gloves and gown for all patient contact and goggles when within 3 feet
- Dedicated equipment
- Airborne precautions in isolated negative pressure rooms and use of N-95 filter respirator

Bioterrorism

Responding to Biologic Agents

Community responses to biologic agents, such as anthrax, smallpox, and influenza, require coordination and planning with public health and other healthcare providers to meet the needs of those infected and to provide information to those who are at risk. Collaborative efforts include planning for:

- Notification of all those involved immediately per telephone/email tree
- Immunization plans, including availability of vaccines, sites for administration, staffing
- Education of the public about signs and symptoms and steps to take to prevent becoming infected or spreading infection
- Training of staff for emergency preparedness/ infection control
- Stockpiling medications and equipment, such as personal protective equipment, respirators
- Facilities plan to accommodate large numbers of patients in isolation rooms, including cohorting
- Environmental monitoring of air and water for contamination
- Establishing procedures with coroner for handling deaths
- Epidemiological studies and surveillance
- Staff assigned to serve as liaison among agencies

Role of the Infection Preventionist

Biological terrorism may result in high rates of morbidity and mortality, depending upon the biological agent disseminated and the method of dissemination. Roles of the IP in biological terrorism include:

- The IP should begin by making a personal plan for family and self so that the professional can be available to provide leadership during the emergency situation.
- The IP must be familiar with emergency preparedness plans and should take an active part in planning with public health officials.
- The IP should know where emergency supplies are stockpiled and the location of points of dispensing, where the general public can go to obtain necessary equipment or immunizations.
- The IP should ensure that hospital supplies and medications are sufficient to deal with a large influx of patients. Necessary supplies and medications may include antimicrobial agents, respirators, PPE, laboratory supplies, and linen. Negative pressure rooms should also be available.
- The IP should identify vulnerable populations (such as children and the elderly) associated with different biological agents.

Preparation for Influx of Patients

The IP and the infection control team should develop specific plans for dealing with different bioterrorism agents and training should be provided to staff. An organized approach should include the following:

- Be on the alert for possible bioterrorism-related infections, based on clusters of patients or symptoms
- Use personal protection equipment, including respirators when indicated
- Complete thorough assessment of patient, including medical history, physical examination, immunization record, and travel history
- Provide a probable diagnosis based on symptoms and lab findings, including cultures
- Provide treatment, including prophylaxis while waiting for laboratory findings
- Use transmission precautions as well as isolation for suspected biologic agents
- Notify local, state, and federal authorities as per established protocol
- Conduct surveillance and epidemiological studies to identify at risk populations
- Develop plans to accommodate large numbers of patients:
    - Restricting elective admissions
    - Transferring patients to other facilities

Anthrax

There are a number of different infections that could be part of a bioterrorism attack. The type of barrier/isolation needed is dependent upon the symptoms and the mode of transmission. Knowledge of typical presenting symptoms and prompt precautions are essential to prevent spread of disease. Anthrax (*Bacillus anthracis*) usually occurs from contact with animals, but as a bioterrorism weapon, anthrax would most likely be aerosolized and inhaled. It is not transferred from person to person. There are three forms of anthrax:

- Inhaled: Causes fever, cough, fever, shortness of breath, and general debility
- Cutaneous: Causes small non-painful sores that blister and ulcerate with necrosis at the center
- Gastrointestinal: Causes nausea, vomiting, diarrhea, and abdominal pain

The inhaled form of anthrax is the most severe with about a 50% mortality rate. The vaccine for anthrax is not yet available to the public. Precautions include:

- Prophylaxis with antibiotics after exposure
- Standard precautions
- Contact precautions for wounds if there are cutaneous lesions

Pneumonic Plague

Yersinia pestis causes pneumonic plague, which is normally carried by fleas from infected rats but can be aerosolized to use as a biologic weapon. There are three forms of plague, but they sometimes occur together and bubonic and septicemic plague can develop into pneumonic, which is the primary concern related to bioterrorism:

- **Bubonic** occurs when a person is bitten by an infected flea.
- **Pneumonic** occurs with inhalation and results in pneumonia with fever, headache, cough, and progressive respiratory failure.
- **Septicemic** occurs when *Y. pestis* invades the bloodstream, often after initial bubonic or pneumonic plague.

Pneumonic plague can spread easily from person to person. There is no vaccine available. Precautions include:

- Immediate antibiotics within first 24 hours are necessary, so early diagnosis is critical
- Prophylaxis with antibiotics may protect those exposed
- Droplet precautions should be used with appropriate barriers, such as surgical mask

Botulism

Clostridium botulinum produces an extremely poisonous toxin that causes botulism. The organism can be aerosolized or used to infect food. There are three primary forms of botulisms:

- **Food borne botulism** results from contamination of food. This type poses the greatest threat from bioterrorism. Symptoms usually appear 12-36 hours after ingestion but may be delayed for 2 weeks and include nausea, vomiting, dyspnea, dysphagia, slurred speech, progressive weakness, and paralysis.
- **Infant botulism** results from *C. botulinum* ingested into the intestinal tract. Constipation, poor feeding, and progressive weakness are presenting symptoms.
- **Wound botulism** results from contamination of open skin, but symptoms are similar to food borne botulism.

Botulism is not transmitted from person to person, but contaminated food has the potential to infect many people, especially if the contaminated food is manufactured and widely distributed.

Precautions include:

- Antitoxin after exposure and as early in disease as possible
- Standard precautions

Tularemia

Francisella tularensis causes tularemia, which is usually transmitted from small mammals to humans through insect bites, ingestion of contaminated food or water, inhalation, or handling of infected animals. Although there is no evidence of person-to-person transmission, *F. tularensis* has the potential to be aerosolized for use as in bioterrorism because it is highly infective and requires only about 10 organisms to infect. Flu-like symptoms appear in 3-5 days after exposure and progress to severe respiratory infection and pneumonia. A vaccine for laboratory workers was available until recently, but the FDA is reviewing it at present, so there is no vaccine available now.

- Prophylaxis with antibiotics within 24 hours may prevent disease
- Standard precautions are sufficient
- Biologic safety measures should be used for laboratory specimens
- Autopsy procedures that may cause tissue to be aerosolized should be avoided

Smallpox

The **variola virus** causes smallpox, which has been eradicated worldwide since 1980, but has the potential for use as a biological weapon because people are no longer vaccinated. Smallpox is extremely contagious and has a high mortality rate (about 30%). Flu-like symptoms appear about 7-17 days after exposure with fever, weakness, vomiting and rash that begins on the face and arms and spreads. The rash becomes pustular, then crusts and scabs over before finally sloughing off, leaving scars. People remain infective from the first rash until all scabs are gone. The disease can spread through contact with infective fluid from lesions or from contact with clothes or bedding. Aerosol spread is theoretically possible. Precautions include:

- Vaccination must be done before symptoms appear and as soon as possible after exposure as vaccination after rash appears will not affect the severity of the disease.
- Maximum precautions should be used, which includes the use of gowns and gloves to enter the room and keeping the patient in a patient or cohorted room.

Viral Hemorrhagic Fevers

Viral hemorrhagic fevers are zoonoses (spread from animals to humans) and comprise a number of different diseases: Ebola, Lassa, Marburg, yellow, Argentine and Crimean-Congo. Some hemorrhagic fevers can spread person to person, notably Ebola, Marburg, and Lassa through close contact with body fluids or items contaminated. Hemorrhagic fevers are extremely contagious multi-system diseases, and those in contact with infected patients are at risk of infection Symptoms vary somewhat according to the disease but present with flu-like symptoms that progress to bleeding under the skin and internally, and some people develop kidney failure and central nervous system symptoms, such as coma and seizures. Treatment is supportive although ribavirin has been used to treat Crimean-Congo hemorrhagic fever. Mortality rates are high. Only yellow fever and Argentine have vaccines. Maximum precautions must be used with full barrier precautions, with care used in any handling of blood and body fluids or wastes.

Employee/Occupational Health

Screening and Immunization Programs

Pre-Employment Screening and Immunizations of Healthcare Workers

There are a number of issues regarding pre-employment screening, such as screening for criminal records and drug use, but among those concerns, screening for immune status is extremely important for all those employed within a healthcare facility because one healthcare worker can infect many patients, and lack of immunity places the healthcare worker at risk as well. Issues to consider include:

- **Proof of immune status**: Will verbal history be sufficient or must medical records be provided to prove immunization? Which diseases must be included? What testing for immune status will be provided?
- **Immunizations**: Will immunizations be required or voluntary? Which immunizations? What forms are necessary?
- **Service area**: How will immunization requirements vary from one service area to another? Will all staff be required to have some immunizations?
- **Special circumstances**: How will screening and immunizations be done for people who are immunocompromised, HIV positive, or pregnant?

Policies and Procedures

Recommended policies and procedures for pre-placement screening of healthcare workers are based on guidelines of the American Hospital Association, the Joint Commission, OSHA, and the CDC:

- Background check and drug testing (required by Joint Commission)
- Worker provides dates of two doses of measles, mumps, and rubella vaccinations (MMR) and verbal report of varicella or submits for serology testing
- Workers in contact with blood, body fluids, or body tissue must provide evidence of positive antibodies to HBV or be offered HBV vaccinations. HBV vaccinations cannot be required but non-immunized staff can be prevented from working in high-risk areas.
- Two-step TB skin testing (recommended by OSHA) 1-3 weeks apart. Chest x-ray is required for positive skin testing.
- Immunizations required for all healthcare facility workers should include: MMR, varicella, HBV, and influenza. Tetanus toxoid should be current.

Screening Programs

While employment pre-screening requirements focuses on new workers, often other healthcare workers were hired before immunization requirements or are in need of retesting and reimmunization, so the IP needs to develop programs for screening. Depending upon the number of workers involved, there are different approaches that can be used:

- **Anniversary date** reviews for all staff can include a health update and screening for infectious diseases and immunizations as needed.
- **Department and/or unit review** of all staff in that area can be done during a prescribed period of time with the department chair or supervisor ensuring that all staff are notified and screened.
- **Screening and immunization drives** can be done for 1-2 weeks periods once or twice a year with notices to all employees to participate.
- **Flu shot drives** can be done yearly prior to flu season. Placing staff and tables near staff lounges or dining areas to provide immunizations reminds staff and saves staff time.

HEPATITIS IMMUNIZATION RECOMMENDATIONS FOR HEALTHCARE WORKERS

Safety of the vaccines can be attested to by the fact that there have been no serious reactions to them even though more than one billion **hepatitis B vaccine** and seven million doses of **hepatitis A vaccine** doses have been given since 1995 in the US. Equally safe is the combined vaccine for both A and B. This is recommended to all healthcare workers. The few mild problems related to vaccination include soreness or moderate fever, neither of which last more than three days. However, injections should be delayed in the event of illness until it has resolved; those allergic to baker's yeast or to a previous hepatitis B shot should not be vaccinated.

SCREENING FOR IMMUNITY TO HEPATITIS B

Immunity to infectious diseases is acquired through vaccinations or antibodies in response to a natural infection. Immunity with vaccinations usually takes 10-14 days, but the length of time varies according to the type of vaccination. Immunity may be almost 100% or much lower, depending upon the type of vaccination and the disease. Natural infections do not always confer immunity, and there is no immunity for some infections, such as HIV. Most people who went to school in the United States received vaccinations as children in order to attend school. Healthcare providers who contact blood or body fluids should be immunized for hepatitis B. The anti-HBc test can identify people who were previously vaccinated or infected with hepatitis B and may have acquired immunity or the chronic form of the disease. Those who test positive for anti-HBc, must also be tested with HBsAg to determine if they have chronic infection rather than immunity.

SCREENING FOR IMMUNITY TO TUBERCULOSIS

Immunity to tuberculosis (TB) is established by regular (upon hire and after possible exposure) TB testing, most often with a tuberculosis skin test (TST), or with the QuantiFERON-TB Gold test, which uses whole blood to test for *Mycobacterium tuberculosis,* including both latent and active infection although it cannot differentiate the two. Positive tests are followed by chest x-rays, sputum cultures, and clinical evaluation. BCG (bacille Calmette-Guérin) is a tuberculosis vaccine routinely administered to children in countries with high incidences of childhood tuberculous meningitis. It is not recommended in the United States because infection with *Mycobacterium tuberculosis* has a low incidence and adult immunization is variable. QuantiFERON-TB Gold test is not affected by prior BCG vaccination but TST can show false positives. Healthcare workers may receive BCG vaccinations if they work with a large number of TB patients with resistant strains of TB, there is ongoing transmission of this disease to healthcare workers, and TB control precautions are unsuccessful.

Screening for Immunity to Measles, Mumps, Rubella, and Influenza

Most children are now immunized against measles, mumps, and rubella through the MMR vaccination at about 12-15 months. Serological testing for rubella should be done for women of childbearing age so they can be offered vaccinations before becoming pregnant. Women should avoid pregnancy for at least 8 weeks after a vaccination. Healthcare workers who do not have immunity and are pregnant should not be assigned to work with patients who may have rubella. Non-immune adults may receive MMR.

Recommendations for Screening for Immunity to COVID-19

Serology tests detect the presence of **antibodies to the COVID** coronavirus, indicating that the person has had a COVID-19 infection. Some tests, but not all, may detect antibodies generated by vaccination. Current vaccines stimulate antibodies to specific viral protein targets, typically the spike protein, but antibody tests may be sensitive to other proteins that are more common with infection. Therefore, the FDA currently states that the tests should not be used to assess the degree of immunity that infection or vaccination provides because research is not adequate to determine how much protection is afforded by the level of antibodies; and relying on the test may make people less careful in avoiding infection. Antibody tests are not recommended for routine use and should only be used by physicians with an understanding of the limitations. Antibody tests may be useful by public health officials to help assess levels of community transmission.

Preventing and Controlling Influenza in the Healthcare Setting

A program for prevention and control of influenza should feature annual influenza vaccination of all eligible patients and healthcare personnel, implementation of standard and droplet precautions for infected individuals, active surveillance, influenza testing for new illness cases, restriction of ill visitors and personnel, administration of prophylactic antiviral medications, and respiratory hygiene/cough etiquette.

All healthcare personnel, especially those in high-risk areas, should be monitored for symptoms of respiratory infection, and rapid influenza tests performed to confirm that the cause of symptoms is influenza. If so, remove the infected workers from direct patient contact duties. They should not provide patient care for 5 days following the onset of symptoms.

Use antiviral drugs for treatment and chemoprophylaxis of influenza, institute droplet precautions, establish cohorts of patients with confirmed or suspected influenza, reoffer influenza vaccinations to unvaccinated staff and patients, restrict staff movement between wards or buildings, and restrict contact between ill staff, visitors, and patients.

Joint Commission Requirements for Internal Control of Influenza

Regarding influenza, the Joint Commission standard requires healthcare organizations to:

- Establish an annual influenza vaccination program to include staff and licensed independent practitioners
- Provide access to influenza vaccinations onsite
- Educate staff and licensed independent practitioners on flu vaccination, appropriate precautions, and diagnosis, transmission, and potential impact of influenza
- Annually evaluate participation and reasons for non-participation in the immunization program
- Take efforts to increase participation in the program

Immunization of Staff Exposed to Influenza

During seasonal outbreaks of influenza, staff may be infected in the community or by contact with infected patients. Prompt immunization of staff can help to curtail outbreaks as staff are commonly exposed and may spread infection to multiple patients if infected. The IP should ensure that all staff, especially those with direct patient contact, receive annual influenza vaccinations. The CDC provides guidelines for immunization of both patients and staff who are not immunized. Those that apply to staff include the following:

- Rapid influenza virus testing for staff with recent onset of symptoms
- Restricting staff movement from outbreak areas
- Administering current season's vaccination to those not immunized
- Providing influenza antiviral prophylaxis and treatment according to most current recommendations. Prophylaxis should be considered for all staff, even those immunized, if the influenza is a variant and not matched by the vaccine.
- Removing infected staff from direct patient care, especially in high-risk areas
- Surgery may be limited to emergency procedures and elective procedures postponed

Determining Risk for Exposure Based on Job Classification/Department

Part of the determination regarding screening and immunization requirements depends upon the risk of **occupational exposure**, and this may vary by job classification and from one department to another. This determination requires careful auditing of positions to determine which ones have direct patient contact that could result in transmission of infection. Staff may be at risk from airborne or droplet transmission even though they are not involved in direct patient care, including environmental and nutritional services staff who enter patient rooms. Ideally, all personnel employed in a healthcare facility would have the basic recommended vaccinations in order to reduce risk. A system should be in place to quickly identify anyone who has had contact with a patient later diagnosed with an infectious disease. All visits to patients' rooms by nursing, laboratory, physical therapy, environmental, respiratory, nutritional, or other services should be by assigned personnel with records maintained regarding contact.

Communicable Diseases and Exposures

Signs and Symptoms of Infection in Employees

Signs and symptoms of infection in employees should be discussed as part of in-service so that employees know the type of symptoms that they should report for potential laboratory confirmation and those for which they should not report to work because of the danger they pose to others. For example, a person with a cough, an active infection, or diarrhea should not work with patients. Additionally, those with open cuts or rashes, such as from eczema, that compromise the integrity of the skin are at higher risk for developing skin infections, such as *staphylococcus aureus,* which may not be obvious at first. Employees should be tested for immunity to infectious diseases and immunized before coming in contact with patients as this will reduce the incidence of infection, but immunity is not possible for all conditions, so infection control policies that are clear and effective are critical.

Monitoring of Those Exposed to Communicable Diseases

Laboratory Monitoring of Patients and Employees

Laboratory results for patients should be evaluated on a daily basis, at least, to check for any organisms that might spread or cause an outbreak:

- *Streptococcus pyogenes*
- *Staphylococcus aureus*
- Vancomycin-resistant enterococci
- *Shigella spp.*
- *Salmonella spp.*
- *Mycobacterium tuberculosis*
- *Pseudomonas aeruginosa*
- *Neisseria meningitidis*
- *Legionella spp.*

Additionally, organisms that might pose particular problems to certain patient populations, such as in the neonatal unit, should be flagged for evaluation. Staff must be alert to the possibility of infection so that cultures or other laboratory tests can be done if there is a suspicion of an infection because lab reports alone are insufficient as some infections may be present without lab tests. Staff with signs of infection or possible exposure should be sent for appropriate lab testing and relieved of work duties if there is likelihood that they pose a risk to patients or other staff.

Issues Related to Monitoring Healthcare Workers

Healthcare worker exposure to communicable diseases can be from droplets, airborne particles, or contact with blood or body fluids. There are a number of issues involved in investigation and follow-up after exposure. The most common exposure is through injury with contaminated sharps, such as needles, putting people at risk for HIV, HBV, and HCV especially. The type of exposure and the disease determine the steps to be taken.

- Immediate reporting of all potential exposure, such as needle stick injuries or infectious diagnoses, must be done so that steps can be taken to determine the degree of exposure and steps to prevent infection.
- Contact investigations may need to be completed, especially for airborne or droplet exposure, to ensure that all those in contact with the infected person are notified.
- Healthcare workers may need to be removed from duty or patient contact during incubation period.
- Prophylaxis, immunizations, or treatment may be initiated.
- Periodic re-testing may be necessary.

Monitoring Healthcare Workers Exposed to HIV

The CDC defines occupational HIV exposure as percutaneous injury with a contaminated sharp or exposure of non-intact skin or mucous membranes to infectious material, such as blood or body fluids. The transmission risk is 0.3% with sharps and 0.09% with other exposure. Prophylaxis is considered 80% effective based on limited studies. Exposure is classified in three ways:

- **Exposure material**: Blood or blood-contaminated fluids have established transmission while other body fluids, such as CSF, urine, stool, and tears or only theoretically or potentially infectious.
- **Exposure type:** A few drops of fluid are less contagious than a major splash, and a superficial or solid needle injury are less contagious than a large bore hollow needle with obvious blood contaminant or deep injury.
- **Exposure source**: Asymptomatic HIV positive with viral load <1500 c/mL is a low risk, but symptomatic HIV positive, AIDS, acute retroviral syndrome, or viral load >1500 c/mL are high risks. Low risk is usually assumed if source cannot be tested.

Post-Exposure Prophylaxis and Serology

Post-exposure prophylaxis (PEP) for HIV should be initiated as soon as possible within 24 hours even for suspected exposure and continued for 4 weeks. If the suspected source proves to be HIV negative, then PEP can be discontinued:

- Low-risk exposure: Usually treated with a 2-drug protocol
- High-risk exposure: Usually treated with a ≥3-drug protocol

The healthcare worker should be re-evaluated at 72 hours, and HIV serology tests should be done initially to establish a baseline, at 6 weeks, 12 weeks, and 6 months. If there is HCV seroconversion, then HIV serology must be done at 12 months as well. Monitoring must be done for evidence of toxicity related to treatment while PEP is administered. Seroconversions must be reported according to guidelines to public health officials. Healthcare workers receiving PEP should be counseled regarding secondary transmission of the virus to others and provided with information about safe sex practices.

Monitoring Healthcare Workers Exposed to Hepatitis B

Hepatitis B (HBV) is highly contagious through blood and body fluids and is easily transmissible through a sharps injury, but transmission has been recorded in healthcare workers without sharp injuries from exposure of mucous membranes or non-intact skin to infective material. HBV in dried blood on environmental surfaces can remain viable for one week. Previously vaccinated adults are usually not tested, but healthcare workers with occupational exposure may be tested to determine serologic response and may be administered additional vaccine. Exposure to blood products that have both positive surface antigens (HBsAg) and e antigens (HBeAG) causes increased risk of infection. HBV post-exposure prophylaxis (PEP) is effective if administered within 24 hours. A combination of passive HB immunoglobulin (HBIG) and active HB vaccination may be used for PEP or a series of vaccinations alone. Healthcare workers who have documented completion of HBV vaccination series but have not had post-vaccination serology should be given a booster.

Monitoring Healthcare Workers Exposed to Hepatitis C

Hepatitis C virus (HCV) is not efficiently transmitted through contact with blood contact with mucous membranes or non-intact skin and has been linked only to sharps injury with hollow-bore needles. Follow-up serology after exposure should be done to determine if there has been transmission of HCV so that early diagnosis and referral can be made. The risk of environmental contamination appears to be very low. There is no post-exposure prophylaxis that has proven effective at this time. Those who convert to seropositive for HCV should receive counseling in a number of areas:

- **Liver protection**: People who are positive should avoid alcohol, non-prescription drugs or prescription drugs that may damage the liver.
- **Transmission risk**: People should not donate blood or tissue and should cover cuts or sores to avoid spreading infection.
- **Evaluation for chronic liver disease**: People should have routine liver function tests.

Monitoring Healthcare Workers Exposed to Tuberculosis

Exposure to tuberculosis (TB) in a healthcare facility is almost always the result of inadequate or delayed diagnosis of active TB in a patient. Upon diagnosis, immediate contact investigation must be done to determine all those who might be at risk of infection, including nursing, laboratory, and housekeeping staff. A two-step PPD skin testing or the QuantiFERON-TB Gold test should be done to determine if those exposed have become infected. Those who test positive must be evaluated to ensure that they do not have active TB. Treatment protocols for latent or active TB must be initiated as soon as possible. Healthcare workers with active pulmonary or laryngeal TB or who stopped treatment must be excluded from work until symptoms subside and 3 sputum tests are negative or treatment is completed.

Tuberculosis Testing and the Booster Phenomenon for Exposed Healthcare Workers

Tuberculosis testing often involves skin testing with the PPD test. A two-step procedure is now recommended because of the possibility of false negatives and to prevent misdiagnosis on the basis of the **booster phenomenon.**

A negative PPD finding can occur with an old infection because sensitivity wanes over time; however, subsequent tests months later might react positively because of the "boost" caused by the first test, suggesting an acute or recent infection and leading to unnecessary treatment. Therefore, with the two-step procedure, a second test is done 1-3 weeks after the first to determine the effect of the first test. If the second test converts to positive in this short period of time, then it is considered evidence of a boosted reaction to a previous infection. If the second test is negative, it is considered a true negative and subsequent changes to positive would be considered new infections.

Monitoring Healthcare Workers Exposed to SARS-CoV

Severe acute respiratory syndrome corona virus (SARS-CoV), first identified in 2002. SARS is highly contagious through airborne means and may present as a case of flu with fever and chills but rapidly causes pneumonia or acute respiratory distress syndrome. Isolation and barrier precautions are adequate protection, but diagnosis may be delayed, posing a threat to family, healthcare workers, and other patients. Staff who have had high-risk exposure, such as to being present in an aerosol-generating procedure, to SARS should be restricted from work and advised to stay at home and avoid contact with others for at least 10 days, the usual incubation time, with vigilant monitoring of fever and signs of respiratory infection with guidance from public health officials. Staff with low-risk exposure, such as contact without adequate barrier protection but without aerosol contamination can continue to work with temperatures taken BID and vigilant monitoring or respiratory symptoms.

Monitoring Healthcare Workers Exposed to COVID-19

Protocols for the monitoring of healthcare workers exposed to COVID-19 patients have varied throughout the pandemic and still continue to do so. Initially, those who were exposed were to quarantine for 14 days, but a huge influx of patients coupled with staff shortages caused a change so that staff in many areas could continue working with daily screening unless the person showed symptoms. With the onset of symptoms, then the staff person quarantined for 14 days. At present, the recommendation remains that those exposed should quarantine for 14 days and be tested before returning to work. Those who developed mild to moderate illness or were asymptomatic should remain out of work for at least 10 days (up to 20 for severe disease) after onset of symptoms or diagnosis if asymptomatic and 24 hours after fever. The protocols that are actually in place depend on the state and the healthcare facility policies. Some states have passed laws that prohibit requiring vaccinations in most work places.

Monitoring Healthcare Workers Exposed to Ebola

There are a number of issues related to the investigation and follow-up for healthcare workers exposed to the communicable disease Ebola. One issue is the type of restriction or quarantine required, and this may vary from state to state. The recommended time for voluntary seclusion is 20 days, during which those exposed should stay at home and avoid contact with others, public places, and public transportation. Some healthcare workers have been kept in isolation in healthcare facilities while others have stayed at home. However, it is not always clear who should be considered exposed and whether that should include all healthcare workers caring for Ebola patients or those showing symptoms, such as elevated temperature ≥38.0 °C (100.4 °F). Cost is another issue. Exposure at work should be covered under Worker's Compensation or facility liability insurance, but healthcare workers volunteering in West Africa may have no resources to cover lost work time after return. Tracing exposure to the general public from potentially-infected healthcare workers who appeared in public places or took public transportation may be very difficult.

Monitoring Healthcare Workers Exposed to Varicella-Zoster Virus

Perhaps it is because of its more common name, chicken pox, that varicella-zoster virus is not given the respect it deserves. It can be lethal to those infected. Before the introduction of the varicella vaccine in 1995, about 4 million cases of the disease were reported annually; there were 4,000 to 9,000 hospitalizations and 100 deaths. Varicella is the greatest vaccine-preventable killer of children in the United States. Children under the age of 10 account for 90 percent of all varicella cases, approximately 60 percent of hospitalizations, and 40 percent of deaths due to varicella.

As of 2019, an estimated 91% percent of American children ages 19-35 months old had received the varicella vaccine. To protect patients from healthcare workers who may carry varicella, healthcare facilities should have a policy of screening employees and offering those who have not had chicken pox inoculation with the vaccine. Upon confirmation of chickenpox in a patient or a healthcare employee, all employees not immune should be furloughed.

Monitoring Healthcare Workers Exposed to Measles, Mumps, or Rubella

All persons who work in healthcare facilities or who have contact with any patients should be immune to measles, mumps, and rubella. If not, immunize them and restrict their contact with patients for 23 days.

If a patient with symptoms has not been previously inoculated with the MMR vaccine, immediate consideration should be given to vaccination if there are no compelling reasons not to. Immediately isolate the patient if there is a rash. Report to Public Health all the contacts the patient has had during the period of communicability; they will contact any congregate settings where the patient has been or where someone who has had contact with the patient has been.

In the case of rubella, if the patient is a pregnant female, particularly if she is in her first trimester, serologically evaluate for rubella-specific IgM and IgG antibodies. If positive, do not inoculate with MMR. There is no treatment for rubella.

Monitoring Healthcare Workers Exposed to Bacterial Meningitis

Neisseria bacterium causes *Neisseria meningitides*, which is transmitted by airborne droplets that bring on nasopharyngeal colonization and spread to other organs via the circulatory system. **Epidemic meningitis**, seen most frequently in college dormitories and military barracks, can underlie an even more serious condition, Waterhouse-Friderichsen Syndrome. This can quickly be fatal if glucocorticoid and mineralocorticoid replacement of salts, glucose, and steroids is not begun immediately. Military recruits and college students are inoculated as a defense with capsular polysaccharides during outbreaks. Patients with suspected *N. meningitides* should be placed on droplet precautions until ruled out or until 24 hours of appropriate antibiotic therapy has been complete. The recommended antibiotics for *Neisseria meningitidis* are third-generation cephalosporins, like ceftriaxone (the treatment of choice), until culture and sensitivities return. If the strain is penicillin-susceptible, the patient can then be switched to Penicillin G. Duration of IV antibiotic therapy is usually 7 days, but some patients may still have nasal colonization after this period and need to take rifampin to prevent subsequent transmission to others.

First Responder Exposure to Infectious Disease

Emergency medical technicians and paramedics regularly come into contact with potential disease carriers. However, certain occupations not ordinarily associated with healthcare do have higher risks for being exposed to infectious disease. These include **firefighters and police officers**. All of them may find themselves working in the dark of night and oblivious to body fluids they cannot see but come into contact with. EMTs ride in ambulances using sharps while attempting to administer first aid in vehicles on the way to the hospital that are bouncing and swerving about. All are exposed to cuts and exposure to bloodborne infections as well as respiratory pathogens.

Facilitating Follow-Up for First Responder Exposure

First responders may be exposed to communicable diseases before a diagnosis is made or may not be informed of a diagnosis, so the IP must have a program in place to monitor, inform, and follow-up exposures. All first responder groups should be identified and a notification system devised, including information about contact persons and healthcare providers for the first responders. When a communicable disease is diagnosed, a contact investigation should include first responders as well as facility staff. Contact should be made immediately by telephone and in writing, especially important if post-exposure prophylaxis is needed. The IP should be the designated contact person at the facility if first responders need to report communicable diseases that might have infected patients on the way to the facility. The IP should coordinate any testing of source patients or providing information that may be necessary to treat exposure in first responders.

Post-Exposure Prophylaxis for First Responders

Avoiding occupational blood exposures is the best way to prevent transmission of the two pathogens of greatest concern to healthcare workers: hepatitis B virus and human immunodeficiency virus (HIV). (Hepatitis C virus does not appear to be a significant risk for bloodborne transmission.)

If the source of the pathogen's social history, adverse clinical symptoms, or positive results on laboratory tests so indicate, an intense response to the situation is justified. That is, **post-exposure prophylaxis (PEP)** should be started as soon as possible in cases of high-risk exposures.

If a percutaneous exposure to Hepatitis B is caught within one week and multiple doses of hemoglobin are administered, there is only a 25% chance the victim will acquire the disease. The chance of passing on HIV through a percutaneous incident is only 0.3% to begin with, and, because infection does not occur immediately, there is a short period during which antiretroviral intervention can halt or modify viral replication.

Duties of the Infection Control Nurse Working with First Responders

The role of an **infection control nurse** is a rather recent one in the area of working with prehospital personnel, coming about in the last 10 years. The duties of an infection control nurse who may be working for a fire department could include:

- Taking care of firemen's immunizations for hepatitis A and B
- Annual TB skin testing
- Flu shots
- Leading classes on bloodborne pathogens
- Serving as liaison with the hospital IP to follow up on a patient who may have had a communicable disease
- Handling all kinds of questions about illnesses and disease
- Instructing on how to use personal protection against threats of bioterrorism

Some first responders now use fanny packs to gain fast access to personal protective equipment (PPE) items such as gloves, plastic eyewear, masks, sanitary wipes, and paper sleeves. It puts these and other essential PPE items within quick and easy reach. They can thereby protect themselves and patients from exposure to infectious agents.

Providing Counseling to Healthcare Workers Exposed to Communicable Diseases

Providing counseling to healthcare workers exposed to a communicable disease is extremely important, especially those exposed to a serious disease, such as HIV or TB. The HCW may face the possibility of medications, side effects, debility, or even death. In some cases, infection might pose a risk to family members or negatively affect relationships. While people react differently to exposure incidents, studies have indicated that over 40% of staff that have exposure incidents report increased stress and depression after the event. Some have reported symptoms consistent with post-traumatic stress disorder (PTSD) with nightmares and panic attacks. Others have left the field of healthcare altogether as a result of exposure. The infection control plan should include plans for counseling for all staff involved in exposure incidents and automatic referrals should be mad with each event. A counselor should be provided free of charge or healthcare plans should provide for counseling.

Occupational Health Issues for Healthcare Workers in Countries with Limited Resources

Workers of many developing countries are caught in a vicious cycle of low productivity, low income, malnutrition, and infectious diseases. These lead to lower work capacity, lower income, and illness. Poor sanitation and lack of public amenities further contribute to ill health.

The king of manual labor typical of these nations produces repetitive trauma in malnourished men, women, and children and leads to a number of health problems. Musculoskeletal disease is one of the most common. Exposure to known carcinogenic chemicals is commonplace; exposure to solvents also increases the risk of spontaneous abortions in women workers. Agriculture workers are commonly exposed to a variety of pesticides and herbicides. There is a need to develop a database on occupational health in developing countries and create awareness among health personnel, NGOs, and labor organizations that chronic occupational diseases are preventable but rarely curable. Even though, in developing countries, health priorities focus more on infectious diseases, improving the health of workers would contribute tremendously to those nations' growth.

Needle Sticks and Splashes

Follow-Up for Healthcare Workers Exposed to Needle Stick Injuries

Needle stick injuries are the most common type of exposure experienced by healthcare workers providing direct patient care as well as housekeeping staff or environmental services workers who may come in contact with contaminated needles. It is estimated that there are anywhere from 600,000 to 800,000 needle stick injuries are suffered by healthcare workers (hospital and non-hospital based) annually, and it is required that they be reported, but the reality is that surveys have indicated that only about 1/5th of injuries are reported for a variety of reasons, such as staff being too busy, being embarrassed, or being unconcerned because the injury did not appear to break the skin. Most injuries are related to the use of syringes even with safety devices. A program to investigate and follow-up needle stick injuries must include a concerted campaign to educate staff on the importance of reporting injuries so that accurate baseline data can be obtained and evaluations of the injuries with necessary interventions can be done.

Procedures to Follow in the Event of a Needle Stick

Whenever potentially infectious human blood enters the body by needle stick, cut, contamination of broken skin, or a splash to a mucous membrane, immediately bleed the puncture or cut and scrub with soap and water. This may prevent the virus from entering tissues. Flush the nose and mouth if they were exposed. Immediately notify the supervisor.

Post-exposure treatment begins once the exposure source is known to be or even suspected of being HIV infected. It also begins if the source status for HIV is unknown and the injury is a deep penetrating blood-contaminated cut or puncture where proper cleaning is not possible. Likewise, if a large volume of blood has contacted non-intact skin or mucous membranes. Prescribed PEP medications taken while awaiting more information on the source can be discontinued later, if warranted, when the exposure risk has been fully defined.

Hepatitis B immune globulin and pre-exposure vaccine treats Hepatitis B, HIV may be prevented with post-exposure antiviral and inhibitor drugs AZT and Lamivudine, taken ASAP. Hepatitis C has no preventive therapy available.

Reducing Risks of Sharps Injuries

OSHA holds that a combination of engineering and work practice controls, personal protective equipment, training, medical surveillance, hepatitis B vaccination, signs and labels, and other requirements should minimize the risk of disease transmission through accidents with sharps.

A wide variety of medical devices have been developed to reduce the risk of needle sticks and other sharps injuries by replacing sharps with non-needle devices or incorporating safety features designed to reduce the likelihood of injury. Many drugs, for example, can now be administered through inhalants, time release pills, or skin patches rather than being injected.

OSHA Standards of Exposure to Blood or Infectious Material

OSHA requires that safeguards to prevent occupational exposure and incidents be a part of infection control policies. Additionally, the FDA has requirements related to the safety of medical devices. Some states have regulations that are more restrictive than those of OSHA. Important elements include:

- An exposure control plan that outlines methods to reduce staff injury/exposure.
- The use of universal precautions at all times with all patients.
- Planning work practices to minimize danger and using newer and safer technologies as they become available, such as needles engineered to prevent injury.
- Sharps disposal methods that prohibit bending, recapping, shearing, breaking, or handling contaminated needles or other sharps. Scooping with one hand may be used if recapping is essential.
- Workers must be trained in use of universal precautions and methods to decrease exposure.
- Procedures for post-exposure evaluation and treatment must be part of exposure control plan.
- Immunization with Hepatitis B vaccine available to healthcare workers.

Trending Occupational Exposure Incidents

Occupational exposure incidents are a major area of concern for any facility. While needle stick injuries are the most common, other incidents may include accidental ingestion or skin contact. The infection control plan must clearly define occupational exposure incidents and part of the staff education must be the understanding that 100% of incidents must be reported immediately by the person involved in the incident or anyone observing the incident. An incident report form, print or electronic, must be available to all departments and staff. The IP monitors all exposure incidents and gathers data about types of incidents and frequency, using analysis to determine if there is an increase or decrease. Monitoring trends in exposure is especially important if new safety measures, such as the use of needle safety devices, are instituted so that effectiveness can be determined.

Case-Control Studies of Occupational Injuries in Medical Facilities

The case-control study retrospectively examines exposures to suspected risk or protection factors in relation to an outcome that is known at the start of the study. Like a cohort study, it compares a group of diseased subjects with another group lacking that disease. Researchers obtain subject histories and data from medical charts and records to isolate the variables. Case-control studies have the advantage that a small study group is permissible and can be used for studying diseases that do not emerge in great numbers in the general population. According to the CDC, studies on occupational injuries in medical facilities have found the following:

- Hospital-based healthcare personnel annually suffer some 385,000 needle sticks and other sharps-related injuries.
- On average, 1,000 sharps injuries occur daily.
- 40% of sharps injuries happen after sharps use (and before their disposal).
- 41% of sharps injuries occur during the use of sharps (i.e., during injections).
- 15% of sharps injuries occur after the sharps have been disposed of.

Identifying Transmission Risks and Safe Work Practices

Assessing Patients and Employees at Risk of Disease Transmission

Patients or staff with suspicious symptoms, such as an unexplained or chronic cough or foul discharge, should be monitored carefully and appropriate lab testing and precautions taken to reduce the **risk of transmission.** Most infections are not easily transmissible, but those in close contact with an infected person have some risk. Prophylaxis may be needed to protect staff and other patients if there is substantial risk of transmission. There are a number of factors that increase risk of transmission to both staff and employees:

- Patient beds in very close proximity, less than 1 meter, increase the chance of cross infection
- Sharing of equipment among different patients can spread microorganisms
- One employee making contact with multiple patients increases the chance of cross infection
- Failure to use adequate handwashing procedures and universal precautions increases the chance of transmitting infection
- Inadequate monitoring of infections and lab reports can lead to outbreaks

Levels of Restriction

Healthcare Workers with Symptoms

Various types of symptoms pose the risk of being associated with infectious diseases and infection control policies should contain guidelines for immediately reporting these symptoms to employee health/infection control and applying work restrictions:

- Diarrhea can be related to infectious processes and any staff with diarrhea, especially those with direct patient contact or food workers should be restricted from duty until symptoms clear.
- Skin rashes can be caused by viral diseases, such as chickenpox or measles, and workers should be restricted from duty according to diagnosis.
- Cough can be caused by viral or bacterial infections and staff should be evaluated and restricted from work until cough clears.
- Dermatitis, especially on the hands, should be evaluated for work restriction and causes, and treatment provided. If a latex allergy is causing the dermatitis, that could pose a serious risk to the staff person as well as leading to infection of irritated skin that can infect others.

Healthcare Workers with Communicable Diseases

On the basis of documented nosocomial transmission, healthcare workers are considered to be at significant risk for acquiring or transmitting hepatitis B, influenza, measles, mumps, rubella, and varicella. All of these diseases can be prevented through inoculation, which safeguards the health of workers and protects patients from becoming infected through exposure to infected workers. The CDC recommends that all healthcare facilities provide such inoculations. It also recommends that they develop a written policy for restricting healthcare workers who are ill and educate staff on that policy. The CDC provides a list of some of the common diseases of personnel in healthcare, saying for each malady whether workers should be released from patient/resident contact, if partial work restriction should be in place, and the duration of time for this restriction.

Healthcare Worker Exposure to Tuberculosis, Pertussis, and Herpetic Whitlow

The level of work restriction for healthcare workers exposed to a communicable disease varies considerably according to the type of infection. Typical restrictions from work include:

- **Tuberculosis** requires restriction of those with active pulmonary or pharyngeal TB until they have had adequate treatment, symptoms subside, and 3 sputum cultures are negative.
- **Pertussis** requires restriction for the first 5 days of treatment after onset of symptoms.
- **Herpetic whitlow** (intense Herpes Simplex infection of the fingers) requires restriction until lesions heal as they may shed virus even with gloves.

Healthcare Worker Exposure to Hepatitis B and Influenza

Some communicable diseases pose a danger to healthcare workers and to patients and others who have contact with an infected healthcare worker. Work restrictions may vary somewhat depending on state and local regulations. The CDC, OSHA, and ACIP provide some recommendations, which include:

- **Hepatitis B:** Healthcare workers with acute or chronic HB who do not perform exposure-prone procedures are only required to always use standard precautions. Those who do perform exposure-prone procedures should be restricted from those procedures until a review panel can determine appropriate restrictions. Healthcare workers should be immunized against HBV.
- **Influenza:** Healthcare workers with influenza should be restricted from contact with patients and others during the period when the disorder is infectious, which usually begins one day prior to onset of symptoms (when the person is unaware of the infection and contagious) and up to 5 days after onset of symptoms. Healthcare workers should receive annual influenza vaccinations.

Healthcare Worker Exposure to Measles, Mumps, Rubella, and Varicella

Restrictions for healthcare workers exposed to measles, mumps, rubella, and varicella are as follows:

- **Measles:** Active disease requires restriction from duty until 7 days after onset of rash and with exposure restriction from duty from the 5th days through the 21st day after exposure and/or 4 days after onset of rash.
- **Mumps:** Active disease requires restriction from duty until 9 days after onset of parotitis and with exposure restriction from duty from the 9th through the 26th day after exposure or until 9 days after onset of parotitis.
- **Rubella:** Active disease requires restriction from duty until 5 days after onset of rash and with exposure restriction from the 7th through the 21st day after exposure.
- **Varicella**: Active disease requires restriction from duty until all lesions are dry and crusted and with exposure restriction from duty from the 10th through the 21st (or 28th if VZIG given) day or until all lesions are dry and crusted if active disease occurs.

Management and Communication

Planning the Infection Control Program

Infection Control Programs

Planning and Allocating Resources

Steps involved in setting up an infection control program plan and allocating resources are as follows:

1. Prepare the written mission statement, goals, measurable objectives, and action plans for the Infection Control Plan; distribute copies to facility staff and officers
2. Incorporate the facility profile (patient population, major services offered, customer needs and satisfaction, number of healthcare workers) in the Infection Control Plan
3. Recommend specific equipment, personnel, and resources
4. Evaluate hardware and software options for computer applications
5. Set up an Infection Control Committee if there is not already one and facilitate committee meetings
6. Participate in special projects (e.g., cost benefit, efficacy study, product evaluation)
7. Prepare the program's budget
8. Monitor the program's revenue and expenditures
9. Recommend changes in practice based on clinical outcomes and financial implications
10. Document cost reduction in the organization through program activities
11. Publish a regular bulletin updating staff on anything having to do with infection control

Designing an Infection Surveillance System

A key component of the Infection Control Program is the formation of an infection surveillance system. Steps involved in designing the **infection surveillance system** are as follows:

1. Develop plan based on population served and services provided
2. Establish method for identifying baseline/threshold rates
3. Structure laboratory reporting system
4. Determine appropriate and feasible facility-specific denominator data for:
    a. Surgical procedures
    b. Device-related infections
    c. Population at risk
5. Identify potential infections resulting from reportable pathogens
6. Set up surveillance software package for infection control
7. Facilitate post-discharge follow-up for exposure to nosocomial communicable diseases
8. Integrate surveillance activities within affiliated healthcare settings (e.g., ambulatory, home health, long term care, acute care), developing referral forms
9. Set up procedures for performing surveillance studies
10. Establish method to identify patients requiring follow-up or isolation
11. Select indicators for use in antimicrobial monitoring and evaluation
12. Review and modify plan as necessary on a continuing basis.

Creating Job Descriptions for Infection Control Positions

Job descriptions are often vague documents that list generalities but do not adequately represent the actual requirements of a position, but in order to get properly qualified staff, a job description should be up-to-date and accurate. Job descriptions for infection control program positions should include the following:

- **General job description** that states the major areas of responsibility. Some infection control positions include other responsibilities, such as employee health or in-service training, and this should be clear. The work schedule (times and days) should be outlined.
- **Qualifications**, including the type of degrees, licenses, and certification that is required. Desired work experience should be included, such as 3 years of experience in infection control. This may also include a section about the ability to demonstrate knowledge, such as "demonstrates knowledge of epidemiology."
- **Salary and benefits**, such as insurance and vacation time.
- **Duties** that are expected. This should be a comprehensive list that lists specific activities, such as conducting surveillance, providing staff training, and preparing the annual report.

Issues Related to Equipment and Resources for the Infection Control Program

Specific equipment and resources for the infection control program may be overlooked in the budget process but are critically important. Resources include not only personnel in the program but consultants to provide additional information or guidance. A valuable resource for IPs is membership in state and national organizations, such as the Association for Professionals in Infection Control (APIC) in order to remain keep abreast of current trends and regulations. The IPs should receive journals, such as *The American Journal of Infection Control* and *The Journal of Hospital Infection.* They must have access to a medical library and reference materials to aid in research and office space and conference rooms for meetings. Basic equipment, such as computers, printers, scanners, and telephones must be available in numbers sufficient for the number of staff. Additional equipment, such as projectors and screens for computer presentations may be needed.

Managing the Infection Control Program

Management of the Infection Control Program requires the IP to set annual goals and develop objectives (the means for obtaining the goals) while building measures of success. An example would be as follows: The goal is to increase staff productivity by discontinuing total house surveillance. An enabling objective would be to develop criterion-based surveillance indicators for the ICU. Resources to support a typical infection control program include one trained IP for every 100 occupied beds, according to the CDC's Delphi Project. Other necessary resources include:

- Information systems (computers, internet access, integrated databases)
- Clerical, analytical, and statistical support
- Laboratory support
- Dedicated budget

Allocate resources based on:

- Population
- Common diagnoses
- High-risk subgroups
- Services
- Type and number of procedures performed

Establish performance improvement teams to implement HAI reduction interventions. Develop focused surveillance measures. Publicize activities by distributing an annual report with program goals for the coming year.

Duties of an Infection Control Committee

The Infection Control Committee's job is to prevent and control healthcare-associated infections. It is generally comprised of members from a variety of disciplines within the healthcare facility: medical, nursing, infection control, risk management, quality assurance, microbiology, surgery, central sterilization, environmental services, etc. It plans, monitors, evaluates, updates, and sets infection control policy through surveillance of healthcare-associated infections, investigation of infection outbreaks and infection clusters, development of infection control procedures for all departments, staff and patient education, product evaluation, medical waste management, etc.

Specific Personnel in the Infection Control Committee

Personnel for the infection control committee vary in number according to the size of the facility and its programs. In 1980, the CDC recommended 1 IP per every 250 patient beds, but this was before the extensive use of outpatient surgery and shortened hospital stays, which make counting just patients in hospital beds non-representative, so current recommendations are for one IP for every 100 patient beds. Most committees include physicians who are infection control specialist and/or epidemiologists, but other personnel should include representatives from different major departments in the facility, such as nursing services, laboratory, and environmental services. Additional personnel that may be necessary in large facilities include biostatisticians, research analysts, computer programmers, and office staff. An effective infection control program must have adequate staff to carry out surveillance, analyze results, disseminate results, and train staff. The number and type of personnel must be considered in light of the demands on their time and the tasks to be accomplished.

Role of the Joint Commission in Development of the Infection Control Program

The Joint Commission, which accredits most healthcare facilities in the United States, established a requirement in 1969 that hospitals have both committees for infection control and isolation facilities in response to growing concern about healthcare-associated infections. One current goal of the Joint Commission is to "reduce the risk of healthcare-associated infections," applying to both patients and healthcare workers. The Joint Commission lists extensive standards for surveillance, prevention, and control of infection to which healthcare facilities must comply. Because these guidelines and the necessity of having an organized infection control program are explicit in the accreditation requirement, many healthcare facilities incorporate Joint Commission wording regarding infections into their infection control mission statement. Hospitals are given an accreditation report that is publicly listed, showing their compliance with goals established by the Joint Commission. Joint Commission International accredits hospitals throughout the world.

Assessing Needs for the Infection Control Program

Number of Healthcare workers

The number of healthcare workers in a facility has a considerable impact on the planning process for an infection control plan because of the need to train and monitor staff compliance with infection control. One IP may be able to personally train a staff of 30, but when the staff numbers are in the hundreds with all different levels of expertise, and then there are many issues related to training and monitoring:

- Training sessions are needed at different times of day for people working on different shifts as well as repeat training sessions to accommodate large numbers of staff
- Different types of training specific to the needs of special areas, such as ICU or HRN, are necessary
- Increased economic resources are needed with large numbers of staff because of costs involved in purchasing or producing training materials and kits
- Infection control staff resources needed to provide training along with associated costs increase with numbers of healthcare workers

Customer Needs and Satisfaction

Customer needs and satisfaction can be difficult to define and relate to the infection control plan because they are very individual. Assessment of satisfaction, including opportunities for feedback, must be built into any plan. The assumption may be that the patient is the customer, but with an infection control plan, there are many customers:

- **Hospital administrators** want a plan that is cost-effective and reduces infections and liability.
- **Physicians** want a plan that provides positive outcomes for their patients and assists them in providing care.
- **Nursing staff** want a plan that is practical, efficient, and can be implemented without increasing the work burden.
- **Patients** want to avoid complications and regain their health without worrying about a plan.
- **Environmental services** want a plan that relates to the resources available in the departments.
- **Accreditation agencies** want a plan that provides documented proof of compliance with standards related to infection control.

Major Services Offered

The major services offered by a facility is of primary importance in developing an infection control plan as some types of service carry much higher risks than others.

- Intensive care units are consistently cited as high-risk areas because of the severity of the patients' condition as well as the need for invasive devices, such as central venous lines and ventilators.
- Transplant units pose special risk because of the immunocompromised status of patients.
- Surgical service, by its nature, involves invasive procedures that pose the risk for surgical site and bloodstream infections.
- Outpatient services bring a wide variety of patients together and make follow-up difficult.
- Clinics, depending upon the type, may bring patients who are very ill or immunocompromised into the facility.
- High-risk nurseries have infants with little resistance to infection.
- Laboratory services facilitate testing and surveillance if on site but also have risk factors associated with bloodborne pathogens. Off-site services may delay testing.

Assessing the Patient Population

The patient population is an important consideration when developing an infection control plan. There are a number of issues that can impact planning:

- **Size** of the population varies considerably according to the size of the facility. A facility that accommodates 100 patients needs a much different plan than one with 1000 patients.
- **Demographic information** may provide information about risk factors:
  - Socioeconomic status may impact general health, compliance with medical treatments, and follow-up.
  - Age variations affect risk factors. Neonates pose different problems for infection control than geriatric patients.
  - Cultural factors, related to ethnicity or country of origin, may pose distinct health problems.
- **Immunocompromised status** poses greater risk of infections. Status may be related to external factors, such as high rates of HIV related to IV drug use, or immunosuppression from drugs related to transplantation, and these types of subgroups represent distinct risk factors.

Information Technology Requirements

Medical Information Systems and Electronic Health Records

Medical information systems are especially important in health care, as health information covers a wealth of data. The patient data relating to patient services kept on file include patient demographics, eligibility, hospital admission, discharge, complaints, pharmaceutical records, treatments, imaging, and so on. Much of that information is now going into computer systems for easier retrieval and the ability to employ it in retrospective studies, so that patient information is now called electronic health records. This, along with computer-based administration functions, make hospitals more efficient and, at least in theory, enable medical personnel to devote more time to patient care.

Electronic Communications Technology

Potentially useful technology includes the **Personal Data Assistant (PDA)/Phone**. This mobile computing device connects via communications satellite to the internet to allow such things as email, calendar maintenance, keeping directories, browsing the Web, and appointment scheduling. A cell phone is included, and some models have cameras built in. Medical uses include entering and tracking insurance data, reviewing lab reports, and writing prescriptions. It differs from handheld PC's because the latter contain keyboards and can perform such desktop applications as word processing. It is likely that, in the near future, features of both will meld into one device.

Information System Configuration

Like spokes in a wheel, satellite computers link via a local area network (LAN) system—wired or wireless—into the hospital's computer servers where programs and databases are stored and central processors where operations are processed. Users access the programs and data from one of the many satellite personal computers located around the facility. With permission, they can access any kind of data in storage and use it for updating records, gathering treatment information, etc. Operators may exchange information with other operators at other nodes, either actively or through email. The same central data system may also be used for various other hospital functions, such as operating the air conditioning and heating systems. Systems may also be hooked in, via internet, to other healthcare facilities and such organizations as the Centers for Disease Control.

Evaluation of Hardware and Software Options

The infection control program must be able to survey, analyze and take action quickly in the event of outbreaks or clusters of infection. Often, infection control is hampered by a lack of integration among existing computer **hardware and software programs**. The laboratory may use one program: nursing, another. In some facilities, record keeping and reporting is still done by hand. Therefore, the problem of deciding what course to take with hardware and software can be difficult. Ideally, all computer systems and software should be integrated, but this can be very costly. If a facility uses a software designer to create a program specifically meeting the needs of an institution, it may not communicate with reporting or other software. Even if programs and equipment are purchased, they may be subject to expensive updates every couple of years. Some programs are web-based, requiring internet capability. In many cases, hiring a consultant with expertise in medical hardware and software to advise about the best solution may be the best option.

Mobile Computer Applications

Mobile computer applications relevant in the healthcare environment include:

- **Alert messaging and communication**: Mobile computing can supply test results and the ability to forward them.
- **Clinical document**: Provides pictures of documents and the ability to make notes about them.
- **Charge capture and coding**: Healthcare workers may record insurance charge data at the time care is given; automatic AMA coding is possible.
- **Laboratory order entry and results reporting**: Lab tests may be ordered on the go and the results viewed anywhere.
- **Prescription writing**: Accessing the patient, medication, and dose records from anywhere, a doctor can write prescriptions any time from anyplace.

Hospital epidemiologists need automated tools for data collection, storage, and analysis, and should choose systems and software accordingly, along with communications abilities.

Recommending Changes to Practice

Recommending Changes Based on Clinical Outcomes and Financial Implications

Interventions and outcomes should be tied to each other. After an initial cost-benefit analysis and institution of an intervention in infection control, outcomes need to be assessed carefully to determine if the intervention is meeting the goal set for it and is cost-effective. If, for example, the hospital is investing $92,000 additionally each year expecting a savings of 5 infections at $135,000 ($43,000 net), but in fact the savings amount to only 2 infections at $34,000, then the added cost to the hospital is $59,000. **Changes in practice**, however, cannot be made only on the basis of monetary figures. Further analysis must be done to determine if other variables affected the outcomes. If the hospital opened a transplant unit with additional surgical patients, then the reduction in 2 infections might be impressive. If there is a *staph* carrier among the staff, then this might account for additional infections. In some cases, a change of practice is required.

Measuring Compliance with Regulations and Standards

There is a maze of regulations and standards that must be reconciled and complied with, and this task falls within the responsibilities of the IP. Various regulating agencies include:

- State and local government regulations may overlap other agencies because most states rely on other regulatory agencies, such as the FDA and CDC for medical standards although standards related to kitchens, food preparation, and sanitation may vary somewhat.
- Hospital Infection Control Practices Advisory Committee (HIPAC) works with the CDC to establish standards and guideline.
- CDC is central to prevention of control of infections and issues standards and procedures for preventing transmission, such as barrier precautions, isolation guidelines, and TB monitoring, and disease reporting.
- OSHA regulates occupational health issues related to exposure to infectious materials.
- FDA regulates medications and medical devices, including recall and reuse issues.
- Joint Commission accredits hospitals and medical facilities and requires extensive documented compliance with standards.

Responsibilities of Infection Control Officer with Regards to Regulations

Regulatory standards responsibilities:

- Comply with infection control regulations and standards
- Assist in obtaining accreditations/licensure and maintaining standards
- Proactively influence policymaking bodies
- Inform management and staff of alterations in infection control regulations and standards
- Report cases of communicable diseases to Public Health authorities
- Anticipate pending legislation in the area of infection control.

Identifying Opportunities for Improvement

Opportunities for improvement may be evident on analysis of indicators (typical causes of infection, such as central venous lines) and outcomes (rates of infection). Through surveillance activities, both numerator and denominator data is produced and these outcomes should be measured against internal benchmarks that have been established, or external benchmarks, such as national rates of infection. Once it is clear where variances lie, then these particular indicators can be targeted for improvement. Additionally, other findings or observations may indicate the need for changes in processes. For example, cost-benefit analysis may show that some procedures or processes are not cost-effective and there may be a number of different solutions that might achieve the same or better results. These procedures or process may be reviewed and alternate solutions sought so that these processes or procedures become a target for reduction in variable costs to a facility.

Assigning Value to Infection Prevention

Arguments for Funding for an Infection Control Program

Arguments for adequately funding an infection control program include the following:

- The functioning program's intent is to improve safety and quality while reducing overall costs.
- Fewer nosocomial hospital stay days for a patient on a prospective payment plan like Medicare means lower costs and better profits; also, some lost opportunity costs would be eliminated by not tying up facilities for treatment of patients with healthcare-associated infections.
- Maintaining regulatory compliance, preventing medical errors, and building a safer environment for patients and staff brings benefits to the organization beyond reducing costs of infection. The absence of a good program can lead to a bad reputation for excessive hospital-associated infections, which leads to losing patients and patient referrals, as well as dissatisfied employees leaving for other jobs. A good program gives hospital staff the ego boost of bragging rights.
- Reduced infections mean reduced use of antibiotics that contribute to drug resistance problems.

Primary Payer for Healthcare-Associated Infections

Even though it is difficult to prove **negligence** and few patients recover damages, patients are inclined to bring lawsuits in an endeavor to recover damages after extended hospital stays resulting from healthcare-associated infections.

However, in most cases, it is an insurer, whether government or private, not an individual patient, paying the bills. Because the majority of such infections can be prevented through greater diligence, insurers contest charges associated with the extended stays, particularly the largest insurer, Medicare.

A study of 33 Medicare patients who developed nosocomial pneumonia found that hospital costs for almost all patients exceeded reimbursements, with a median net loss of $5,800 per case to the hospital. The authors of the study concluded that hospitals have substantial financial incentives for implementing cost-effective measures for preventing nosocomial pneumonias.

Impact of Healthcare-Associated Infections on the Nation

Healthcare-associated infections have nationwide impacts that are important to consider when justifying expenditures for infection control programs:

- They are in the top five leading causes of death in the US.
- They cause or contribute to about 99,000 deaths a year.
- At any given time, 1 in 31 patients in the hospital setting is infected with a healthcare-associated infection.
- They cause an excess length of hospital stay of 10.4 days per patient.
- They cause excess hospital expenses of $7 billion to $15 billion per year in the US, and societal expenses of up to $12 billion per year.
- Mean cost per case attributed to bloodstream infections is anywhere from $18,000 to $95,000.

Justifying Expenditures

Cost-Effective Analysis, Efficacy Studies, and Product Evaluations

Each year, about 2 million healthcare-associated infections result in 99,000 deaths and an estimated $7 billion to $15 billion in additional health costs. From that perspective, decreasing infections should reduce costs, but there are human savings in suffering as well, and it can be difficult to place a dollar value on that. A **cost-effective analysis** measures the effectiveness of an intervention rather than the monetary savings. If each infection adds about 12 days to hospitalization, then a reduction in infection by 5 would be calculated:

$$5 \times 12 = 60 \text{ fewer patient infection days}$$

Efficacy studies may compare a series of cost-benefit analyses to determine the intervention with the best cost-benefit. They may also be used for **process or product evaluation.** For example, a study might be done to determine the infection rates of 4 different types of catheters to determine which type resulted in the fewest infections, thus saving the most money (and infection days).

Incremental cost-effectiveness ratio is the ratio of cost change to outcome change.

Cost-Benefit Analysis

Surgical site infections result in an average of 9.7 additional days of hospitalization and costs $25,000 to $90,000. (In actuality, the cost may vary widely from one institution to another; so local data may be used.) A **cost-benefit analysis** uses average cost of infection and the cost of intervention to demonstrate savings. For example, if an institution were averaging 10 surgical site infections per year, the annual cost would be:

$$10 \times \$27{,}000 = \$270{,}000$$

If the interventions include new software ($10,000) for surveillance, an additional staff person ($65,000), benefits ($15,000) and increased staff education, including materials ($2000), the total intervention cost would be:

$$\$10{,}000 + \$65{,}000 + \$15{,}000 + \$2000 = \$92{,}000$$

If the goal were to decrease infections by 50% to 5 infections per year, the savings would be calculated:

$$5 \times \$27{,}000 = \$135{,}000$$

Subtracting the intervention cost from the savings gives us the net annual benefit:

$$\$135{,}000 - \$92{,}000 = \$43{,}000$$

Utility and Patient Preferences as Related to Health Outcome Analysis

Cost-effective analysis compares the cost of alternative approaches to obtaining a common objective such as healthcare-associated infection control, while **cost-utility analysis** looks at the cost of alternatives while adjusting outcomes to consider patient preferences. The most common cost-utility approach is termed **quality adjusted life years (QALYs),** which combines patient longevity and individuals' preferences about different levels of health-related quality of life into a single measure. An example might be taking a strict, infection-controlled, antimicrobial approach to surgery and comparing its effectiveness against standard surgical practices for the same procedure. One might do that by comparing the quality adjusted post-operative life years of patients on the assumption that the controlled approach will show greater longevity.

Quality of Life Years as Related to the Health Outcome Analysis

Quality-adjusted life years are a measure that is most often associated with medical interventions where the patient's potential benefits for a risky procedure must be balanced against remaining in a state of poor health. In the area of public health, recommendations may have to be made on trade-offs between one set of conditions that may prove injurious to health and another set of conditions that may have its own drawbacks. For example, a dose response model weighted by quality adjusted life years saved may be used to make recommendations on eating fish that are beneficial to coronary health but also contain trace amounts of mercury.

Where infection control is concerned, cost benefit analysis of investing in better healthcare-associated infection disease control is rarely used because society does not like placing a monetary value on states of health. Only when there are no expected mortality differences between interventions, simply morbidity differences which can be expressed as quality adjusted life years are cost utility analyses useful.

Barriers to Measuring Increased Costs of Healthcare-Associated Infections

About 10% of hospitalized patients acquire an infection after admission, meaning the patient's stay will be prolonged. They therefore occupy what may be a scarce bed and require additional diagnostic and therapeutic interventions. An estimate of the cost of these infections in 2002 is $7 billion to $15 billion per year. Usually, the patient's insurance company bears the expense, but increasingly, they are rebelling against it.

However, different statistical methods may be used to determine the impact on the attributable cost of nosocomial infection, and the methods yield different results in attempts to control such cost variables as relative severity of illness, duration of surgery, gender, obesity, congestive heart failure, diabetes, etc. One statistical method is to compare the costs of infected and uninfected patients by a t-test in a matched and unmatched comparison, another involves regression analysis, and a third uses a two-stage method.

Documentation of Cost Reduction from Infection Control Activities

Many costs associated with infection control are fixed and realistically cannot be recouped; however, infection control is mandated, not optional, so the goal of an infection control program is to use resources as efficiently as possible to lower the infection rate to the point of diminishing returns where there is acceptable reduction of infection rates but further investment is not cost-effective. **Documentation** requires extensive statistical analysis that includes cost-benefit and cost-effectiveness. Calculations should document monetary savings based on fewer infections and reduction in infection days, theoretically opening the rooms to other patients and increased income, referred to as opportunity costs, which must also be calculated. Any variable costs associated with opportunity costs must be considered. Targeted analysis of specific interventions that show outcomes can help to evaluate the effectiveness of the infection control program. Cost reduction should be demonstrated with graphs, charts, and explanatory text.

Communication

Communication Aspects of the Infection Control Program

Some elements that should be included in the communications aspects of an infection control program include:

- Identifying healthcare workers' responsibilities to prevent and control infections
- Distributing infection control findings and recommendations
- Disseminating pertinent regulatory policies and procedures, guidelines, consensus statements, position papers, and standards to applicable departments
- Providing consultation on issues relating to infection control
- Preparing an annual summary of Infection Control Program activities
- Consulting with risk management in the investigation of claims
- Serving as an infection control liaison with public health authorities
- Serving as an infection control liaison among healthcare facilities, medical staff, and community
- Marketing/Promoting the Infection Control Program within and outside the facility
- Advising administrative staff on the infection control implications of architectural design and renovation
- Advising site contractors on the infection control implications of architectural design and renovation
- Supervising infection control aspects of facility construction projects

Role of the Infection Control Professional as a Liaison

The role of **liaison officer** is an integral part of the IP's responsibilities, especially with the increase of outpatient surgery and short hospital stays, sending patients home or into extended care facilities. Communication among the different agencies and facilities caring for patients is necessary if infection control surveillance and preventive methods are to be accurate and effective. It is especially important that the IP serve as liaison to feeder institutions, such as small hospitals that transfer patients into a larger facility and extended care facilities to which discharge patients are transferred. Having an assigned IP to serve as liaison and to meet regularly with other agencies/ facilities allows the IP to serve as a consultant so that shared goals and objectives can be developed. Maintaining a close working relationship with the public health department is necessary because of reporting requirements and the need for cooperation in the event of outbreaks or pandemics.

Internal Communication

Information Exchange Between Occupational Health and the Infection Control Department

Occupational/employee health and infection control departments must work closely together because employee health and exposure issues are in the purview of the IP. In some facilities, the IP is in charge of both areas, and in a small facility, this might be efficient, but only part of employee health issues relates to infection control, so this may not be the best utilization of expertise. The director of the employee health program and the IP should attend each other's meetings when possible and should establish guidelines for the sharing of information so that both departments work cooperatively. While privacy issues are a matter of concern, staff should be provided with release forms that clearly state that all matters related to infection control would be shared between the departments. The infection control and employee health departments should collaborate on the development of policies, new employee orientation and infection control education.

Facilitating Meetings of the Infection Control Committee

Facilitating meetings of the infection control committee requires preplanning as well as active guidance during the meeting. Focusing on one or two issues of the action plan may be more productive than trying to discuss all goals and objectives:

- Send reminders to committee members, including date and time and a clear outline of what is expected of the member at the meeting, such as giving a report or providing information.
- Review task lists from prior meetings to ensure that all issues are covered.
- Prepare an agenda based on the action plan and task lists, to guide the group discussion.
- Review surveillance data and prepare reports of any outbreaks or clusters of concern.
- Copy all pertinent documents and data reports for committee members.
- Reserve any necessary equipment, such as computers or projectors, and arrange for them to be set up and available in the meeting room.
- Monitor time and ensure discussions are balanced and each person contributes.

Information to Include in the Annual Summary of the Infection Control Program

The **Annual Report of the Infection Control Program**, prepared by the Infection Control Committee and issued by the head administrator, provides the facility and the public with information activities of the infection control team over the past fiscal year. It highlights achievements of the team, presents progress made toward objectives it has set, updates new developments for the past year, and previews the proposed Infection Control Annual Program for the coming year. An annual report can also be useful for demonstrating to The Joint Commission the scope and actions of the infection control program.

Presenting the Annual Summary

The annual summary is an important tool for the IP because it clearly outlines the progress (or lack) in infection control over the year. Since outcomes are of primary importance, the summary should utilize the infection control plan and be organized in the same way, listing the goal, the objectives (actions), and the specific outcomes related to those objectives. Each goal and objective should be included, even if no action took place. Statistical analysis should be completed prior to beginning the annual summary, and the analyses should be included in the document. Charts, graphs, and diagrams, such as line and bar graphs, flow charts, decision trees, and cause and effect diagrams should be part of the summary. The summary should highlight achievements and list ongoing or potential goals for the following year. A separate timeline that gives a brief summary of action month by month may also be included.

Distribution of Findings to Committees, Departments, and Units

Infection control findings are the result of surveillance activities that may target particular units or in some cases individuals. For this reason, there may be some restriction to access of some or all reports. Part of establishing an infection control program is to determine the reporting tree: who gets which report and how. Typically, all members of the infection control committee would have access to all reports, as would the administration. Reports that related to the entire facility, such as overall infection rates, would be distributed widely. For more sensitive reports, at the next level department chairs would receive reports and recommendations related to their own units and would then disseminate the information as appropriate. Any individual findings, such as surgical site infections for individual surgeons, are usually provided to the department chair and the individual. Dissemination may be in print or by password protected internet or Intranet postings.

Providing Consultation on Issues Related to Infection Control

Infection control is central to patient safety and any changes in a facility, whether it is a change of product or procedure or a renovation project, has the potential to increase transmission of disease; therefore, an IP should be a standing member available for **consultation** of any committee or group whose actions may impact patient care. The IP should be knowledgeable about the issues and be prepared to research and provide guidance. Risk management professionals protect the institution from liability related to patient injury, including infections, and it is critical that risk management have as clear an understanding of causes related to an infection as possible. The IP may use tracer methodology to identify possible sources of transmission and to determine if processes were used correctly in an effort to prevent infection because this information can help to support or deny liability, allowing risk management to make decisions about a case.

Consultation on Occupational Infections and/or Exposures

The IP consults with management regarding the **Exposure Control Plan** for occupational infections/exposures. OSHA defines occupational exposure as "reasonably anticipated skin, eye, mucous membrane, or parenteral contact with blood or other potentially infectious materials" resulting from performance of duties. Further, any employer with employee(s) with such occupational exposure must have a written Exposure Control Plan, which aims to minimize or eliminate danger to the employee(s). This plan must include:

- Documented input from staff involved in direct patient care
- A schedule and methods of compliance, such as Hepatitis B vaccination programs
- Methods of communicating hazards to staff
- Record keeping
- Procedures for investigating exposure incidents that might result in infection
- Annual review and update to reflect technology changes or safer medical devices
- An exposure determination that includes listing of all job classifications with exposures and the types of exposures

Collaborating with Staff to Reduce Risks of Infection

The IP can work with healthcare staff to reduce the risk of infection to patients through the following:

- When setting up an infection control program, address the risks of transmitting infections between patients and healthcare workers.
- Recommend to Human Resources the type of screening for disease risks of healthcare workers advisable prior to hire or placement.
- Screen healthcare workers for communicable disease history and infections.
- Assess risk of occupational exposure to infectious diseases by job classification or department and respond accordingly.
- Investigate and provide necessary assistance to healthcare workers exposed to communicable diseases, including follow-up for exposed emergency-response personnel.
- Assist with analysis, determine trends in occupational exposure incidents.
- Collaborate on immunization programs for healthcare workers.
- Recommend work restrictions for infected healthcare workers.

Communicating Needs to the Administration

In an era of increasing medical costs and decreasing reimbursement, communicating infection control resource needs to administration requires careful planning and statistical analysis to support the need and the cost-effectiveness of the resources, outlining exactly how the resources are going to improve infection control. Strategies include:

- **Statistical support**, including cost-benefit and cost-effectiveness analysis to demonstrate value of the resource in controlling infection. The use of charts and diagrams is effective as a tool to present information clearly.
- **Research support** can include a literature review and summary of reports and research supporting the use of the resource.
- **Demonstrations** that allow the administration to see the resource and view its use can be persuasive.
- **Staff support** from other healthcare workers, such as physicians or nurses, who recognize the need may bolster an argument in favor of a resource.

External Communication

Liaison with Public Health Authorities, Healthcare Facilities, and the Community

The day-to-day activities of a **Public Health Liaison**, for those facilities that have one on staff, may include interacting with Infection Control regarding nosocomial diseases; with the Emergency Department staff to review admissions and track reportable diseases; with the lab to review reportable conditions from laboratory testing; attending meetings of the hospital's IC, ED, Emergency Preparedness, Safety and Microbiology Departments; filing mandatory reports with the state on communicable disease cases; fielding phone calls from other public health agencies; and providing information and education on public health, as requested by hospital staff.

In the case of a breakout, the liaison could be getting patient histories to determine where they may have acquired their infection, reviewing lab results rapidly, and submitting as soon as possible a report for follow-up by the state to prevent potential widespread infection. Facilities with a public health liaison are able to establish more effective communication regarding emergency preparedness in breakouts of infection as well as situations such as bioterrorism or a pandemic.

Reporting Communicable Diseases to the Appropriate Health Authorities

Mechanisms for **reporting of communicable diseases** vary somewhat from state to state, but there are city, county, state, national, and international reporting regulations. The IP will normally notify the local and state authorities of communicable diseases, and the state, in turn, notifies the CDC, which may notify WHO for internationally reportable diseases, such as smallpox or polio. The CDC maintains a reportable disease list, which is upgraded and revised as necessary and reissued July 1 of each year. It includes infections of concern, such as HIV and HBV. Each state also maintains a reportable disease list, which may or may not be identical with that of the CDC, so the IP must be familiar with all reportable disease requirements. Much data at the state and local level is confidential name-based information, but data collected at the CDC is without names or personal identifying information. Some states require reporting of healthcare-associated infections.

Marketing and Promoting the Infection Control Plan

Providing an infection control plan is only the beginning of **marketing and promoting**, which must be ongoing endeavors. Some marketing strategies include:

- Patient information sheets telling patients about infection controls standards and procedures and what they should expect from the staff, such as handwashing before and after every contact.
- Maintaining a high profile by visiting different departments and units, talking to staff, asking and answering questions.
- Monthly or weekly promotions, such as slogans, posters, and flyers about hand washing throughout the facility.
- Joint activities and promotions with other agencies/facilities in the area.
- Mini-conferences with speakers about infection control issues and vendor displays.
- Regularly scheduled training sessions for staff and other healthcare workers in the area.
- Events with participative activities, such as handwashing contests with glow in the dark powders or solutions to determine effectiveness of handwashing technique.
- Infection control crossword puzzles or games.
- Newsletters to staff and community about infection control issues.

Sentinel Events

A sentinel event, any unexpected occurrence of healthcare-associated infection, can include the risk of death or actual death, serious physical injury, or psychological injury. It also includes any process variation for which a recurrence would carry a significant chance of a serious adverse outcome, including loss of limb or function. Such events are called "sentinel" because they signal the need for immediate investigation and response. The event indicates an unhealthy work environment as a result of avoidable disease, disability, or untimely death and points to an absence of, or poor application of, preventive measures. Sentinel events, in number and type, are taken into consideration when healthcare facilities come up for accreditation.

An infection is considered a sentinel event if it is determined that the death or injury would not have occurred without the infection. Each case must be dealt with individually, and, if defined as sentinel, a root cause analysis that defines the problem through gathering evidence to identify what contributed to the problem must be done. Once a root cause has been determined, an action plan that identifies all the different elements that contributed to the problem is recommended and instituted. The theory is that finding the root cause can eliminate the problem rather than just treating it. Thus, finding the source of an infection would be more important than just treating the infection.

Medication Errors and Medical Errors

A **medication error** is any preventable event that may cause or lead to inappropriate medication use or patient harm. One common source of medication error is the verbal communication of prescription or medication orders. Others include mistakes in:

- Prescribing
- Monitoring
- Transcribing
- Dispensing
- Administering
- Compliance
- Drug Age
- Documentation
- Dose/IV Flow Rate: Wrong dose, dosing at the wrong time
- Labeling
- Patient Identification
- Authorization
- Issuing Wrong Drug
- Specifying Wrong Route/Site
- Using Wrong Administration Technique

The National Academy of Sciences' Institute of Medicine describes a **medical error** as a mistake made by a healthcare provider that results in a patient being injured by or dying of that mistake rather than from the medical condition he or she checked into the hospital with. The mistakes include an inappropriate method of care or choosing the correct course of care but carrying it out incorrectly so that it kills the patient. It also includes misdiagnosis, drug interactions, and wrong site surgery. Probably half of adverse reactions to medicines are the result of medical errors.

Advising on Construction and Renovation Planning

Construction and renovation pose serious risks to both patients and staff because of the danger of dust and water contamination; therefore, the administration must be advised of all the implications when these projects are undertaken as there are often considerable expenses beyond construction costs in preventing transmission of disease. The American Institute of Architects (AIA) Academy of Architecture for Health publishes guidelines that are used by the CDC and states as minimum standards for construction and renovation in a healthcare facility. These guidelines require input from the IP at all stages of construction, including planning that includes an infection control risk assessment (ICRA). The IP helps to identify support structures that will be needed during construction. Based on the ICRA, a comprehensive plan for renovation and construction should be developed that includes all of the necessary elements to carry out the project while ensuring infection control monitoring and patient safety.

Issues Related to Construction

The IP and administration must deal with a number of issues related to construction:

Preventing environmental contamination:

- Construction areas must be sealed off with heavy plastic or drywall.
- Negative pressure must be maintained in construction area.
- Foot traffic should be directed around construction.
- Cleaning of construction site and removing debris must be done daily.

Protecting patients:

- Patient units may be closed.
- Patients, especially those at high risk, may be transferred away from construction areas.
- Patient transportation should be limited.
- Additional surveillance may be required.

Incorporating infection control into construction design:

- Walls, floors, and surfaces should be easy to clean and resistant to disinfectant and water damage.
- Adequate handwashing facilities and space for sharps disposal must be available.
- Positive and/or negative pressure airflow should be planned as needed by the type of construction project.

Implementing and Monitoring Policies and Procedures

Implementing Changes in Policies, Procedures, or Working Standards

Changes in policies, procedures, or working standards are common and, the IP is responsible for educating the staff about changes related to infection control, which should be communicated to staff in an effective and timely manner:

- **Policies** are usually changed after a period of discussion and review by administration and staff, so all staff should be made aware of policies under discussion. Preliminary information should be disseminated to staff regarding the issue during meetings or through printed notices.
- **Procedures** may be changed to increase efficiency or improve patient safety often as the result of surveillance and data about outcomes. Procedures changes are best communicated in workshops with demonstrations. Posters and handouts should be available as well.
- **Working standards** are often changed because of regulatory or accrediting requirements and this information should be covered extensively in a variety of different ways such as discussions, workshops, and handouts so that the implications are clearly understood.

Communicating Changes in Regulations and Standards

Communication of changes in regulations and standards must be made in a timely manner and disseminated widely, especially in the changes result in differences in processes or procedures. The IP is often the first person to receive information about pending changes and should begin early to make plans to communicate to others. There are a number of ways to **communicate changes**:

- Infection Control Plan should be updated on an annual basis to include all information related to changes in regulations and standards
- Consulting with administration about impending changes and courses of action
- Staff meetings with department heads and staff who are directly impacted by changes to outline changes
- Print materials, such as documents, fliers, and posters should be prepared to provide the necessary information
- Email communications can quickly alert staff to changes
- Training classes that cover new standards should be provided as quickly as possible

Influencing Policymaking Bodies

The IP is in a unique position to influence policymaking within an institution, but even more important is the ability to influence policymaking at a state or national level. The IP should take an active role in national organizations that promote the development of consistent standards and participation in the political process. Three organizations have cooperated to create model legislation that can serve as a template for state legislatures adopting regulations regarding collecting and reporting of data regarding healthcare-associated infection:

- *The Association for Professionals in Infection Control and Epidemiology (APIC)* (15,000+ members), open to physicians, epidemiologists, nurses, laboratory technicians, and others involved in reducing the risk of infection.
- *The Infectious Disease Society of America (IDSA)* (12,000+ members), open to scientists, physicians, and others specialize in infectious diseases.
- *The Society for Healthcare Epidemiology of America (SHEA)* is open to physicians and others who work in infection control in a healthcare field. Various levels of membership are available based on the individual's education, experience, and professional relationship with infectious disease and epidemiology.

Implications of Pending Legislation

When healthcare-associated infections first became reportable, confidentially was a cornerstone, protecting the reporting institution from liability; however, in response to morbidity, mortality, and costs associated with healthcare-associated infections, increasingly states are passing **new laws** requiring public reporting. Because there is no national standard, the laws, including definitions and types of reporting, vary considerably. In response, APIC, SHEA, and IDSA have proposed legislation to try to standardize reporting requirements. As reports become public, in some cases with hospital specific data, there is tremendous pressure on the IP to reduce rates of infection. The IP must be familiar with current or pending legislation and keep the administration appraised, taking early steps toward compliance.

Quality Performance Improvement and Patient Safety

CONTINUOUS QUALITY IMPROVEMENT (CQI)

Continuous quality improvement (CQI) emphasizes the organization and systems and processes within that organization rather than individuals. It recognizes internal customers (staff) and external customers (patients) and utilizes data to improve processes. CQI represents the concept that most processes can be improved. CQI uses the scientific method of experimentation to meet needs and improve services and utilizes various tools, such as brainstorming, multivoting, various charts and diagrams, storyboarding, and meetings. Core concepts include:

- Quality and success are meeting or exceeding internal and external customer's needs and expectations.
- Problems relate to processes, and variations in process lead to variations in results.
- Change can be made in small steps.

Steps to CQI include:

1. Form a knowledgeable team.
2. Identify and define measures used to determine success.
3. Brainstorm strategies for change.
4. Plan, collect, and utilize data as part of making decisions.
5. Test changes and revise or refine as needed.

MULTIDISCIPLINARY QUALITY/PERFORMANCE STRATEGIES

Continuous quality improvement (CQI) is a **multidisciplinary management** philosophy that can be applied to all aspects of business, whether related to infection control, purchasing, or human resources issues. The skills used for epidemiologic research (data collection, analysis, outcomes, action plans) are all applicable to analysis of non-infectious events because they are based on solid scientific methods. Multi-disciplinary planning can bring valuable insights from various perspectives, and strategies used in one context can often be applied to another. Increasingly, infection control must be concerned with cost-effectiveness as the costs of medical care continue to rise, so the IP is not in an isolated position in an institution but is just one part of the whole, facing similar concerns as those in other disciplines. Disciplines are often interrelated in their functions. For example, Human Resources hires personnel, but the IP monitors and trains them for compliance with infection control standards. Purchasing may order catheters, but the type may affect infection rates.

QUALITY MANAGEMENT

TOTAL QUALITY MANAGEMENT (TQM)

Total quality management (TQM), a comprehensive and structured approach to organizing problem solving, decision making, and progress measurement, is strongly customer-centered. Though it originated in the manufacturing sector, it has been adapted for use in virtually every type of organization. Its mission is to improve the quality of the organization's offerings to its publics through ongoing refinements to its operations in response to continuous feedback. TQM requirements may be defined separately for each organization or may choose to adhere to established and published standards, such as the International Organization for Standardization's ISO 9000 series. It is marked by staff participation in problem-solving, using metrics to determine whether an objective has been obtained, and documenting and disseminating results.

Baldrige National Quality Program and the EFQM Excellence Model

A part of the National Institute of Standards and Technology's *Baldrige National Quality Program* (the Institute being a part of the US Department of Commerce) for furthering management effectiveness, the *Baldrige Award for Healthcare Criteria* is annually awarded to organizations that are improving healthcare outcomes and delivering the highest quality healthcare service.

Award recipients, having put an emphasis on healthcare performance results that have led to rapid improvements in patient care, are credited by the award committee for providing superior healthcare quality and value to their patients. The recipients become models for the healthcare industry to follow.

The *EFQM Excellence Model* is a European version of the Baldrige Awards; it also includes healthcare organizations under its award umbrella and is equally focused on developing standards for use in self-assessment of quality management.

Six Sigma and Balanced Score Card

Six Sigma, a quality control program originated in the 1980's at Motorola, uses statistics to measure and improve a company's operational performance. A move to improve quality output, it created a new standard along with the methodology and cultural change needed to implement it. It exported the program to a variety of other organizations, including some hospitals.

Developed by two Harvard professors in the 1990's, the **Balanced Score Card (BSC)** management system translates mission and strategy into objectives and metrics that are organized into four different perspectives: Financial, customer, internal business processes, and learning and growth. They use statistical feedback to inspire employees toward achievement of specified outcomes. BSC gives healthcare providers, for example, the ability to make informed decisions about service quality through, among other measures, the analysis of clinical outcomes.

Role of the IP in Quality Control, Education, and Research

Roles of the IP in quality control, education, and research include:

- Coordinating the organization's quality/performance improvement activities as they relate to infection control
- Seeking out opportunities to improve the Infection Control program
- Participating in multidisciplinary quality/performance improvement initiatives
- Reporting quality improvement initiatives and improvements resulting from initiatives
- Assessing healthcare worker educational needs pertaining to infection control
- Developing educational offerings, including goals, strategies, measurable objectives, and lesson plans, to meet staff needs
- Gathering appropriate published educational materials and prepares homemade materials and handouts
- Presenting and/or coordinating training sessions on a variety of infection control topics
- Evaluating the effectiveness of education
- Participating in the facility's orientation program for new employees
- Disseminating information facility-wide on infection control
- Instructing patients/families in methods to prevent and control infections
- Delivering lectures on infectious illness topics to the community
- Keeping current on literature of infection control

Root Cause Analysis

Root cause analysis (RCA) is a retrospective attempt to determine the cause of an event, often a sentinel event such as an unexpected death, or a cluster of events. **Root cause analysis** involves interviews, observations, and review of medical records. Often, an extensive questionnaire is completed by the IP doing the RCA, tracing essentially every step in hospitalization and care, including every treatment, every medication, and every contact. The focus of the RCA is on systems and processes rather than individuals. How did the system break down? Where did the problem arise? In some cases, there may be one root cause, but in others, the causes may be multiple. The RCA also must include a thorough review of literature to ensure that **action plans** based on the results of the RCA reflect current best practices. Action plans without RCA may be non-productive. If, for example, an infection was caused by contaminated air, action plans to increase disinfection of the operating room surfaces would not be effective.

Environmental Inspections

Environmental inspections to evaluate infection control practices and hazards requires a multi-faceted approach that includes:

- Surveillance reports regarding the incidence of infection
- Feedback of reports to staff
- Observation of clinical practice

In all facilities, environmental inspections should be ongoing, but in large facilities, observing all staff for compliance with infection control practices can be difficult if not impossible, so utilizing surveillance reports to target areas of concern may be more time and cost effective. Once an area is targeted, feedback should be provided to staff and comprehensive inspections should include direct observation of staff during clinical work rather than staff demonstrations. The IP or designated team members should participate in the investigation. Environmental culturing may be done as well as staff cultures when indicated. Questionnaires may be used to solicit information about staff compliance, understanding of infection control, and satisfaction with training.

Patient Safety Performance Improvement Activities

Patient safety performance improvement activities are those that are designed as campaigns to reduce error or improve patient outcomes, such as reduction in infection. Often the activities are targeted to one group (such as physicians) or one type of patient, but they may also be broader. Because performance improvement and processes are central to the Joint Commission's accreditation standards, those standards make a good starting point to look at possible improvement activities as well as the data that has been collected. Many problems are multidisciplinary and may involve, for example, both environmental services and infection control, such as the need to increase hepatitis B vaccinations in housekeeping staff. Teams must decide what to measure, collect data, determine solutions, and then implement solutions in a concerted effort. Patient safety performance activities may include such activities as monitoring air flow to negative-pressure rooms or placing hand antiseptics in every room.

Performance Improvement Charts and Diagrams

Pareto Chart

A Pareto chart is a combination vertical bar graph and line graph. Typically, bar graph values are arranged in descending order. For example, if incidences of bloodstream infections were being plotted by unit, the unit with the largest number would be first on the left. A line graph superimposed over the bar graph usually shows what accumulated percentage of the total is represented by the elements of the bar graph. Thus, if 50 infections occurred in ICU and that represented 30% of the total, the line graph would start at 30%. If 40 infections occurred in the transplant unit (24% of total), the line graph would show 54% at the bar for the transplant unit. The Pareto chart helps to demonstrate the most common causes or sources of problems and has given rise to the 80/20 rule: 80% of the problem often derives from 20% of causes.

Ishikawa "Fishbone" Diagram

The Ishikawa "fishbone" diagram resembling the head and bones of a fish, is an analysis tool to determine causes and effects. In infection control, it is used to help identify root causes. Typically, the "head" is labeled with the problem (the effect). Then, each bone is labeled with a category (causes), traditionally M (used for manufacturing), P (used for administration and service), and S (used for service).

- M: methods, materials, manpower, machines (equipment), measurement, mother nature (environment).
- P: people, prices, promotion, places, policies, procedures, product.
- S: surroundings, suppliers, systems, skills.

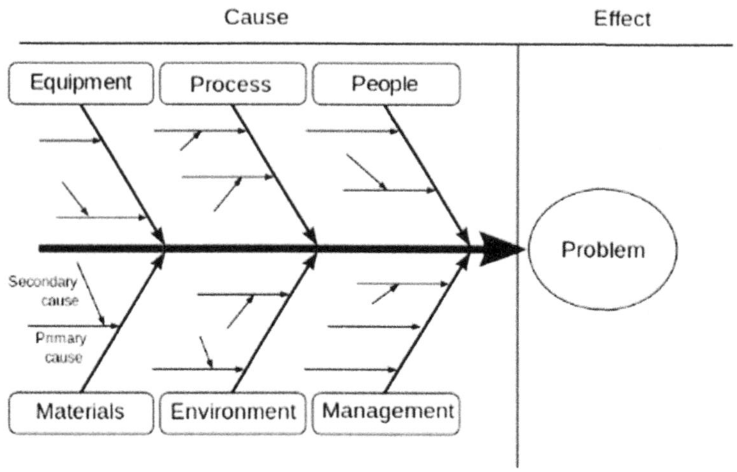

The categories serve only as a guide and can be selected and modified as needed. For example, if the effect is urinary tract infections, then all possible causes, derived from brainstorming, would be listed on the "bones": people, places, product, surroundings, material Then, each category listed would be questioned: "What are the issues affecting this category?" "What is the problem?" "Why is it happening?"

Flow Charts

A flow chart is a tool of quality improvement and is used to provide a pictorial/ schematic representation of a process. It is a particularly helpful tool for quality improvement projects when each step in a process is analyzed when searching for solutions to a problem. Typically, the following symbols are used:

- Parallelogram: Input and output (start/end)
- Arrow: Direction of flow
- Diamond-shape: Conditional decision (Yes/No or True/False)
- Circles: Connectors with diverging paths with multiple arrows coming in but only one going out.

A variety of other symbols may be used as well to indicate different functions. Flow goes from top to bottom and left to right. Flow charts are particularly helpful to help people to visualize how a process is carried out and to examine a process for problems. Flow charts may also be used to plan a process before it is utilized.

Education and Research

Education

Professional Development of Infection Control Personnel

Identifying goals for professional development and ongoing education of infection control personnel requires a commitment on the part of the infection control professional to remain current and on the part of the facility administration to provide financial support or incentives, such as advancement in pay for those who continue their education, tuition assistance, and release time. The goals of both professional development and ongoing education are for staff to be knowledgeable and informed with expertise in the area of infection control and epidemiology. Professional development can include membership in national organizations, attending regional or national conferences, or taking courses in traditional classes or through the internet. One goal of any infection control program should be for staff to complete certification for infection control professionals. If not already required as a qualification for the job of infection control professional, completing this certification within a year or two may be a condition of hiring.

Education Standards for Healthcare Workers

The Joint Commission is the oldest and largest national healthcare accrediting body in the United States and accredits about 19,000 healthcare organizations. As a response to efforts by the American College of Surgeons to protect patients undergoing hospital-based surgery from death unrelated to the course of their illness, it created the Hospital Standardization Program shortly after the turn of the century. In its continuing concern for protecting patient safety, it has been on a campaign since 2005 to educate healthcare workers in the necessity for strict hand hygiene. It expects the organizations it accredits to carry out training in this and other areas of infection prevention in their employee training. This includes new employee orientation and continuing education programs.

Minimum Required Training in Handling Bloodborne Disease Risks

Required training must provide the following:

- Explanations of the epidemiology, symptoms, and modes of transmission of bloodborne diseases
- A review of the facility's exposure control plan
- A discussion of what tasks present higher risks
- Methods of preventing or decreasing exposure
- Review of protective gear, including disposal of used protective coverings
- Information regarding the Hepatitis B vaccine
- Details of what to do in the event of an exposure
- Proper actions to take and individuals to contract should an emergency arise involving blood or other possibly infectious materials
- Post-exposure evaluation and follow up
- Signs, labels, and/or color coding required with regard to blood or other possibly infectious materials
- An opportunity for an interactive question and answer session with the individual(s) conducting training

Educational Opportunities on Infection Control

Since its founding, the primary priority of the Association for Professionals in Infection Control and Epidemiology (APIC) has been education, and it remains their main priority today. APIC chapters periodically run workshops and specialized training courses in various states and regions and also grants certification in infection control (CIC).

The Society for Healthcare Epidemiology of America (SHEA), in collaboration with the CDC, offers training programs in medical epidemiology for physicians.

Area Health Education Centers (AHEC) provide regional programs providing continuing education across the United States.

Developing Goals, Objectives and Lesson Plans

Once a topic for infection control education has been chosen, then goals, measurable objectives with strategies, and lesson plans must be developed. A class should stay focused on one area rather than trying to cover many things. A sample may be as follows:

Goal: Increase compliance with hand hygiene standards in ICU.

Objectives:

- Develop series of posters and fliers by June 1.
- Observe 100% compliance with hand hygiene standards at 2 weeks, 1 month, and 2 months after training is completed.

Strategies:

- Conduct 4 classes at different times over a one-week period, May 25-31.
- Place posters in all nursing units, staff rooms, and utility rooms by January 3.
- Develop a slide show presentation for class and intranet/internet for access by all staff by May 25.
- Utilize handwashing kits.

Lesson plans:

- Discussion period: Why do we need 100% compliance?
- Slide show: The case for hand hygiene.
- Discussion: What did you learn?
- Demonstration and activities to show effectiveness
- Handwashing technique

Assessing Educational Needs of Healthcare Workers

There are a number of different methods that the IP can use to assess the educational needs of healthcare workers pertaining to infection control:

- Review job descriptions to determine the educational qualifications/ certifications for all different levels of staff to determine what, realistically, they should be expected to know about infection control.
- Review job orientation and training materials to determine what staff has been taught about infection control.
- Conduct meetings with staff in different departments to brainstorm areas of concern and potential training needs.
- Meet with team leaders and department heads for their input about the need for infection control education.
- Administer short infection control quizzes to staff asking about standard infection control methods, such as barrier precautions and hand washing to determine basic knowledge.
- Provide questionnaires to staff to obtain information about their own perceptions of what they know or need to know about infection control.
- Make direct observations of staff.

Identifying Learner Outcomes

When the IP plans an educational offering, whether it be a class, an online module, a workshop, or educational materials, the IP should identify **learner outcomes,** which should be conveyed to the learners from the very beginning so that they are aware of the expectations. The subject matter of the educational material and the learner outcomes should be directly related. For example, if the IP is giving a class on decontamination of the environment, then a learner outcome might be: "Identify the difference between disinfectants and antiseptics." There may be one or multiple learner outcomes, but part of the assessment at the end of the learning experience should be to determine if, in fact, the learner outcomes have been achieved. A survey of whether or not the learners felt that they had achieved the learner outcomes can give valuable feedback and guidance to the IP.

Participating in the Facility's Orientation Program for Healthcare workers

The IP's participation in the facility's orientation program for healthcare workers is extremely important because it signals the administrative commitment to infection control. Because of that, the IP presentations should not be relegated to just standalone infection control orientation classes but should be integrated with other presentations so that the new hires understand how infection control is a multidisciplinary focus of the institution. Certainly, hand hygiene and use of barrier precautions must be covered in detail as well as information about surveillance and indicators. They must understand the processes in place for both patient and staff safety, but healthcare workers also need to know what action Human Resources will take if new staff is out of compliance with infection control measures. They should also know, for example what housekeeping does to control infection and what precautions maintenance and food workers use.

Principles of Adult Learning

Adults come to work with a wealth of life and employment experiences. Their attitudes toward education may vary considerably. There are, however, some **principles of adult learning** and typical characteristics of adult learners that an instructor should consider when planning strategies for teaching. According to these principles, and generally speaking, adult learners are:

- Practical and goal-oriented:
    - Provide overviews or summaries and examples
    - Use collaborative discussions with problem-solving exercises
    - Remain organized with the goal in mind
- Self-directed:
    - Provide active involvement, asking for input
    - Allow different options toward achieving the goal
    - Give them responsibilities
- Knowledgeable:
    - Show respect for their life experiences/ education
    - Validate their knowledge and ask for feedback
    - Relate new material to information with which they are familiar
- Relevancy-oriented:
    - Explain how information will be applied on the job
    - Clearly identify objectives
- Motivated:
    - Provide certificates of professional advancement and/or continuing education credit when possible

Educational Considerations

Audience Size

There are a number of issues related to audience size that must be considered when planning presentations.

- Class participation is more difficult in a large class because there may not be time for all to speak individually. Breaking the class into small groups or pairs for discussion for part of the class time can increase participation, but there must be a focused purpose to the discussion so that people stay on task.
- In small groups, placing chairs in a circle or sitting around a table allows people to look at each other and have more active discussions than if they are sitting in rows.
- Online virtual classes can vary considerably in size, depending upon the type of presentation and whether or not scores and replies are automated or posted by the instructor. If a large group is taking an online course, setting up a chat room can facilitate exchange of ideas.

Physical Environment

The physical environment is a major consideration when planning presentations, especially when using audiovisual material.

- First, everyone in the room must be able to hear and see. In a small room, a television screen may suffice, but in a large space, a projection screen must be used.
- Another issue is lighting. Some projectors have low resolution and the lights need to be turned off /dimmed or windows covered. Turning lights on and off a dozen times during a presentation can be very distracting. A small portable light at a speaker podium or an alternate presentation can be used.
- Text size for presentations is another issue: Slide show or other presentations that include text must be of sufficient font size to be read from the back of the room.

Use of Handouts

Handouts are a fixture in classes, but many end up in the wastebasket without ever being used, so thought should be given to providing handouts that are useful:

- Handouts that simply copy a slide show presentation or repeat everything in the presentation are less helpful than those that summarize the main points.
- Giving out handouts immediately prior to a discussion ensures that most of the class will be looking at the handout instead of the speaker. Thus, handouts should be placed in a folder or binder and passed out before class so people can peruse them in advance or passed out at the end of class.
- Handouts can be used to provide guidance or worksheets for small group discussions.
- Poster-type handouts (with drawings or pictures) that can be placed on bulletin boards are useful.
- Handouts should be easily readable and not smudged copies of newspaper articles or small print text.

Reviewing Prepared Educational Tools and Audiovisuals

It is impractical to believe that the IP can produce all educational materials originally, but careful consideration must be given to a number of issues:

- Prices may range from free to hundreds or even thousands of dollars for educational materials, which may be handouts, videos, posters, or entire courses or series of courses available online. The IP must first consider the budget and then look for material within those monetary constraints. Government agencies, such as the CDC, often have posters and handouts as well as slide show presentations and videos available for download online at no cost.
- Quality varies considerably as well. The IP should consider the goal and objectives before choosing materials, and the materials should be evaluated to determine if they cover all needed information in a clear and engaging manner.
- Currency must be considered as well. If material will soon be outdated because of changes in regulations, then it will have to be replaced.

Dissemination of Pertinent Information and Literature

Dissemination of pertinent information and literature on infection control should be an ongoing scheduled process, at least monthly. The easiest way to disseminate this type of information is through newsletters, either print or electronic.

- **Print newsletters** involve costs that must be considered as part of operating expenses. There is also staff time involved in preparing the document as well as copyright considerations. Most government publications are copyright exempt and can be reproduced, but articles of interest from journals require permission, which may be difficult to obtain for new material. An alternative method is for someone to write a review of an article or articles, including a summary of the main points. Use of pictures adds expense, especially if they are in color.
- **Electronic newsletters** involve staff time but are considerably less expensive. Additionally, links to online articles and color pictures can be easily inserted into the newsletter.

Dissemination of Policies, Procedures, Guidelines, Statements, and Standards

Policies, procedures, guidelines, consensus statements, position papers, and standards apply to all staff and should be widely disseminated to all departments. Many institutions now make these types of information available to the public as an ongoing effort to educate the public about infection control and demonstrate the institution's commitment to patient safety. Methods of dissemination include:

- **Print**: Infection control manuals are routinely produced each year and disseminated to all departments and used for staff orientation and training.
- **Internet**: Manuals are now posted on the internet in facility web pages for easy access. In some cases, the complete manual is posted, but in others, only parts. Some areas of the manual may be password protected to limit access.
- **Email**: Both intranet and internet email can be used to send reports.
- **Intranet**: Facilities that have an internal intranet routinely post the infection control manual on the intranet so that it can be easily accessed within the facility to be used for reference and training.

Preparing, Presenting, and Coordination Educational Activities

There are many approaches to teaching, and the IP must prepare, present, and coordinate a wide range of educational workshops, lectures, discussions, and one-on-one instructions on a variety of infection control topics. Planning time for classes should be made as part of the infection control plan, but allowing for flexibility to contend with unexpected needs. All types of classes will be needed, depending upon the purpose and material:

- **Educational workshops** are usually conducted with small groups, allowing for maximal participation and are especially good for demonstrations and practice sessions.
- **Lectures** are often used for more academic or detailed information that may include questions and answers but limits discussion. An effective lecture should include some audiovisual support.
- **Discussions** are best with small groups so that people can actively participate. This is a good for problem-solving.
- **One-on-one instruction** is especially helpful for targeted instruction in procedures for individuals.
- **Computer modules** are good for independent learners.

Patient/Family Education

Assessing Needs

There are a number of ways to assess educational needs of patients/families regarding infection control. Using multiple strategies provides the most accurate results:

- Consult with the public health department about community issues of infection, such as rates of HBV, HIV, and TB, to determine shared educational needs.
- Conduct mail surveys either of the general populace or targeted surveys of former patients and families. Mail survey return rates are often low, so a large number of surveys must be prepared.
- Conduct telephone surveys of the same groups, usually with better response and lower costs, but they are time-consuming and may require hiring temporary staff.
- Conduct onsite surveys for both inpatients and clinic patients, including both patients and family members. When surveys are requested by staff directly, return rates are good.
- Conduct interviews for inpatients, clinic patients, and families, giving the chance for people to elaborate but requiring much staff time.

Methods of Instruction

Methods to instruct patients and families to prevent and control infections depend on many variables, which may include:

- **Goal**: Instruction should be provided keeping the purpose in mind, whether it is to increase handwashing or promote vaccinations.
- **Necessity**: If the patient has a wound or invasive device that requires home care, then intensive one-on-one demonstration and observation is required, but if the need is more general, then fliers or handouts might be sufficient.
- **Educational background**: If most of the hospital population is from an affluent well-educated group, then detailed print information may be indicated. If there is a large illiterate or poorly educated population, then posters or handouts with pictures and little text might be more appropriate.
- **Language**: If there are sufficient populations of non-English speakers, then instructive materials may need to be produced in Spanish, Russian, Chinese, or other languages, or with primarily pictures/drawings.

Public Education

The IP is in a unique position to serve as a **consultant and educator for the community** regarding infectious illness. There are many avenues that the IP can explore:

- **Schools and universities** present many opportunities from demonstrating handwashing to small children in elementary school to speaking with students in medical fields to giving lectures on infectious diseases in university classes or public seminars.
- **Service organizations** often invite speakers to discuss topics of interest, and this presents an opportunity to discuss infectious disease issues and to enlist the aid of other organizations in spreading information.
- **News media** is especially interested in information during times of outbreaks, but they may also be willing to interview or allow reports on a regular basis.
- **Job fairs** present an opportunity to speak to a wide range of people about the field of infection control.
- **Unions** may be interested in field-related information about infection control.

Evaluating Effectiveness of Education

Education, like all interventions, must be evaluated for effectiveness. Two determinants of effectiveness are measures of **behavior modification and compliance rates.** Behavior modification involves thorough observation and measurement, identifying behavior that needs to be changed and then planning and instituting interventions to modify that behavior. Procedures an IP can use include demonstrations of appropriate behavior, reinforcement, and monitoring until new behavior is adopted consistently. This is especially important when longstanding procedures, and habits of behavior, are changed. Compliance rates are often determined by observation, which should be done at intervals and on multiple occasions. Outcomes is another measure of compliance; that is, if education is intended to improve patient safety and decrease infection rates and that occurs, it is a good indication that there is compliance. Compliance rates are calculated by determining the number of events/procedures and degree of compliance. This may be determined through observation or record review.

Research

Development and Testing of a Hypothesis

A **hypothesis** should be generated about the probable cause of the disease/infection based on the information available in laboratory and medical records, epidemiologic study, literature review, and expert opinion. A hypothesis should include the infective agent, the likely source, and the mode of transmission: "Surgical site infections with *Staphylococcus aureus* were caused by reuse and inadequate sterilization of single use irrigation syringes used during the operations in surgery room A."

Hypothesis testing includes data analysis, laboratory findings, and outcomes of environmental testing. It usually includes case control studies, with 2-4 controls picked for each case of infection. They may be matched according to age, sex, or other characteristics, but they are not infected at the time they are picked for the study. Cohort studies, whose controls are picked based on having or lacking exposure, may also be instituted. If the hypothesis cannot be supported, then a new hypothesis or different testing methods may be necessary.

Types of Studies

Cohort Studies

Any study in which there are measures of some characteristic of one or more cohorts at two or more points in time, where cases and controls are observed and data emerges in real time, is considered a cohort analysis. There are a number of subtypes.

- **Prospective cohort studies** choose a group of patients without disease, assess risk factors, and then follow the group over time to determine (prospect for) which ones develop disease. This is typical of general surveillance studies for surgical site infections. Results are often demonstrated in 2 x 2 tables that show presence of disease and exposure/risk. Data is used to calculate relative risk, or risk ratios.
- **Retrospective cohort studies** are initiated after infection develops and data is collected retrospectively from medical records to evaluate whether members of the cohort selected had exposure and developed disease.

Issues of Bias in Retrospective Studies

Retrospective studies ask respondents to recall facts from weeks, months, or years ago and then assume the recollections are accurate. Chances are the responses are guesses, which will be pooled with the questionable guesses of other respondents to create data that is questionable. In fact, respondents are as likely to provide responses they think the investigator would like to hear. This is recall bias.

Misclassification bias could as easily be called the "little white lie" response because a respondent may lie to an investigator if he or she thinks the correct answer would make the researcher think less of him or her.

Unless the data is verified, information gathered from surveys should be considered highly suspect.

Case Control Studies

The case control study starts with an outcome that has already occurred such as an usually large number of deaths from liver cancer reported in a given area.

The preferred research tool would be a randomized double-blind study that would follow a large number of people to see which of them contract a disease and why. But this is expensive and lengthy. The case control method instead takes a small cohort who already has the disease and matches them person-for-person with another cohort similar in all respects except for being free of the disease. Then the task is to isolate factors that might account for the one group's prevalence of that disease and the other's low incidence.

The advantage of case control studies is the ability to determine the association between potential cause and effect on an individual basis. Conclusions reached may not be pinpoint, but they come fast, and speed is usually of the essence in epidemiology.

Cross-Sectional Studies

A cross-sectional study assesses both disease and exposure at the same time in a target population, evaluating the presence of disease at a point in time. For example, a group of people with infections may be assessed for a particular type of exposure or exposures to determine if the exposure(s) are the cause of the infection. Cross-sectional studies can evaluate the effect of multiple variables and how they relate. Cross-sectional studies can be constructed and analyzed similarly to case control when sampling involves cases and a random selection of controls, yielding prevalence odds ratio.

Cross-sectional studies offer epidemiologists a quick way to determine whether there is a problem which warrants further study. Because it is difficult without using control groups to determine whether any given exposure actually causes a given disease, they are not as useful as analytic studies for establishing cause and effect.

A cross-sectional study can also be considered an ecological or correlational study in which information is collected on a group rather than on individual members. In this case, care must be taken not to draw conclusions about individuals using group data and commit an error of reasoning (ecological fallacy). If constructed as a cohort cross-sectional study with an entire group being studied at one time, a 2x2 table can be used and calculations would provide a prevalence ratio. Cross-sectional studies often look for the same types of data as cohort studies but require less time and are less expensive.

Observational Descriptive Studies

Whether to use analytical or descriptive (observational) approaches to study relationships between given risk factors and outcomes largely depends upon the study objectives. Hypotheses useful in constructing analytical studies for producing statistically tested results can be developed through the collection of descriptive data. Observational approaches include the following:

- **Case reports** describe an unusual feature or unusual association between the disease and some exposure factor, often raising questions of new health hazards or clinical syndromes.
- **Case series** are grouped case reports with common elements and suspected common exposures reported in sequence. While these may produce valuable early evidence for diseases which can later be studied in more detail, their lack of control groups may result in false leads and wasted energy and resources.
- **Cross-sectional studies** are surveys that collect information on individual health status, health-related behaviors, and other exposure factors to estimate whether selected exposures are linked to diseases.

Observational Studies vs. Controlled, Randomized Trials

There are three major **disadvantages to controlled, randomized trials** that affect their accuracy:

- Strong subject biases may preclude the recruitment of sufficient patients or clinics into a randomized experiment. For example, consider an experiment that requires the subject to have blood drawn twice a day for three weeks. It would probably be impossible to recruit sufficient patients into a controlled trial.
- Because women, elderly people, and minority ethnic groups are often excluded from randomized trials, patients enrolled are often not representative of the average patient seen in clinical practice.
- Such trials are often carried out by university hospitals – which differ from the settings where most patients are treated.

Therefore, results from observational analyses may seem more relevant and more readily applicable to clinical practice.

Accurate Data in Medical Research

Observational studies often rely on existing administrative data such as insurance claims. Such studies provide a fuzzy picture and allow for only very general comparisons of outcomes across different cohorts of patients. As researchers began to supplement administrative data with patient self-reported data or medical record review, limitations in the validity of these easily obtainable data sets began to emerge.

For example, what were once thought to be global problems in the quality of breast cancer care appear to be largely the result of imprecise measurement. Data about a disease and its treatments collected for epidemiological studies can tolerate less-than-complete accuracy, as treatment decisions are not likely to be made on the basis of these results alone. This is particularly true if the data collected are primarily used as control variables and the accuracy does not vary across the groups being compared. If data accuracy does vary with the groups being compared, though, the potential for bias should be explored.

Precise Data in Medical Research

The randomized controlled trial is the principal research design in the evaluation of medical interventions, and a controlled experiment must be repeatable to validate the test results. However, etiological hypotheses cannot generally be tested in randomized experiments. It is impossible to do a controlled experiment on, say, the effect of second-hand tobacco smoke on the human body. Besides being non-repeatable, epidemiological research suffers from the problems of confounding and selection bias that often distort findings from observational studies. Applying statistics is seldom of any help because there is a danger that meta-analyses of observational data, while the analyst may produce very **precise** results, they may well be simply producing tight confidence intervals around spurious results. Research in epidemiology usually has a great deal of wiggle room; data does not have to be that precise, so, given its drawbacks, statistically combining data should not be a prominent component of observational studies. The researcher in epidemiology should concentrate on consistency, integrity, validity, timeliness, completeness and relevance, and hope that his or her data is also accurate.

Time Series Analysis of Epidemiology Research

As the name implies, a time series analysis of epidemiology research is a way of organizing and looking at a sequence of observations made over time. Examples from public health might be weekly admissions to hospital OR's or monthly mortality counts. In research using regression analysis, time series models are needed for making valid inferences by virtue of spotting correlations in data which has been collected to represent specific time periods. Temporal studies are usually based on large databases so that even weak associations may be detected.

Agencies involved in setting standards for the collection and analysis of agents of disease:

- The United States Pharmacopeia (USP) specifies protocols for the monitoring of microbiological concentrations on surfaces and air in areas where sterile pharmaceutical compounding takes place.
- The Food and Drug Administration (FDA) provides regulatory requirements and recommendations for the drug manufacturing industry.
- The American Conference of Governmental Industrial Hygienists (ACGIH) specifies practices to achieve accurate monitoring of indoor airborne microbial concentrations.

Resources and Databases

The Global Infectious Disease and Epidemiology Network (GIDEON) is a private, for-profit subscription service with an interactive and comprehensive internet web-based knowledge management tool that provides quick access to a large knowledge database. It is used for diagnosis and reference in the fields of tropical and infectious diseases, epidemiology, microbiology, and antimicrobial chemotherapy covering diagnosis, epidemiology, therapy, and microbiology in four modules that include much of the world's medical literature in those areas.

The CDC sponsors several surveillance and data collection services that compiles databases on the health and wellness of Americans. These include the following:

- The National Health and Nutrition Examination Survey (NHANES), which surveys adults and children, collecting data on their health and nutrition status.
- The National Health Interview Survey, which collects various health-related data through the use of home visits and phone calls.
- The National Hospital Care Survey, which focuses on healthcare facilities, collecting data on resource utilization, mortality rates, and quality of care.

Literature Reviews

Conducting Literature Searches

While there is still a place for research in a medical library that has the latest journals and materials, the reality is that almost all current information can be obtained with an online search; however, access to some journals may require membership in organizations or online subscriptions, and these should be included in the infection control budget for resources because research is critical if the IP is to stay current and anticipate trends. Information sources include:

- Journals sponsored by national or other organizations:
    - Clinical Infectious Diseases (IDSA)
    - The Journal of Infectious Diseases (IDSA)
    - American Journal of Infection Control (APIC)
    - Infection Control and Hospital Epidemiology (SHEA)
    - Journal of the American Medical Association (AMA)
    - *New England Journal of Medicine* (Massachusetts Medical Society)

- Government websites with information of interest include:
  - State websites for Departments of Health
  - CDC: https://www.cdc.gov/
  - FDA: http://www.fda.gov/
  - OSHA: http://www.osha.gov/
  - NiOSH: http://www.cdc.gov/niosh/

Steps of Critical Reading

There are a number of steps to **critical reading** to evaluate research:

1. Consider the source of the material. If it is in the popular press, it may have little validity compared to something published in a juried journal.
2. Review the author's credentials to determine if a person is an expert in the field of study.
3. Determine the thesis, or the central claim of the research. It should be clearly stated.
4. Examine the organization of the article, whether it is based on a particular theory, and the type of methodology used.
5. Review the evidence to determine how it is used to support the main points. Look for statistical evidence and sample size to determine if the findings have wide applicability.
6. Evaluate the overall article to determine if the information seems credible and useful and should be communicated to administration and/or staff.

Questions to Consider When Reviewing a Study

Questions to consider when reviewing a study include the following:

- Was the approach to investigation well thought out and researched? Were the hypotheses relevant to the topic of research? Was the approach followed?
- What methods of investigating were chosen? Were they appropriate? If not, might there be better methods that would have led to different results?
- Were known major risk factors (confounders like age, race, or smoking habits) accounted for?
- Was sensitivity analysis performed and adjustments made to control for unmeasured potential confounders?
- Did the authors push a stated or implicit objective by selectively choosing what results to report or making inappropriate use of methods?
- Were confidence intervals provided?
- Were major results related to the *a priori* hypothesis?
- Were the strengths and limitations of study design, execution, and data adequately discussed?
- Was note taken of competing causes of mortality or morbidity that might influence findings?
- Were contradictory or implausible results satisfactorily explained?
- Were alternative explanations for the results seriously explored and discussed?
- What are the public health implications of the results?

Issues and Barriers in Medical Research Studies

Common Errors Made When Reading Medical Studies

Common errors made when reading medical studies include the following:

- Assuming that correlation between two things proves that one causes the other. For instance, it was believed many years ago that multiple pregnancies had a protective effect against breast cancer, an early epidemiological finding. Later research noted that women with many children usually begin having them earlier. Preventive effects were not, therefore, tied to family size but to a woman's age at the time of her first pregnancy.
- Epidemiology never proves (or disproves) anything because it cannot establish a cause-and-effect relationship.
- Studies involving sample sizes of less than several hundred should be considered highly suspect, though a large sample size is no guarantee of accuracy if the study is poorly done.
- Recall bias and misclassification bias skew results on retrospective studies. Unless the data is verified, information gathered from surveys should be considered highly suspect.
- Beware of conclusions that seem biologically implausible, such as "smoking causes hair loss."

Constraints in the Development of Epidemiologic Studies

Major constraints encountered in developing epidemiologic studies of infectious diseases include:

- One of the biggest problems in pursuing research data, oddly enough, has been telemarketing. Dinner time calls from salespeople pretending to be researchers has put a major crimp in population-based research by destroying the public's goodwill toward strangers calling them and asking if they would be willing to answer a few questions.
- The problem of disappearing funding for any kind of social programs, meaning that agencies have had to allocate what used to be their research dollars into basic program support. As a result, researchers have not been able to provide reliable data on various populations, and this has seriously reduced the reliability of existing surveillance systems.
- Advances in computer technology: The same technology that has made it easier to mine data from patient records has made the records' gatekeepers, citing the need for heightened patient confidentiality, more wary of attempts to get at those records, including attempts by those doing legitimate epidemiological research.

Risk Stratification and the Likelihood Ratio

Risk stratification is a way of accounting for the fact that, in any kind of medical research, it is impossible to match all the characteristics (age, sex, medical history, etc.) of one control cohort against those of an experimental cohort, much less match all of the conditions affecting each group. Life is not like a laboratory. If what we are looking at is a single variable – perhaps hand hygiene – having to do with surgery infection rates, for example, one way this could be sorted out would be to compare infection outcomes for both groups after compensating for totaled or averaged risk factors for members of each group. That is, say, if one group had 12 people over 60 and at greater risk for infection and the other group had only 6, a risk factor would be entered to account for that.

INCORPORATING RESEARCH FINDINGS INTO PRACTICE

Incorporating research findings should be central to all work of the IP and should be routinely disseminated as part of practice, education, and consultation. Any time the IP gives a presentation or provides written material, references should be made to research findings because this provides supporting evidence and lends credence to the information the IP is providing. Often research can provide guidance for surveillance or interventions and give valuable insights. References that are used or referred to should always be properly cited so that the work of researchers is credited. If a presentation is given orally, then the IP should prepare a list of references. Newsletters and email or internet reports and communications should include research highlights or summaries of current studies of interest, with links to online articles provided, when possible, to encourage people to read the research for themselves and become more knowledgeable about issues of infection control.

Environment of Care

Environmental Safety

Environmental Reservoirs

Environmental reservoirs are places (other than humans or animals) that can cultivate the accumulation and growth of infectious particles. Some environmental reservoirs in the healthcare setting include:

- **Soiled hospital linens**: The process of handling soiled hospital linens presents not only a risk to unprotected staff but also contributes to airborne contamination.
- Hospital fungal infections strongly correlate with **construction projects**; preparing for construction in medical care settings includes:
  - Containment of affected areas
  - Monitoring the passage of workers through them
  - Disinfecting worker clothing
- **Food products** (whether raw and cooked): Temperature sensitive food must be kept refrigerated or frozen at required temperatures until ready to be served or cooked. Internal temperature of meat and fish on the stove and in warmers must be checked to assure it the items are thoroughly cooked through.
- **Plants**: The soil in which plants are rooted are reservoirs, as are cut flowers and the water in their vases.
- **Air**: Microbial aerosols float on the breezes, so careful consideration should be given ventilation and air-conditioning systems
- **Building materials**: Carpeting can act as microbial reservoirs.
- **Water**: Contaminated unit water lines supply water as a coolant to equipment and produce a fine spray which can then be inhaled by both the patient and the staff.
- **Infant Formula**: Powdered infant formula has been implicated in outbreaks of *Salmonella* and *E. sakazakii* infection. Mortality rates are 50 percent or more.
- **Surfaces**: Any surface in a medical care environment is a potential source of infection.

Modifying Inanimate Environmental Reservoirs

Measures to contain inanimate reservoirs consist almost entirely of removing them before they represent a hazard. These reservoirs include food items, intravenous infusates, or medical devices. In addition, sewage and waste may have to be handled in a more rigorous fashion, aseptic techniques may be strengthened or modified, and chemical or physical means may be used to destroy the slightest traces of the agent. The Centers for Disease Control report that healthcare infections and pseudo-outbreaks can be minimized by:

- Effective use of cleaners and disinfectants
- Proper maintenance of medical equipment (e.g., automated endoscope reprocessors or hydrotherapy equipment)
- Adherence to water quality standards for hemodialysis
- Adherence to ventilation standards for specialized care environments (e.g., airborne infection isolation rooms, protective environments, or operating rooms)
- Prompt correction of water intrusion into the facility

Except for water quality determinations in hemodialysis settings and other situations where sampling is directed by epidemiologic principles and results can be applied directly to infection control decisions, routine environmental sampling is not usually advised.

Modifying Animate Environmental Reservoirs

Measures to contain animate reservoirs include:

- Restricting the movement of exposed patients to isolation areas for the full incubation period.
- Keeping personal hygiene of hospital patients to a high standard. The causative bacteria for healthcare-associated infection pneumonia have been found in teeth of hospitalized patients with poor oral hygiene especially if they have difficulty in getting to a sink in their hospital room. Possibly due to the patient's exposure to antibiotics that suppress the normal defensive flora, teeth can become super-infected by pathogenic bacteria. Pathogens in the mouth then may be aspirated into the lower respiratory tracts of the lungs of very ill patients with poor cough reflexes, bringing on such infections as pneumonia.

Additional Environmental Factors that Influence the Spread of Infection

The kind of setting conducive to disease transmission depends upon such factors as:

- Cleanliness vs. filth
- Closed room vs. outdoors
- Slum housing vs. clean room
- Immediate population: *Vibrio cholerae,* an aquatic bacillus, attaches itself to zooplankton. This attachment sustains the environmental survival of *Vibrio* by both providing a rich source of carbon and nitrogen and protecting the bacillus from numerous environmental dangers. On ingestion by humans, some serogroups of *V. cholerae* cause cholera.

Ventilation

HVAC Systems

HVAC systems include all air-handling elements: heating, ventilation, and air conditioning. Generally, centralized HVAC systems have an air-handling unit that is typically located on the roof or in a separate room. Whereas HVAC systems in a home are intended to keep the home at a comfortable temperature, in a healthcare facility, the HVAC system must improve air quality (such as by eliminating dust and odors), prevent the spread of airborne disease, as well as provide patient comfort; therefore, the healthcare HVAC system is held to higher standards. Additionally, the healthcare HVAC system must be able to restrict airflow between different departments and support different temperature and humidity requirements for different areas. Air movement, including direction, may need to be controlled. For example, in operating rooms and other specialty areas, the air enters a room from ceiling registers and exhausts through registers 6 inches above the floor so that clean air flows from the top to the bottom of the room.

Types of Ventilation Systems

There are a number of different types of **ventilation systems** that are used in medical facilities. Heating, ventilation, and air conditioning (HVAC) systems must not only circulate air but also exhaust the stale air to reduce contaminants and provide filtration.

- **Central air conditioning** is relatively inexpensive but does not allow for separate control of temperature in different areas.
- **Dual duct system** has separate heating and cooling systems with two ducts that feed into mixers, allowing for thermostats in individual rooms.
- **Filtration** is needed in addition to other HVAC systems to remove small particles. Filters are rated for efficiency and must be changed regularly. Outdoor air is often filtered by 20-40% efficient filters, mixed with recirculating air, and then refiltered with 90% efficient filters.

Special Hospital Ventilation Systems

Special hospital ventilation systems are designed to prevent the acquisition and/or spread of healthcare-associated infections in operating theatres and patient care areas such as isolation areas for severely immunocompromised patients.

Rooms intended to house patients with suspected or known airborne infectious diseases – pulmonary tuberculosis, chickenpox, or measles, for instance – should be designed with special ventilation and seals permitting them to be maintained at negative air pressure. This minimizes opportunities for infectious pathogens to escape from the room. The opposite should be true for operating theatres as well as rooms that will house immunocompromised patients, where positive air pressure and seals should be used to impede infectious pathogens in the surrounding atmosphere from coming inside the area.

Certain aerosolized medications such as pentamidine, given for conditions like pneumonia associated with AIDS, must be administered in rooms with increased ventilation, as must certain chemotherapy drugs, because they could otherwise contaminate the immediate environment.

Ventilation Requirements for Patient Care Facilities

Ventilation requirements for patient care facilities include the following:

- **Air movement**: In most areas, air moves in from adjacent areas to prevent contamination of the adjacent areas, but in a few cases, air moves out to prevent contamination of the space: protective environment room, delivery room, operating/procedure rooms, trauma room, medication room, clean workroom, pharmacy, and clean laundry room.
- **Air changes of outdoor air per hour**: In most cases, the minimum number is not specified or it is two, but in some cases, the minimum number is 3 (such as the delivery room, operating/procedure rooms, and trauma room).
- **Total air changes per hour**: Varies from 2 (patient corridor) to 15 (operating room), so EPA guidelines must be reviewed. Two is sufficient to remove odors, but patient comfort generally requires 6.
- **All air is exhausted to the outside**: Required for toilets, airborne isolation room, isolation alcove, bronchoscopy room, triage room, ER waiting room, endoscopy processing room, all laboratories, darkroom, and rooms where washing of supplies and equipment or laundry is done including sterilization rooms.

Hospital Ventilation Hazards

One of the most common ventilation hazards is failure to clean or change air filters in the ventilation system. This is an important task in that filters are an ideal location for fungus to grow. In one study, 9 of 11 air filters that had been in use less than 1 month showed fungal growth on them.

Another maintenance error is replacing dirty filters with incompatible new filters. Price considerations or product improvements may have caused the hospital to change filter suppliers. It is possible the new filters may not fit the filter rack originally installed in that supply fan. The size of the filter, the seal on the housing and spacers installed for fit may all contribute to assuring that airflow passes through the filter media and not around the filter media. If the filters do not fit the rack, they do not remove critical particles that could be infectious.

Impact of Water Damage on Hospital Ventilation Systems

Water damage to building materials produces molds that distribute their spores on airborne routes throughout a medical facility. These organic substances include mycotoxins that can produce idiopathic pulmonary hemosiderosis, cytotoxicity, cognitive impairment, immunosuppression, cancer, nosebleeds, cough, joint ache, headache, fatigue, and irritation of the eyes, skin, or respiratory tract. Opportunistic infections occur in persons with lowered resistance to infections, mainly patients with a compromised immune system such as diabetic patients, AIDS patients, or patients undergoing chemotherapy or involved in organ transplants.

Organic dust toxic syndrome, which can produce flu like symptoms, is a condition that arises from a massive single exposure to materials heavily contaminated with mold growth.

Environmental Concerns for Ventilation

Environmental concerns relating to ventilation include the following:

- **Humidity**: Although not specified for many areas, humidity should be maintained between 30% and 60% in specialty areas, such as the newborn nursery and neonatal intensive care unit (NICU), labor and delivery rooms, operating and procedure rooms (including endoscopy rooms), and sterilization room.
- **Temperature**: Usually maintained between 70 °F and 75 °F in most patient care areas, but specialty areas may require a lower or higher temperature (e.g., protective environment room and treatment room 75 °F, newborn nursery 72-78 °F, NICU 72-78 °F, delivery room and operating room 68-73 °F, bronchoscopy room 68-73 °F).
- **Airflow**: Airflow relates to air changes per hour (ACH) and pressure, but these can easily be disrupted if windows or doors are left open or if seals allow air leaks. Doors that are intended to be closed should never be propped open.

Use of Negative Pressure Rooms

Negative pressure rooms are devised as isolation rooms to protect those outside the room from airborne pathogens. In these rooms, air flows from the outside (clean) into the room (dirty) and then to the exterior of the building so that it does not recirculate. If recirculation is necessary, it must be through a HEPA filter. Air exchanges are ≥ 6 in renovated rooms or ≥ 12 in new construction. Windows must remain sealed and doors closed as much as possible to maintain negative pressure. Negative pressure rooms are more difficult to engineer than positive pressure rooms. Negative pressure rooms are used primarily for active infections with *Mycobacterium tuberculosis* (TB) causing a cough with aerosolized infectious particles. Patients who have TB and are immunocompromised, such as those co-infected with HIV pose particular problems. In some cases, a positive pressure room is inside a negative pressure room. Another solution is a freestanding positive pressure facility with the air exiting through filters into the fresh air.

Use of Positive Pressure Rooms and Laminar Air Flow Rooms

A positive pressure room creates a protective environment for patients who are immunocompromised. In these rooms, the pressure is positive within the room so that clean air flows out of the room to the dirty area of the hallways, protecting the patient from pathogens. Air exchanges are >12 per hour, and filtration is by 99.97% HEPA filters. Windows should be sealed for protection and the room outfitted with self-closing doors. Positive pressure rooms are used for those who are immunocompromised:

- HIV/AIDs patients with reduced immunity
- Oncology patients with bone marrow suppression
- Solid organ transplant patients

Laminar air flow (LAF) rooms provide more protection than a positive pressure room because one entire wall is composed of HEPA filters and fans blow air at high velocity through the filters with >100 air exchanges per hour, creating drafts and noise. Staff should work down wind of patients, who are severely immunocompromised such as bone marrow transplant patients

Ventilation in the Operating Room

In an operating room, a positive pressure environment must be maintained with the area of the operating table and the patient considered "clean." Filtered air in large volumes washes over the table from the ceiling and then is drawn to the air returns around the margin of the room. Air displacement must assure that any pathogens shed by the operating room personnel are moved away from the patient by the force of air. Windows should remain sealed and doors closed to maintain the proper pressure and air flow. Air exchanges are 15-25 per hour and 90% filters are used. It is also very important that barriers, such as masks and gowns, be used by all staff to prevent the shedding of bacteria into the operative area and that all surfaces be clean. Local exhaust and filtration systems to capture odors or aerosols generated during operative procedures may be used in addition to the room filtration system.

Designing Airborne Isolation Rooms

The IP must consider the patient population and past history of infectious disease in the community as well as potential risks when helping plan for the design and number of **airborne isolation rooms (AIRs)**. At least one AIR is required in acute care facilities. The direction of airflow is critically important because airborne isolation rooms require negative air pressure to protect staff and visitors from infection. AIRs must include a mechanism for measuring the direction of airflow daily. Air in the AIR must be exhausted to the outside of the building or, if that is impossible, filtered through a HEPA filter and recirculated. AIRs must be sealed (floors, walls, ceilings) and have 12 or more air changes per hour. A handwashing and gowning station must be directly outside or immediately inside the entry door, and doors must contain self-closing devices. Separate toilet, bathing, and handwashing facilities are required for each AIR.

Specific Considerations for Designing Protective Rooms for the Immunocompromised

Immunocompromised individuals, especially those receiving bone marrow transplants or solid-organ transplants require **protective environments (PEs)** to protect them from contamination, especially from aspergillosis. Requirements include the following:

- Positive air pressure in relation to adjacent areas to protect the patient from contamination: The amount of HEPA-filtered air provided must be greater than that exhausted to the corridor.
- The pressure differential must be a minimum of 0.01-inch water gauge.
- HEPA-filtered air must be 99.7% efficient for particles 0.3 microns in diameter.
- 12 air exchanges per hour.
- Sealed windows and tight ceilings and walls.
- Self-closing devices on doors.

Handwashing/gowning stations should be available immediately outside or inside the entry door. At least one PE must be available with an anteroom with positive pressure to protect staff during handwashing and gowning and the patient when the staff enters the room for those patients who require both PE and AIR.

Waste Management

Health Implications of Medical Waste

Source reduction focuses on the fact that medical waste can be toxic and consumes a great deal of handling and landfill space through its sheer quantity. One of the biggest problems generated from medical waste is accidental contact by healthcare workers and waste handlers with blood contaminants through skin puncturing cuts from used needles or sharp instruments. This can be dealt with in part at the source by eliminating the use of needles or sharp components wherever feasible, substituting for them newer, less dangerous methods of medication delivery like inhalants. Toxicity can be dealt with by eliminating the need for the materials that make up the waste in the first place or at least finding benign substitutes for it. The quantity issue may be approached by changing the design or use of products to minimize the amount of waste generated when they are discarded.

Safer and Easier Handling of Medical Waste

Ways to make medical waste safer and easier to handle include:

- Decontaminating infectious waste within the facility where the waste is generated, thus exposing fewer people to it when disposing of it.
- Redesigning the workplace and procedures posing risks to workers' health and safety.
- Eliminating to the maximum extent possible direct contact with waste during routine or maintenance activities; unpackaging untreated waste in sharps containers and red biohazard containers; shredding untreated waste; using aerosols on infectious agents, and compacting sharps containers, whether untreated or treated. Anticipate and prevent incorporating high-risk activities into maintenance tasks.
- Segregating and packaging medical waste, avoiding mixing solid waste with medical waste, for example.
- The long-term solution to mercury emissions from steam autoclaves is for waste generators to prevent the introduction of mercury into the medical waste stream.

Treatment Options for Medical Waste

Hospitals generate more than two million tons of solid waste each year. Many hospitals used to mix all their waste streams together, from outpatient lounge trash to operating room waste. They would then either send the combined load to landfills to be buried without treatment or they had it burned in incinerators, releasing toxic materials like dioxin, mercury, lead, and other pollutants into the air.

Simply dumping untreated waste into landfills means contaminants can leach out and get into the water table. Today, a typical process consists of having a contractor pick up segregated waste from the medical facility, hauling it to a large processing plant such as a large autoclave where the trash is steamed until it is no longer toxic, then compacted, and taken to a landfill.

Mechanical Processes for Disposing of Medical Waste

A mechanical process is supplementary to other methods of rendering medical waste non-hazardous and cannot therefore be considered a treatment process in and of itself. Unless shredders, rams, and other mechanical destruction processes are an integral part of a treatment system that is completely enclosed, they should not be used before the waste is decontaminated. Otherwise, workers and possibly the public would be exposed to pathogens released to the environment by mechanical destruction.

Mechanical destruction can render waste unrecognizable when required. It safely destroys needles and syringes so as to minimize injuries or to render them unusable. Waste can be mechanically shredded, ground, hammered, mixed, agitated, compacted, conveyed via auger, rams, or conveyor belts, and solids separated from liquids to improve the rate of heat transfer or expose more surfaces to chemical disinfectants in preparation for other treatment processes.

Rendering Medical Waste Unrecognizable

Some states require that, before going into a sanitary landfill, all treated medical waste be rendered unrecognizable, something usually accomplished through mechanical destruction processes. Other states insist only that body parts be unrecognizable. Many states also require that sharps be broken (or ground up), made unusable, and/or packaged in puncture-resistant containers.

States are, in fact, likely to have long lists of what are acceptable and unacceptable procedures for disposing of waste, lists that may vary depending upon how the waste is classified and whether it will be incinerated on site or disposed of by other means. For instance, in Michigan, "pathological waste" (human body parts) may be incinerated, buried in a cemetery, cremated, processed for landfill, or ground and flushed into a sanitary sewer.

Radiation or Biological Processes

Disinfecting waste with radiation, biological, or mechanical processes can be done with the following measures:

- Irradiation-based technologies involve electron beams, Cobalt-60, or UV irradiation. Irradiation does not alter the waste physically, so a grinder or shredder is needed to render the waste as unrecognizable as many landfills require.
- Electron beam irradiation showers waste with high-energy electrons to produce chemical dissociation; this ruptures microorganisms' cell walls and thereby destroys them. The effectiveness of this method is contingent upon how well electron energy is absorbed by the mass of waste; this, in turn, is related to density of the waste and whether the energy source is powerful enough to handle it.
- Biological processes: Only a few nonincineration technologies for processing waste have been based on biological processes, which employ enzymes to destroy organic matter.

Thermal and Chemical Processes

Various treatment options for medical waste utilize thermal and/or chemical processes:

- **Low-heat thermal processes**: Thermal energy decontaminates the waste at temperatures that are not high enough to cause chemical breakdown or to support combustion or pyrolysis. Autoclaves may or microwave heaters may apply wet heat (steam) disinfection or dry heat (hot air) disinfection may be employed wherein the waste is heated by conduction or convection or by infrared heat.
- **Medium-heat thermal processes**: Heating waste at temperatures of 350-700 °F chemically breaks down organic material.
- **High-heat thermal processes**: Operating at temperatures ranging from around 1,000 °F to 15,000 °F or higher, these processes produce chemical and physical changes to both organic and inorganic waste resulting in total destruction.
- **Chemical processes**: Exposure to strong disinfectants.
- **Encapsulating compounds**: Sharps, blood, or other body fluids are sealed within a solid matrix prior to disposal.
- **Ozone treatment.**
- **Catalytic oxidation.**
- **Alkali**: Hydrolyzes tissues in heated stainless-steel tanks.

All methods involve mechanical rendering of some sort somewhere in the process.

Infection Control Strategies for Medical Waste Disposal

Medical waste management is mandated by Federal and state laws, which require that certain types of medical waste be separated from others. This regulated medical waste (RMW) is eventually packaged, transported, and disposed of according to specific regulations for the type of waste material. Separate trash containers, lined with red plastic bags or containers and labeled as "Biohazard," must be provided for RMW, which includes:

- **Sharps** include needles, syringes, small vials, pins, probes, and lancets.
- **Blood and body fluid** contaminated material that can drip fluid: sponges, specimen containers, drainage bags (such as Hemovacs), and contaminated tubing.
- **CDC Bio-safety Class 4-associated waste**, such as those related to Marburg hemorrhagic fever.
- **Laboratory materials**, including cultures, infectious agents, and contaminated materials.
- **Animal waste** related to medical research.
- **Human tissue** includes body parts removed during surgery or autopsy.
- **Chemotherapy** waste containing over 3% antineoplastic drugs.

Infection Control Strategies for Sharps Disposal

Injuries, especially needle-sticks, related to medical instruments such as scalpels and needles **(sharps)**, are very common but pose a serious risk of infection. Care should always be used when sharp instruments or needles, and assistance should be obtained when using sharps with people who are confused or uncooperative, increasing the chance of injury. The following guidelines should be used:

- A special sealed sharps container should be available in every room where treatment is done (patients' rooms, clinics, operating rooms).
- Disposable needles should not be removed, recapped, or touched but deposited immediately into the sharps container. If recapping cannot be avoided, the scooping method of recapping using only one hand must be used.
- The sharps container must be checked daily and removed for disposal when about 3/4 full and a new container provided.
- Any non-disposable sharps must be placed in a covered container that is leak and puncture proof and returned to the central supply department for cleaning and sterilization.

Disposal of Biohazardous Waste

Guidelines for the disposal of biohazardous waste:

- All biological waste (blood bags, dirty dressings, disposable needles, etc.) must be stored and disposed of in a safe fashion to minimize risk to staff and the community.
- Staff should sort waste where it is created and as they are discarding it.
- Soak small amounts of infected waste in a hypochlorite solution for at least 12 hours before burying. Place larger quantities in pits with sodium hypochlorite and cover immediately.
- A puncture proof, watertight, and break resistant container for disposable "sharps" such as scalpel blades or needles should be:
  - Clearly labeled in as many languages as necessary
  - Secured to a surface to ensure stability yet removable for disposal, and with an opening large enough to accept needles and scalpel blades, but never large enough for someone to reach into.

Water Management

CDC Recommendations for Air and Water Quality Management

The CDC and the Healthcare Infection Control Practices Advisory Committee (HIPAC) provide recommendations for **air and water quality** in healthcare facilities. While air quality is a major concern, there is little evidence of contaminated air resulting in surgical site infections (although spores of *Aspergillus* in the environment have been implicated in infections). Environmental services maintain both negative and positive pressure rooms and monitors air flow and filtration. Recommendations include:

- Ensuring that heating, ventilation, and air-conditioning (HVAC) filters are installed properly and maintained without leaks or dust overloads
- Engineering humidity controls in the HVAC system to ensure adequate moisture removal
- Ensuring air intakes and outputs are located properly and maintained to ensure operation
- Providing portable HEPA filter units to augment room filtration
- Using airborne sampling tests to evaluate integrity of barriers
- Maintaining water temperatures in the correct range (according to state requirements), with constant recirculation of hot water in patient areas
- Testing water and water equipment for microbes

SOURCES OF WATER-ASSOCIATED INFECTIONS

Sources of water-associated infections include the following:

Source	Considerations
Cooling towers and water distribution systems	Cooling towers may be a source of aerosolized water, increasing the risk of dispersing organisms such as *Legionella* or group A streptococcus, which can then spread through the water distribution system. Fungal contamination can occur from condensation around pipes or from leaking, broken pipes. Stagnant water may lead to development of biofilms.
Water features	Open water features may pose the risk of spread of infection, such as *Legionella,* because they may aerosolize organisms or allow for pools of stagnant water.
Sinks and toilets	Drains and aerators may become contaminated, but the greatest risk is from splashing of contaminated water onto supplies. Aerators should be avoided or routinely decontaminated. Basins should be deep enough to prevent splashing, and they should be located at a safe distance from the point of care. Tap water should be avoided for wound or tracheostomy care. Vacuum toilets may decrease environmental contamination.
Eyewash and drench shower stations	Because these stations are rarely used, they may become contaminated; therefore, they should be routinely cleaned and flushed for at least 3 minutes each week.
Ice machines and storage chests	Ice machines may become contaminated, so they should be routinely emptied, cleaned, and monitored (weekly or monthly).
Water baths/devices	These older systems used to warm blood products or IV solutions may harbor microorganisms, so the manufacturer's directions must be carefully followed, leak tests done, and routine cleaning carried out. Plastic overwraps may help reduce contamination.
Whirlpools	Drains and agitators may become contaminated and cause cross-contamination among patients; therefore, adequate cleaning of equipment and drains is essential.
Patient care equipment	Any equipment rinsed in tap water, such as nebulizers, can pose a risk of infection if water standards are not met. This is especially a risk with reprocessing medical devices.

Design Issues for Handwashing Stations

Handwashing stations should be in each patient room, outside a patient's cubicle curtain, and in the toilet room. Handwashing stations must contain a sink adequate to contain splashes and hand drying material. If space is insufficient (such as in old facilities), then a waiver to place a hand-sanitation station (for alcohol rub) may be obtained by the state, although they are not equivalent because hands must be washed with soap and water to remove residues. Surfaces next to sinks must be nonporous to discourage the growth of fungi. The area beneath a sink cannot be used for storage to reduce the risk of contamination. Built-in refillable soap dispensers should be avoided because of the risk of contamination. Hand-drying materials must be provided and should ideally be dispensed without the need to touch the dispenser. Aerators should be avoided. Ideally, sink controls should be the "no-touch" type, if possible, but state codes vary in their requirements. Elbow-operated handles should be at least 6 inches long. Hands-free electronically controlled faucets have a preset water temperature.

Disruption of Water Services and Boiled Water Advisories

In the event of a disruption of water service or boiled water advisory (BWA), an agreement should be in place with a local vendor to deliver at least a 24-hour supply of water, and the facility's water supply should be outlined and documented. Tap water for consumption requires boiling for 5 minutes and cooling for 10–15 minutes. When the advisory is in effect, signs must be placed on all water facilities and ice machines. Hand hygiene products (such as alcohol gels) must be readily available. Sterile bottled water should be used for wound irrigations. Bottled water or no-rinse bathing cloths should be available for bathing. During a BWA, surgical instruments can be washed and rinsed with the water because the sterilization process will destroy any organisms that remain. If water is shut off so that toilets do not flush, buckets of water should be obtained from a water source to manually flush the toilets.

Environmental Cleaning

Housekeeping Policies

Typical housekeeping policies as they relate to infection control include the following:

- All containers used by housekeeping will meet OSHA labeling requirements and comply with the OSHA Bloodborne Pathogens Standard.
- Detergents or standard disinfectants may be used to disinfect any environmental surfaces or noncritical instruments or devices; high-level disinfectants or liquid chemical sterilizing solutions may not. Alcohol will not be used to disinfect large environmental surfaces.
- Clean and disinfect "high-touch" surfaces (e.g., doorknobs, bed rails, light switches, and surfaces in and around toilets in patients' rooms) on a more frequent basis.
- Prepare cleaning solutions daily or as needed; replace with fresh solution frequently.
- Change mop heads at the beginning of each day and after cleaning up large spills of blood or other body substances; allow them to dry before reuse or use single-use, disposable mop heads and cloths.
- Equip vacuums with HEPA filters for use in areas where patients are at risk.
- Avoid unnecessary exposure of neonates to disinfectant residues.

HOUSEKEEPING POLICIES RELATIVE TO ISOLATION PATIENTS

Housekeeping policies for patients on isolation precautions due to confirmed or suspected communicable disease include the following:

- Housekeeping chores consist of cleaning and disinfecting surfaces not involved in direct delivery of patient care, such surfaces as floors, walls, ceilings, tabletops, and non-medical appliances.
- A proper program of housekeeping is coordinated and even integrated into a facility's infection control program.
- The Infection Control Officer has final approval on EPA compliant housekeeping supplies and procedures, prioritizing effectiveness, product safety, and cost effectiveness in that order.
- Housekeeping employees should be trained and continually updated in procedures and safe handling of cleaning supplies and waste as well as special procedures surrounding patients with communicable diseases.
- Where infectious patients are concerned, housekeeping employees must be alerted to any needs for protective clothing.
- Patient isolation areas should be promptly cleaned and disinfected upon discharge or transfer of the patient. Otherwise, cleaning standards that apply to isolation areas also apply to the entire facility, as every area that patients come into contact with are vulnerable to contamination.

STRATEGIES FOR PREVENTING AND CONTROLLING THE TRANSMISSION OF INFECTION

Strategies for preventing and controlling transmission of infection in environmental services in housekeeping are important because VRE and *Aspergillus* infections have been linked to environmental sources. Daily cleaning strategies include:

- Gloves for all cleaning
- Damp mopping all floors, with disposable mop cloths if possible
- Waste baskets emptied and relined with plastic bags
- Horizontal surfaces, such as bedside stands, cleaned with a disinfectant solution approved by the EPA
- Bathrooms thoroughly cleaned, including vector surfaces, such as faucet handles and doorknobs
- Soap and alcohol antiseptic dispensers checked and refilled
- Terminal cleaning includes disinfecting all parts of the bed and equipment and all room furniture, disposal of non-reusable equipment, disinfecting and/or sterilization of reusable equipment

Infection Control Strategies for Linen Services

Linen is frequently contaminated with blood and body fluids and serves as a source of contamination. Control strategies include:

- Manipulating linen as little as possible, avoiding fanning linen
- Gloves or other barrier precautions worn for contact with contaminated linen or sorting
- Sort/rinse linen away from patient care areas (except for rinsing fecal material from linen in dirty hopper utility room)
- Bag soiled linen at source location
- Leak-proof linen bags in use
- Linen chutes cleaned on scheduled basis and as needed
- Ventilation system should preclude exchange of air from laundry to patient areas
- Soiled laundry area should be separate from patient care areas and storage area for clean linen
- Low temperature washing may be used with controlled amounts of bleach as per established guidelines
- Transportation of clean and dirty linen must be separate

Classification of Environmental Surfaces and Zones of Care

Environmental surfaces include the following:

- **High-touch surfaces**: These are surfaces that are frequently touched and must be cleaned often because of the risk of cross-transmission of microorganisms. High-touch surfaces include doorknobs, knobs on equipment (such as cardiac monitors), call lights, blood pressure cuffs, pulse oximeters, overbed tables, light switches, and computer keys.
- **Low-touch surfaces**: These are infrequently touched surfaces, such as walls, windows, window curtains, floors; they pose a lower risk of cross-transmission.

Zones of care include the following:

- **Patient zone**: The environment and things within easy reach of the patient, including the patient bed and many high-touch surfaces. The patient zone often serves as a reservoir for microorganisms that can be easily spread to patients.
- **Healthcare zone**: All of the surfaces and things outside of the patient zone, including other patients and their patient zones. Microorganisms in the healthcare zone are foreign to the patient and may be introduced into the patient zone, causing infection.

Additional Cleaning Considerations for Specific Areas/Circumstances

Additional cleaning considerations for different areas/circumstances include the following:

Area/Circumstance	Considerations/Procedures
Dusting	Should be done before cleaning floors with chemically treated or microfiber dusters to prevent aerosolizing spores. High areas should be dusted with specially designed high dusters.
Walls, windows, and doors	High-touch areas should be cleaned daily, and spot cleaning should be done to walls, windows, and doors with complete cleanings being done on a regular schedule.
Horizontal surfaces	Horizontal surfaces should be wiped at least daily and when soiled, but cleaning should be done more often during disease outbreaks.

Area/Circumstance	Considerations/Procedures
Pillows and mattresses	Moisture-resistant covers are cleaned with an Environmental Protection Agency (EPA)-registered disinfectant, and fabric covers are laundered between patients and when soiled.
Privacy curtains	Privacy curtains should be changed and cleaned on a regular schedule and when soiled. If using contact precautions, change these when the patient is discharged.
Window treatments	Window treatments should be cleaned on a regular schedule and when soiled.
Bathrooms and commodes	Bathrooms and commodes must be cleaned daily and when soiled, increasing to three times daily with diarrheal outbreaks. Ceramic tile must be checked, and mold should be removed (diluted bleach). The commode must be completely decontaminated before moving it from the room.
Carpets and floors	Must be cleaned last, starting from the back of the room to the front. Hard floors may be cleaned with detergent or disinfectant. Mop and bucket cleaning requires a change of the mop and solution every hour, every three patients, or immediately after cleaning body fluids. Microfiber pads are best for cleaning, especially if using detergent, but they may not access small areas. Carpets should be vacuumed daily but can retain spores, so they are not recommended for intensive care units (ICUs), procedure rooms, and high-traffic areas. Carpets should be deep cleaned on a regular schedule, but they must be dry within 72 hours.
Waste removal	Wastes must be collected daily or after each patient, and receptacles should be lined (usually with plastic). Waste should be placed in biohazard and non-biohazard containers.
Linens	Clean linens and soiled linens must be kept separate. Soiled linen must be placed in covered containers or bags (not on the floor), and labeling or color-coding should be provided for linens soiled with blood or other body fluids.
Dialysis unit	High-touch areas must be decontaminated with disinfectant after each patient. Blood must be cleaned with a disinfectant that is effective against tuberculosis, hepatitis B virus (HBV), and human immunodeficiency virus (HIV) or bleach (1:100).
Examining rooms	Disposable items must be discarded, and high-touch surfaces and items must be wiped with disinfectant. Provide a thorough cleaning at day's end.
Operating rooms and ambulatory surgery center	Damp dusting should be done before the first case, a thorough disinfection done after each case, and thorough disinfection at the end of the day including wet vacuuming of floors with an appropriate disinfectant. If using a mop and bucket, a clean head must be used after each case. Cleaning progresses from high to low and clean to dirty, using only dedicated cleaning supplies.
Procedure rooms	Similar to operating rooms.
Laboratories	Require daily cleaning with counters decontaminated after each shift and when spills occur. Thorough cleanings should occur when the laboratory is closed or when convenient for a 24-hour laboratory.

INFECTION CONTROL ISSUES WITH SURFACE MATERIALS AND ANTIMICROBIALS

Issues associated with surface materials and antimicrobials include the following:

Wall surfaces	Vinyl wall coverings may allow moisture to condense, increasing the risk of fungi. Smooth, painted-surface walls are easier to clean and decontaminate than are textured surfaces. Smooth tile walls (such as in the operating room) should have epoxy-based grout.
Floor coverings	Easily cleanable materials should be used. Carpets are harder to clean, easier to stain, and can harbor pathogens and allergens. Additionally, the frequent vacuuming required of carpets contributes to noise pollution. Carpets saturated with water may serve as a reservoir for *Aspergillus* species and other fungi. If carpeting is used, it should not be placed in areas likely to incur heavy soiling, such as in operating rooms.
Textiles (curtains)	Impregnating textiles with antimicrobials has not proven more effective than routine cleaning methods.
Ceiling tiles/Porous surfaces	If porous tiles, such as acoustic tiles, incur water damage and cannot be completely dried within 48 hours, they must be replaced.

MONITORING FOR ENVIRONMENTAL PATHOGENS

MICROBIOLOGIC MONITORING

Environmental microbiologic monitoring involves ensuring that housekeeping staff maintains a clean environment, but routine sampling of walls, floors, other surfaces, and air in a medical institution is usually not indicated unless an outbreak presents, as the environment is rarely the cause of infection except in those who are immunocompromised. Studies have shown that visual assessment of cleanliness is not always supported by testing. A quick test for contamination is the adenosine triphosphate bioluminescence test; however, finding large numbers of organisms is common, depending upon the number of people in a room, activity, airflow, and other factors. Total bacterial counts generally do not correlate with infection risk. Valid testing requires cultures and quantitative results, with results reported as the number of organisms per area or volume so that swabbing a large area is not compared to swabbing a small area. Sampling methods may include swabbing with a moist sterile swab, a moist gauze, or HEPA vacuum sock. Dry swabs are less efficient at identifying spores.

MONITORING FOR LEGIONNAIRES DISEASE

CDC RECOMMENDATIONS ON DISCOVERING A SINGLE CASE

When a single case of laboratory-confirmed, healthcare-associated **Legionnaires Disease** is definitely identified, or if two or more cases of laboratory-confirmed, possible nosocomial Legionnaires Disease occur during a 6-month period, the CDC recommends that local or state health departments or the CDC be contacted and a combined epidemiologic and environmental investigation be conducted to determine the source(s). If evidence of continued nosocomial transmission is not revealed by retrospective evidence, an intensive prospective surveillance should be continued for at least two months after the date surveillance was initiated.

FINDING EVIDENCE OF TRANSMISSION

If evidence of continuous healthcare-associated transmission is present:

- Save and subtype isolates of *Legionella sp.* obtained from patients and the environment
- Collect and analyze water samples from potential sources of aerosolized water

If a source is not then identified after these analyses, continue surveillance for new cases for at least two months, and, depending on the scope of the outbreak, decide either to defer decontamination pending identification of the source(s) of *Legionella sp.* or proceed with decontamination of the hospital's water distribution system, with special attention given to the specific hospital areas involved in the outbreak. Decontaminate any source of infection found.

Finding Evidence in the Hospital's Heated Water or Cooling System

When evidence of Legionnaires Disease is found in the hospital's heater water system or cooling system, the CDC recommends the following:

- Decontaminate either by running superheated water through the system or hyperchlorinate it. Post warning signs at each outlet being flushed to prevent scald injury to patients, staff, or visitors.
- Clean the hot-water storage tanks and water heaters to remove accumulated scale and sediment.
- Restrict immunocompromised patients from taking showers, and have them use only sterile water for their oral consumption until *Legionella sp.* becomes undetectable by cultures of the hospital water.
- If cooling towers or evaporative condensers are implicated, decontaminate the cooling-tower system. Collect specimens for culture at 2-week intervals for 3 months. When *Legionella sp.* are not detected in cultures during that period, collect cultures monthly for another 3 months.
- Install drift eliminators on operational cooling towers, if this has not already been done, and regularly use an effective biocide. For new construction, always design and place cooling towers so that the tower drift is minimized and directed away from the hospital's air-intake system.

Infection Control Strategies for Recalled Items

The FDA maintains regulates procedures and **recall** regarding contaminated equipment and supplies a website entitled MedWatch to provide safety information for drugs and medical equipment. MedWatch provides electronic listing service to medical professionals and facilities for the following:

- Medical product safety alerts
- Information about drugs and devices
- Summary of safety alerts with links to detailed information

The Safe Medical Practices Act (1990) requires manufacturers and medical device user facilities to report problems with medical devices, including deaths or serious injuries (defined as requiring medical or surgical intervention), within 10 working days. Facilities must also file semiannual reports on January 1 and July 1. User facilities must maintain records for 2 years and must develop written procedures for identification, evaluation, and submission of medical device reports (MDR). MedWatch provides:

- **Reporting forms** (downloadable) for voluntary and mandatory reports
- **Recall and safety information** about recalls, market withdrawals and safety alerts, organized by months and years.

Monitoring Elements for a Safe Care Environment

CDC and HIPAC Rating Categories for Policy and Procedure Recommendations

The CDC and the HIPAC make recommendations about policies and procedures for environmental infection control in healthcare facilities. These recommendations are categorized according to the scientific evidence available to support the recommendations as well as existing state and federal laws. While the recommendations are voluntary, they are often used as a basis for state and federal regulations.

- **Category IA** is well supported by evidence from experimental, clinical, or epidemiologic studies and is strongly recommended for implementation.
- **Category IB** has supporting evidence from some studies, has a good theoretical basis, and is strongly recommended for implementation.
- **Category IC** is required by state or federal regulations or is an industry standard.
- **Category II** is supported by suggestive clinical or epidemiologic studies, has a theoretical basis, and is suggested for implementation.
- **Unresolved** means there is no recommendation because of a lack of consensus or evidence.

Monitoring and Outbreak Investigations Related to the Environment

Environmental monitoring includes the following:

- Conduct a record review to identify postsurgical site infections that might involve the operating room or other environmental factors.
- Perform visual monitoring of construction, renovation, and monitoring for airborne contamination.
- Create contractual agreements regarding HVAC specifications.
- Conduct routine air sampling and culturing from various areas of the facility.

Outbreak investigation includes the following actions as they relate to the environment:

- Confirm the outbreak.
- Determine patient care activities that may be implicated.
- Plan for the types of surveillance activities that are needed.
- Select appropriate environmental sampling and culturing methods (only of items that may be possible vectors or reservoirs for organisms). Sampling may include measuring total particulates or bioaerosols. Media needed for culturing may vary. Electronic monitors or particulate counters may be used.
- Review air standards and bioaerosol threshold standards (baseline levels of spores, organisms to use as comparison). Although no absolute bioaerosol standards have been developed, levels should be kept as low as possible.

Collecting and Culturing Air Samples

Pharmacy Cleanrooms

Rules for collecting and culturing air samples taken in pharmacy cleanrooms are as follows:

- Check engineering controls, gather baseline data with microbiological sampling prior to activating unit when commissioning a cleanroom
- Conduct air sampling on regular basis to check for cleanroom microflora that have penetrated barriers
- Collect samples on nutrient media and incubate them to promote microbial growth
- Attempts should be made to control or eliminate these variables as much as possible:
    - Media selection and storage
    - Plate handling (temperature extremes during shipping to culture labs)
    - Incubation temperature
    - Species viability
    - Species competition

Collecting and Analyzing Airborne Agents in an Industrial Setting

One prominent protocol requires that sampling be done with an impaction type sampler that is calibrated before and after each study. Air samples are taken at multiple times during the day; they are taken at the outdoor air intake of the building and at indoor sites where there have been occupant complaints and, if possible, in at least one area not associated with occupant complaints.

A set of 7 plates exposed at each sampling site comprises two plates of Rose Bengal Agar (RBA) for isolating fungi, two plates of R2Ac agar with Cycloheximide (R2Ac) for detection of environmental-type bacteria, two plates of Heart Infusion Blood Agar (BA) to enhance growth of human commensal bacteria, and one plate of Tryptic Soy Agar (TSA) to detect thermophiles.

Incubation times and temperatures vary for each type of microorganism sampled.

Infection Prevention in Construction and Renovation Projects

Infection Control Risk Assessment (ICRA)

Planning for renovation and construction should include an **infection control risk assessment (ICRA)** and development of a plan to continuously monitor construction activities because construction can result in risk of injury and exposure to microorganisms because spatial separation is often inadequate. Plans should be made to safely transfer patients from one area to another (such as from a patient room to the radiology department). Barriers erected around construction/renovation projects must be sufficient to avoid air and water contamination. Infection control must include environmental testing, including air sampling. The ICRA should also outline design features that are necessary for infection prevention, such as the correct air handling and ventilation for operating rooms and isolation rooms. Considerations should include placement of immunocompromised patients, patient relocation, standards for barriers, specific hazards likely to be encountered, impact of disrupted services (such as power outages, water breaks), and training of staff.

Risk Control for Construction Projects

Construction can release air or waterborne infective organisms into the environment, so all construction should be planned with the IP and other team members in order to minimize contamination. Risk control includes:

- Procedures for approval of projects
- Protocols for reducing dust and debris exposure during construction
- Clear outline of responsibilities for supervision of all aspects of the building process to ensure compliance with safe air/ water standards
- Plan for environmental services to clean work areas, new construction, and renovated areas as well as inspection when project completed
- Identification of high-risk patients and relocation if necessary
- Restriction of admission of immunocompromised patients during construction if necessary
- Staff training regarding dangers of construction to patients
- Evaluation of risk and environmental testing and cultures, including air sampling
- Final inspection prior to admitting patients to new or renovated areas

Advising Contractors on Infection Control Implications of Construction

The IP must work very closely with contractors to assure that they understand infection control implications of construction and that they follow guidelines, including the construction of adequate plastic or drywall barriers. Often the IP and contractor will work together with a consultant who is an expert in medical construction, and the IP must ensure that recommendations are followed. The IP must regularly monitor the construction site for compliance or problems. Agreements about construction cleanup both during and after construction should be made. The CDC advises that mandatory adherence agreements for infection control be part of construction contracts. Contractors must understand what the penalties are for noncompliance and what steps they must take to correct problems. Additionally, the IP and contractor should review plans for construction worker safety and OSHA guidelines, ensuring that workers are protected from potential danger and infection during demolition or construction.

Primary Concerns During Internal Construction/Remodeling

Dust

During a hospital construction/remodeling project, the primary infection control concern are dust and debris. The IP must work with contractors to establish a protocol for reduction of dust and outline their responsibilities for compliance with safe air and water standards. Construction/Renovation can result in large amounts of dust, which can spread *Aspergillus* species and other pathogens and can accumulate in filters in the ventilation system.

Admission of immunocompromised patients may need to be restricted from some areas during construction. A plan must be in place for environmental services to clean all areas, including work areas and newly renovated areas. Dust-producing activities, such as construction work (including new construction work as well as demolition and remodeling) have been associated with a number of outbreaks of aspergillosis. Patients who are immunocompromised are especially at risk and may need to be moved away from construction sites or treated with chemoprophylaxis if this is not possible. Most outbreaks have been traced to contaminated air in the facility, so air quality must be carefully monitored and vacuuming and dry mopping should be restricted.

Additional Concerns

Barriers	The placement and type of barriers must be determined as well as signage. Barriers should be airtight, sealed, and fire-rated.
Filtering	Decisions include use of fresh or recirculated air in construction/renovation area, the types and numbers of filters needed, and whether vents need to be covered and sealed. Filters should be changed more frequently during construction.
Ventilation	The construction zone should have negative airflow and continuous monitoring for the construction site and those areas affected.
Debris	The use of a debris chute with HEPA-filtered negative air machines is better than transporting debris in an elevator, but the chute opening should be sealed when not in use. Debris should be removed each day rather than it being allowed to accumulate. Debris should be moved in carts during hours of low activity with covers that fit tightly to reduce dust. The carts should be cleaned daily.
Noise/ Vibration	These may contribute to noise pollution and stress, but they may also dislodge dust and damage plumbing.
Air sampling	Staff should be educated about risk factors (visible dust, loose ceiling tiles, wet tiles, opened doors), and the types of environmental sampling and monitoring should be determined.
System balancing	The ventilation system should be balanced after construction/renovation is completed and filters examined or replaced, and ducts, vents, and induction units should be inspected and cleaned as needed.
Plumbing	All water lines in the newly constructed or renovated area and adjacent areas should be flushed because vibration caused by construction may have dislodged scale or caused corrosion and leakage.
Cleanup (contractor)	At the end of the project, the contractor should be responsible for removing equipment, debris, partitions, and barriers and should be responsible for cleaning and disinfecting.
Cleanup (staff)	Before returning the area to service, routine cleaning and disinfection of surfaces should be carried out.
Environmental cleaning	Because of increased dust in the air, areas adjacent to the construction site will require more frequent cleaning.
Air handlers/ changes	Some dampers adjacent to the construction site may need to be closed. The air handling system should be checked to ensure it can adequately handle air changes. The ventilation system will need to be cleaned and balanced at the end of construction.
Gas/Electricity	With power interruptions, dust, which may carry pathogens, may be dislodged when the power is reestablished, so running air out of the ducts may be necessary to flush systems before returning the area to service.
Final preparations	Once construction is completed, the site must be thoroughly cleaned and decontaminated prior to the installation of furniture, curtains, and clean supplies and before patient admission.

Infection Control Issues Related to External Excavations

External excavations can generate large amounts of dust, and the more frequently outside doors are opened, the more that dust and unfiltered air will enter the facility and the ventilation system. Therefore, excavation should ideally be conducted during off hours when there is less traffic (although the noise generated may pose another type of pollution) and the air handlers can be more easily adjusted. Accumulation of dust may cause ventilation systems to malfunction, and dust and debris may carry *Aspergillus* species. Appropriate dust-containment barriers must be in place and openings (doors, windows) close to the excavation site should be sealed and barred from use. A schedule for the wetting of soils to keep dust down should be established, and over-wetting, which may promote increased fungi, should be avoided. Workers must be educated about proper hygiene requirements before entering the facility. Materials stored outside should have protective coverings, such as being shrink-wrapped.

Preventing Airborne Infections During Mold-Removing Renovations

Mold removal should be conducted only by licensed health and safety professionals employing trained abatement contractors. All sensitive people, be they patients or staff, should be removed from the area. Workers need to wear disposable protective coveralls and use full face respiratory protection with HEPA filtration providing 99.97 percent removal of particles 0.3 microns in size. There should also be, going into and out of the work site, general filtration of air using negative pressure exhaust equipped with HEPA filtration, air locks, and decontamination chambers. Entire work sites should be insulated with plastic sheeting.

Waste needs to be washed and bagged prior to removal from the work area, and the work area thoroughly cleaned upon the job's completion. Air should be sampled for clearance before the enclosure is dismantled.

Infection Control Issues from Floods or Disasters

Issues associated with water damage from a flood or disaster should be addressed through the following measures:

Survey	A complete survey of the water-damaged site should include looking under carpets and inside cabinets and assessing all furnishings.
Monitoring	A moisture meter or infrared camera should be used to assess moisture in drywall, hardwood floors, and other surfaces. Monitoring may continue during cleanup stages.
Wet materials	Wet materials should be removed within 24 to 48 hours to prevent the spread of pathogens. Damaged wall areas must be opened with cove base removed so that spraying can reach all water-damaged surfaces.
Decontamination	All water-damaged areas, including hardwood, must be sprayed with diluted bleach or chlorine-based mist and left to dry. Staff conducting the spraying must use appropriate personal protective equipment, and the area should be well ventilated. Opened wall areas and then the total area are decontaminated with a 1:9 dilution of copper-8-quinolinolate compound and a pressurized sprayer. Surface soil is removed by scrubbing with a detergent, such as 1:200 trisodium phosphate, followed by 1:10 bleach. Hard surfaces are cleaned with undiluted bleach and are not rinsed.
Ventilation	The area should be sealed, and the ventilation system should be balanced to cause a negative-pressure state of the area. Mobile HEPA-filtering machines may need to be placed in the water-damaged area.
Ceilings	Wet ceiling tiles should be removed, and ceilings should be vacuumed with a HEPA-filtered vacuum cleaner, left to dry, and then covered with standard ceiling materials.
Wall vinyl/ drywall	Vinyl must be stripped because it can harbor fungi. Water-damaged drywall and insulation must be removed, and intact drywall should be cleaned. Note: Water-damaged areas must be removed to 12 inches above the water mark.
Furnishings	Upholstered furniture usually must be discarded, but if only steam damage has occurred, then they may be dried. Hardwood with intact laminate may be decontaminated with bleach solution, but if the laminate is over particleboard, then the item should be discarded because particleboard retains moisture.

Cleaning, Disinfection, Sterilization of Medical Devices and Equipment

Cleaning, Disinfecting, and Sterilizing Practices

Infection Control Strategies for Cleaning

Cleaning involves mechanical removal of contaminants and includes both pre-cleaning and cleaning. Disinfection and sterilization procedures should be preceded by cleaning in order for them to be effective because many chemicals deactivate in the presence of organic or inorganic materials:

- **Pre-cleaning** includes wiping down of equipment with disposable cloths, usually dampened with detergent solution, to remove secretions, dirt, and debris. Parts should be detached so that cleaning materials can reach all surfaces. Tubes and syringes should be flushed with air or solution. Pre-cleaning should be done as quickly as possible after use to prevent an increase in microbial count.
- **Cleaning** includes washing with detergents or enzyme solutions (used for organic material because they promote protein lysis), often involving soaking for prescribed periods of time. Ultrasonic cleaning, which uses high-energy sound waves to dislodge debris, may be used for instruments that are difficult to mechanically clean.

Cleaning Items and Surfaces Prior to Sterilization or Disinfection

Prior to processing items used in patient care, cleaning must be done with detergent and water or enzymatic cleansers and any foreign residue should be removed because the residue may interfere with sterilization and disinfection. Detergent solutions should be neutral or near neutral. Enzymes (proteases) are used to work on proteins. Solutions may also contain lipases to break down fat and amylases to address starches. Materials dried on items are difficult to remove, so presoaking or rinsing of items contaminated with body fluids is recommended. Manual cleaning (done for items without a mechanical unit) should include adequate friction (often with a brush) or fluidics (fluid under pressure) to ensure cleaning. Automated washer-disinfectors, similar to a dishwasher, should be loaded according to the manufacturer's directions, with hinged instruments opened and items disassembled if possible. Automated washer-disinfectors should adequately clean, disinfect, and dry solid and hollow medical equipment. Washer-sterilizers cleanse with water and detergent and hot steam. Ultrasonic cleaners may be used to remove foreign residue.

Clean vs. Aseptic Techniques

Clean technique is a form of medical asepsis in which clean and disinfected rather than sterile technique and equipment is used. The purpose is to minimize the risk of transmission of pathogens from the person and environment to the patient. However, sterile gloves should be used with sterile dressings as well as avoiding touching (the no-touch approach) the sterile dressings directly. A clean gown should be used to prevent contamination of clothing if indicated by the type of wound.

Aseptic technique is a form of medical asepsis in which maximum effort is used to keep an area, wound, and supplies free of pathogens and to prevent the spread of infection. The CDC recommends sterile technique for the first 24–48 hours for all wounds with primary closure, and the American

College of Surgeons recommends sterile technique for all surgical wounds for the first 24 hours. Aseptic technique requires the following:

- Barriers: Sterile gloves, gowns, masks, and drapes
- Sterile supplies and clean or sterile equipment as appropriate
- Hand hygiene and skin antisepsis
- Appropriate environmental cleaning and disinfection

Clean and Aseptic Techniques for Medical Procedures

Both clean and aseptic techniques require hand hygiene for all medical procedures, including before and after applying gloves (whether clean or sterile). Procedures are as follows:

- **Wound cleansing**: Clean gloves and personal protective equipment (PPE), but sterile supplies (irrigant and irrigating device) are used with clean technique.
- **Dressing change (routine):** Clean gloves and PPE if needed, and sterile supplies are used with clean technique.
- **Dressing change with wound debridement (chemical, enzymatic, mechanical)**: Clean gloves and PPE if needed and sterile supplies with clean technique.
- Dressing change with sharp wound debridement at bedside: Sterile gloves, PPE, supplies, and technique.
- **Dressing change (central line):** Sterile gloves to remove dressings and a second pair of sterile gloves (or use of double-gloving technique) to apply new dressing as well as surgical mask and all sterile supplies.
- **Tracheal suctioning (for suctioning a catheter without a protective enclosed sheath):** Sterile gloves, use of PPE including face shield or facemask while suctioning. Sterile catheter and other supplies with clean technique.
- **Tracheostomy care/suctioning**: Clean gloves and PPE including face shield and facemask. Sterile supplies with clean technique.

Infection Control Strategies for Disinfection

Properties of the Ideal Disinfectant

Properties of the ideal disinfectant include the following:

- Inexpensive
- Non-caustic and non-corrosive
- Environmentally safe, will not harm other forms of life (except for pathogens)
- Effective

Ideal disinfectants do not exist. Even if they could meet the other conditions, all disinfectants, without exception, are potentially harmful and even toxic to humans or animals. A "sure kill" rate on bacteria, molds, funguses, and viruses cannot be obtained without using a compound also harmful to higher forms of life.

Besides, bacteria reproduce rapidly and evolve over relatively short periods, so any bacteria that survive a chemical attack will go on to give rise to the next generation. Over a period of a few years, a new "super race" of the bugs emerge that develop, over many generations, resistance to hostile chemicals. Creating and maintaining conditions not conducive to bacterial survival and multiplication is, as an alternative to killing them with chemicals, an idea now getting a great deal of attention.

Limitations of Various Disinfectants

A wide range of disinfectants must be used in a hospital because different ones have specific purposes and they are not interchangeable. Mechanical cleaning should precede disinfection. Some disinfectants have toxic fumes, some degrade materials, some are irritating to skin, so there are many considerations when choosing the correct disinfectant.

- **High level disinfectants** include those that are sporicidal, such as glutaraldehyde and hydrogen peroxide, but are not used on housekeeping surfaces. These chemical sterilants are often deactivated by organic and inorganic materials, and guidelines for time, temperature, concentration, and use must be followed precisely.
- **Intermediate level and low-level disinfectants** include alcohol, which is a good general-purpose disinfectant that is compatible with other disinfectants. Iodophors are unstable at high temperatures. Chlorine compounds (bleach) are effective against blood or body fluids but deteriorate rapidly when stored and are corrosive of many surfaces. Phenolics deteriorate rubber, are irritating to skin and eyes, and cannot be used on food surfaces.

Spaulding Criteria for Choosing Disinfectants

Critical Items

Earle H. Spaulding developed a three-category classification system for different levels of sterilization/disinfection based on the type of item (instrument and/or equipment) and its use. Referred to as the **Spaulding Criteria**, the categories include critical, semicritical, and noncritical. While not applicable in all situations, this system is often used for reference.

Critical items are those that enter sterile tissue and carry a high risk of infection if they are contaminated with any type of organism or spores. These items are usually purchased as sterile in special packaging, or they are sterilized, preferably with steam heat. Critical items include surgical instruments, implants, catheters, and ultrasonic probes intended for use inside body cavities. Chemical sterilants should only be used for heat-sensitive items because they pose a number of problems in sterilization. First, the item to be sterilized must be thoroughly cleaned for the sterilization to be effective, and the concentration and contact time must be exactly as required. Furthermore, the item may need to be rinsed of the sterilant after processing (increasing the risk of contamination) and then placed in sterile packaging. The more steps that are involved, the more likely contamination is to occur.

Semicritical Items

Semicritical items are those that are used on nonintact skin and mucous membranes and carry a risk of infection if not adequately disinfected. These items should be free of bacteria, viruses, and fungi but may still contain a small number of spores because the respiratory tract and gastrointestinal tract are usually resistant to spores but not to other pathogens. **Semicritical items** include anesthesia equipment, various types of scopes (bronchoscope, endoscope, laryngoscope, cystoscope), various types of probes (vaginal, anal, esophageal manometry, prostate biopsy), and coagulation devices (infrared). Semicritical items require at least high-level disinfection, which may require rinsing. Semicritical items are often reprocessed for reuse, and a number of outbreaks have occurred because standards of reprocessing were not met. Reprocessing is often done by third parties rather than in house because of the difficulty in meeting standards.

Noncritical Items

Noncritical items are those that only come in contact with intact skin and do not touch mucous membranes or open wounds. **Noncritical items** include environmental equipment such as the bed, side rails, and bedside stands, overbed table, chairs, linens, and the floor. Noncritical items also include medical equipment such as blood pressure cuffs, pulse oximeters, walkers, bedpans, canes, and crutches. There is little direct risk of infection to the patient from appropriate contact with noncritical items. Noncritical items are usually disinfected in the room with low-level disinfection, or they are transported to another area of the facility (such as the laundry) for cleaning. One problem with noncritical items is that they have a role in secondary infection, such as when a healthcare provider fails to use proper hand hygiene and carries pathogens or spores on the hands from noncritical items of one patient to another or multiple other patients.

Classes of Chemical Disinfectants

The four classes of chemical disinfectants are clear soluble phenolics, hypochlorites, alcohols, and aldehydes.

- Hycolin, a **clear soluble phenolic**, will kill most bacteria but do not perform all that well against viruses.
- Presept and Milton, **hypochlorites**, generally effective against bacteria, fungi, viruses, and bacterial spores, are commonly used to decontaminate areas where there has been blood spillage, even though organic matter (such as blood) inactivates them. They decay in storage and are corrosive to metals.
- **Alcohols** like methanol, ethanol, and isopropanol should be used only after all visible surface dirt has been removed from the area to be disinfected. When an area is clean, alcohols have a good record going up against bacteria and viruses.
- Though active against bacteria, viruses, and fungi, the two **aldehydes**, glutaraldehyde and formaldehyde, work slowly against tubercle bacilli and have the added disadvantage of irritating skin and eyes.

Issues Related to Surface and Air Disinfection

Surface and air disinfection have been a matter of debate among healthcare providers because of costs, toxicity, and the possibility of increasing antimicrobial resistance. Studies have indicated that there is little difference in healthcare-associated infection rates with detergent use for noncritical surfaces as opposed to disinfectant use. Noncritical surfaces are those that come in contact with intact skin and contribute minimally to infections, such as floors and walls. Some surfaces, such as bedside tables, may potentially become contaminated with blood or body fluids and should be disinfected. Some argue that floors should be disinfected because they can become contaminated and in turn contaminate detergent solutions used to clean; however, studies have shown that bacterial counts return to pre-disinfection rates within a few hours. Detergent solutions can become contaminated, but the trend toward use of pre-moistened disposable mop heads rather than bucket solutions reduces this concern. Air disinfection with aerosols is not recommended in the United States.

Disinfection of Noncritical Equipment and Environmental Surfaces

Environmental contamination is a key factor in transmission of many healthcare-associated infections, so thorough decontamination of noncritical medical equipment and all environmental surfaces should be done when surfaces are soiled, when patients are discharged, and according to a routine schedule (e.g., daily or 3-5 days a week). Studies have shown that many surfaces that may carry pathogens are often left uncleaned or insufficiently cleaned. Contact time with low-level disinfection should be at least 1 minute (many products are labeled for a 30-second to 2-minute contact time), although some disinfectants are labeled for longer periods (such as 10 minutes) even though the longer period is essentially unworkable because it would require repeated application or immersion. In some cases, a disinfectant labeled as being effective for nonenveloped viruses (norovirus, adenovirus, poliovirus) must be used if these infections or Ebola is suspected or confirmed. The manufacturer's directions regarding dilution must be followed. Wet mops and cloths have the potential for contamination; therefore, disposable microfiber pads are safer.

Justifying the Use of Surface Disinfectants on Noncritical Surfaces

Though it does not mean they should not be disinfected along with critical surfaces, noncritical surfaces in the hospital or clinic, by definition, carry a low risk of transmitting a pathogen to patients. Low risk or no, there are always opportunities for people to make skin contact with these surfaces and thereby transfer any contaminants from them.

Noncritical surfaces of medical equipment (such as blood pressure cuffs and stethoscopes) are, after all, repeatedly touched by medical staff and may also become contaminated with patient material. Disinfectants should periodically be applied. Bed rails, bedside tables, and such are considered housekeeping surfaces, and while they seem to play an insignificant role in transmitting disease, they should also get attention through the application of either disinfectants or detergents at appropriate intervals.

Range of Activity of Disinfectants Against Various Agents

The range of activity of disinfectants against various agents include the following:

- **Mycobacteria and spores**: Relatively resistant. Whereas non-enveloped viruses (e.g., Coxsackie) tend to be more resistant, enveloped viruses (e.g., HIV) can be killed by most disinfectants.
- **Fungal spores**: Easily killed.
- **Bacterial spores like *Clostridia***: Resistant to most of the more common disinfectants.
- **Tubercle bacteria**: More resistant to chemical disinfectants than other bacteria can be killed by exposure to 2% alkaline glutaraldehyde solution (trade name, Cidex) for one hour.
- **Viruses causing rabies, Lassa fever and other hemorrhagic fevers**: High resistance, inactivated by Cidex, as are hepatitis B virus (HBV) and HIV, in 1-2 minutes, though soiled items should be placed in a 2% glutaraldehyde solution for 30 minutes just to be on the safe side. Exposure to 70% alcohol solution for 10 minutes is also effective.

Disinfection Considerations and Procedures

Disinfection considerations and procedures include the following:

Circumstance/Area	Considerations/Procedures
Blood/Body fluids	Some disinfectants are inactivated by organic material. For large spills, an absorbent material (such as powder) should be placed on the spill before pouring a disinfectant directly on the spill and then cleaning. Decontamination requires a disinfectant that is effective against the hepatitis B virus (HBV) and human immunodeficiency virus (HIV), a tuberculocidal disinfectant, or a bleach solution (1:100 for nonporous surfaces and 1:10 for porous surfaces).
Clostridium difficile	A bleach solution (1:10) or a sporicidal agent will kill some spores. Spores are most common in the patient zone, the floor (especially carpeted floors), and bathrooms. Terminal cleaning with UV light or hydrogen peroxide vapor will further reduce the spore count.
Norovirus diarrhea	High-touch areas are cleaned and disinfected three times daily (with quaternary ammonium compounds [QACs or "quats"] or a bleach solution), and low-touch areas are cleaned and disinfected two times daily while wearing a gown and gloves. Privacy curtains should be changed upon transfer or discharge of the patient; carpets and upholstered furniture should be steam cleaned.
Mycobacterium tuberculosis	Disinfectant must be Environmental Protection Agency (EPA)-registered as a tuberculocidal, and the manufacturer's recommendations for contact time must be followed.
Nursery	Patient zones must be thoroughly cleaned and disinfected, but infants are removed from beds during the process and are returned after surfaces are dry. Quaternary ammonium compounds (QACs or quats) are recommended. Alcohol may cloud plastics.
Severe acute respiratory syndrome (SARS)	Thorough cleaning and disinfecting are required daily and on patient discharge with virucidal disinfectant or bleach (1:100), wearing gloves, gown, mask, and protective eyewear.
COVID-19	Same as for SARS.
Multidrug-resistant organisms (MDROs)	MDROs are killed by most disinfectants, but rigorous cleaning is required using contact precautions. Privacy curtains are changed on patient discharge.
Isolation rooms	Same as for MDROs.
Bedbugs	The patient's belongings should be placed in secured plastic bags, clutter removed, area vacuumed with HEPA-filtered vacuum, and reusable equipment thoroughly cleaned while wearing gown and gloves. Insecticide may be needed per an exterminator.

Infection Control Strategies for Sterilization

Sterilization is a process that completely destroys microorganisms, including spores. Sterilization may be done physically by different methods, including steam pressure, dry heat, or ethylene oxide gas. Chemical sterilants, registered by the FDA, may be used, but manufacturer's directions must be followed. In some cases, the difference between chemical sterilization and disinfection relates to the length of time the process takes. For example, many chemicals require 10-20 minutes (and some up to 12 hours) for effectiveness, but this may be impractical for cleaning of surfaces, such as floors. Sterilization can be influenced by a number of factors:

- Pre-sterilization cleaning may be inadequate, resulting in proteins or other debris that interfere with sterilizing
- Packaging may prevent adequate contact of sterilizing agent with item
- Loading of sterilizer must be done properly to ensure contact of sterilizing agent with all items
- Time and temperature of sterilizer must be sufficient to kill organisms

METHODS OF STERILIZATION

STERILIZATION METHOD BASED ON ITEM TYPE

Methods of sterilization include the following:

- **High temperature**: Used for heat-tolerant critical/semicritical items for patient care, including surgical instruments. May use steam heat for 40 minutes or dry heat for 1-6 hours (varies according to temperature).
- **Low temperature**: Used for heat-sensitive critical and semicritical items for patient care. May use ethylene oxide gas for 15 hours, hydrogen peroxide gas plasma for 28-52 minutes, ozone for 4 hours, or hydrogen peroxide vapor for 55 minutes.
- **Liquid immersion**: Used for heat-critical/semicritical items that tolerate immersion. Chemical sterilants include >2% glutaraldehyde for about 10 hours, glutaraldehyde (1.12%) with phenol (1.93%) for 12 hours, hydrogen peroxide (7.35%) with peracetic acid (0.23%) for 3 hours, hydrogen peroxide (1%) with peracetic acid (0.08%) for 25 minutes, hydrogen peroxide (7.5%) for 30 minutes, chlorine (650–675 ppm) for 10 minutes, peracetic acid (>0.2%) for 12 minutes (at 50–56 °C), or ortho-phthalaldehyde (0.55%) for 15 minutes.

STEAM STERILIZATION (AUTOCLAVING)

Steam sterilization (autoclaving) is commonly used to sterilize medical equipment and supplies. The temperature settings are usually 121 °C for 30 minutes or 132 °C for 4 minutes, although sterilization times may vary according to the type of item. Steam sterilization is nontoxic and rapidly kills pathogens. Steam sterilization is the least affected by foreign residue of any sterilization process, and it is able to effectively penetrate device lumens as well as fabrics and packaging. Steam cycles are relatively easy to control, and the cycle time is rapid. However, there are some disadvantages:

- Steam sterilization can only be used with heat-tolerant items.
- Microsurgical instruments may be damaged over time with multiple exposures.
- Because items are frequently not dried adequately, the moisture may result in rusting of the instruments.
- Over time, scopes (such as the laryngoscope) may have a lower ability to transmit light.
- As with any source of heat, there is a potential of burns.

FLASH STERILIZATION

Flash sterilization is a form of steam sterilization done for unwrapped items, generally at 27–28 pounds of pressure. Flash sterilization use temperatures of 132 °C for 3-10 minutes, depending on the type of steam sterilizer used (gravity displacement, prevacuum, or steam-fluid pressure-pulse) and the type of items being processed. For example, medical instruments with no lumens require 3 minutes but rubber or plastic items or those with lumens require 10 minutes with gravity displacement and 4 minutes with pre-vacuum. The steam-flush pressure pulse sterilizer requires 4 minutes for all types of items. Items are usually placed in an open tray, so there is no protective packaging in place after the procedure is completed. Therefore, flash sterilizers are usually placed close to where the items will be used, such as next to an operating room. Some manufacturers provide reusable sterilization containers so that the item remains sterile until the container is opened, reducing the time the item is exposed to the air. Instruments are hot and could burn staff or patients.

Hydrogen Peroxide Gas Plasma Sterilization

Hydrogen peroxide gas plasma sterilization can be used on most medical devices, but it cannot process paper, linens, or liquids, so synthetic packaging must be used. In this low-temperature process (<50 °C), hydrogen peroxide is vaporized under high pressure and diffuses through the chamber, and an electrical field is used to produce gas plasma (charged particles), which produces microcidal free radicals that disrupt the metabolism of microorganisms. This process inactivates pathogens including vegetative bacteria, fungi, yeasts, viruses, and bacterial spores. Hydrogen peroxide gas plasma sterilization is environmentally safe and is used for heat- and moisture-sensitive items, such as plastics, metal alloys that may corrode, and electrical devices. The cycle time is about 28 minutes, and no aeration time is required after sterilization. The hydrogen vapor may not penetrate all lumens (such as on an endoscope), so the manufacturer's directions must be consulted.

Stages

There are five stages to the hydrogen peroxide plasma gas sterilization process:

1. **Chamber evacuation** creates a vacuum with reduced internal pressure.
2. **Peroxide injection** into the chamber causes the solution to evaporate and disperse throughout the chamber, killing bacteria on contact.
3. **Diffusion of peroxide** throughout chamber sterilizes items and then chamber pressure is reduced.
4. **Electromagnetic field** breaks apart peroxide vapor and creates a low-temperature plasma cloud, producing ultraviolet light and free radicals. Components then recombine into oxygen and water. Stages 1-3 repeat.
5. **Venting** of chamber equalizes pressure so chamber will open.

Vaporized Hydrogen Peroxide Sterilization

Vaporized hydrogen peroxide sterilization is a low-temperature method that can be used to sterilize heat- and moisture-sensitive medical devices with some limitations based on lumen size. Vaporized hydrogen peroxide kills all forms of microorganisms and bacterial spores (including anthrax). The vapor is produced from a solution composed of hydrogen peroxide and water. Vaporized hydrogen peroxide cannot be used to sterilize linens, liquids, powder, or paper materials and requires synthetic packaging. Vaporized hydrogen peroxide is environmentally safe and leaves no toxic residue, so no aeration time is needed upon completion of the sterilization process. The cycle time is about 55 minutes. However, hydrogen peroxide is irritating to the skin, eyes, and respiratory system if an individual is exposed to the vapor. Concentrations greater than 75 ppm are dangerous to humans. Vaporized hydrogen peroxide can also be used to decontaminate enclosed and sealed areas, such as an isolation room.

100% Ethylene Oxide (ETO) Sterilization

The most common chemical sterilant, 100% ethylene oxide (ETO) sterilization, can be used for critical and semicritical heat- or moisture-sensitive medical devices; however, the gas is absorbed by many different materials, so items must be aerated after sterilization. ETO is a flammable, explosive gas, and occupational exposure can cause cancer, hematological disorders, genetic disorders, tissue burns (from residue left on medical devices, genetic disorders, and spontaneous abortion). Emissions from the equipment are regulated by the states. ETO inactivates all microorganisms, although bacterial spores are more resistant, so a biological indicator that is sensitive to *Bacillus atrophaeus* is essential. ETO may not adequately penetrate all lumens, so it is not commonly used to reprocess endoscopes. The exposure time needed is 1-6 hours depending on the concentration of gas (450-1200 mg/L), the temperature (37-63 °C), and the humidity (40-80%). Higher temperatures and higher gas concentrations decrease the exposure time. Many ETO blends have been phased out because the hydrocarbons used in the blends damaged the ozone layer.

Peracetic Acid Sterilization

Peracetic acid sterilization is a low-temperature (50 °C) method commonly used to sterilize medical, dental, and surgical instruments, including endoscopes and arthroscopes (rigid and flexible). Peracetic acid is effective in the presence of organic material. Peracetic acid sterilization inactivates Gram-positive and Gram-negative bacteria, yeasts, fungi, and viruses as well as bacterial spores. During the process, a diluted solution of peracetic acid is pumped through the devices and scopes for 12 minutes. Connectors allow direct flow through endoscopes, but the correct connector must be used. Following the sterilization process, the peracetic acid is discarded to the sewer and the devices are rinsed four times with filtered water to remove all peracetic acid residue. Biological monitors must be used during the process (*Geobacillus stearothermophilus* spore strips).

Ozone Sterilization

Ozone sterilization (generated from oxygen and water), developed in 2003, is a nontoxic, low-temperature (30-35 °C) form of sterilization used for heat- and moisture-sensitive medical items, including metal and plastic instruments, with some limitations on lumen size. Ozone sterilization should not be used with natural rubber, latex, fabrics, some metals (copper, brass, bronze, zinc, and nickel), and items that are sensitive to a vacuum, such as flexible endoscopes and liquids. Ozone is a gas that transforms into oxygen when in contact with a catalytic agent. Ozone sterilization kills all forms of microorganisms and bacterial spores. Additionally, some studies indicate that ozone sterilization may deactivate prions. Ozone sterilization is relatively inexpensive and lacks many of the dangers associated with other sterilizing procedures; however, the chambers tend to be relatively small, and the time needed for sterilization is long, usually about 4 hours and 15 minutes, although no aeration is necessary because there is no toxic byproduct.

Ionizing Radiation, Dry-Heat Sterilization, and Microwaves

Ionizing radiation is a low-temperature method of sterilization and involves the use of cobalt 60 gamma rays or electron accelerators. It can be used for a variety of medical devices as well as transplantation tissue, but it is costly and is used primarily for large-scale commercial operations.

Dry-heat sterilization is used for moisture-sensitive and heat-tolerant devices. Dry heat is inexpensive, nontoxic, and noncorrosive, and it penetrates materials well. Dry-heat sterilizers may have static air or forced air, although forced air provides a more uniform temperature. Dry-heat sterilization is slow compared to many other methods with the time required corresponding to the temperature: 170 °C requires 60 minutes, 160 °C requires 120 minutes, and 150 °C requires 150 minutes.

Microwaves are used for the limited sterilization of compatible medical devices, such as dentures, urinary catheters (for self-catheterization), contact lenses, and dental instruments. Microwaves vary widely in wattage and megahertz and should be tested for effectiveness, but 5 minutes at 600 W/2450 MHz is usually effective against pathogens, including spores.

Chemical Sterilization

Chemical sterilants include the following:

Chemical	Advantages	Disadvantages
Glutaraldehyde	Compatible with most materials and relatively inexpensive.	Slow mycobactericidal activity, coagulates blood and fixes organic material, is irritating to the skin and respiratory system.
Hydrogen peroxide	Enhances removal of organic material and inactivates *Cryptosporidium*. No activation is needed.	Incompatible with brass, zinc, copper, nickel/silver plating.
Improved hydrogen peroxide (2%)	No activation needed. Works quickly within 8 minutes at 20 °C. 12-month shelf life and 14-day reuse.	Data limited concerning material compatibility and organic material resistance.
Ortho-phthalaldehyde (OPA)	No activation needed, works rapidly, does not coagulate blood or fix organic material, and is compatible with most materials.	Slow sporicidal activity, stains protein on tissue, clothing, and environmental surfaces. May cause eye irritation or anaphylactic reaction.
Peracetic acid/hydrogen peroxide	Requires no activation and has no significant odor or irritant.	Incompatible with lead, brass, zinc, and copper.

Ultraviolet Radiation and Hydrogen Peroxide Vapor for Room Decontamination

Room decontamination with **ultraviolet (UV) irradiation** is effective at reducing vegetative bacteria within 15-20 minutes and *Clostridium difficile* within 35-100 minutes, although effectiveness is reduced if environmental surfaces are not within the line of sight of the irradiation equipment. The presence of organic material reduces effectiveness, so cleaning prior to UV irradiation is essential.

Room decontamination with **hydrogen peroxide (HP) vapor** is very effective in eradicating multiple pathogens, including methicillin-resistant *Staphylococcus aureus* (MRSA), *Mycobacterium tuberculosis*, and *C. difficile* spores. However, decontamination with HP vapor requires about four times longer than standard cleaning. UV irradiation and HP vapor systems are costly, and decontamination requires removing patients and staff from the rooms, so these methods are effective only for terminal decontamination. The downtime is greater than for standard cleaning. In comparison, UV irradiation is faster, but HP is more effective at destroying spore-forming organisms.

Single-Use and Reprocessed Devices

Reuse of Single-Use Devices

Single-use devices (SUD), such as surgical drills, catheters, and endotracheal tubes, are manufactured for one-time use, but the reality is that for many years SUDs were reused with little regulatory oversight regarding methods of disinfecting/sterilization to determine if the SUDs were safe for use. Many hospitals reprocessed their own devices although some sent them to third party reprocessors. In response to concerns about this practice, the Medical User Fee and Modernization Act (MDUFMA) was issued in 2002, with requirements for reprocessing, including applications for 510(k)s and validation data demonstrating that the reprocessed SUD is essentially equivalent to the original SUD. Reprocessed devices are classified as critical (in contact with sterile tissue), semicritical (in contact with mucous membranes), or noncritical (topical contact with skin only). The process of validation includes procedures for cleaning and sterilization, the types of materials, and product testing. Studies have shown that properly reprocessed SUDs are equivalent in safety to the original.

Reprocessing Endoscopes

Endoscopes of all types are used are used to look inside the body and should be airtight. **Steps to reprocessing** include the following:

1. **Leak testing**: The leak tester is attached to the endoscope, and the endoscope is submerged in water. Water should be used for the pressure test, and all parts of the endoscope should be examined during the test for evidence of leaks (bubbles) for at least 90 seconds.
2. **Clean the endoscope**: Water and an enzymatic cleanser are used to flush and brush external surfaces and all channels.
3. **Disinfect**: Immerse the endoscope in a high-level disinfectant or chemical sterilants, and ensure that all surfaces and channels are in contact with the disinfectant/sterilant and that exposure matches that recommended by manufacturer. (Alternatively, use another sterilization method, such as ozone sterilization.)
4. **Rinse with sterile or filtered water**, making sure that the water rinses all the external surfaces and channels.
5. **Rinse with 70-90% alcohol** and dry with forced air.
6. **Store** the endoscope by hanging it vertically to encourage drying and limit recontamination.

Issues with Reprocessing Medical Devices

Reprocessing of medical devices requires that a separate area or room be available other than where procedures are carried out. This area must have sufficient space and ventilation for the type of disinfection/sterilization process that will be used. Costs are a consideration, and many choose to use a third-party reprocessor rather than carrying out the reprocessing on site. A log must be maintained for reprocessed endoscopes and other medical devices in case an outbreak occurs. The log must contain the date, the patient's name, the procedure, the physician's name, and the type of reprocessing (including the use of an automated endoscope washer-disinfector [AEWD]) that was done as well as the serial number of the device. Personnel involved in reprocessing must be trained in the biological and chemical hazards associated with the disinfection/sterilization process and must have access to appropriate personal protective equipment (PPE). Infections associated with reprocessed devices should be reported to the physician, infection control person, appropriate public health entity, Centers for Disease Control and Prevention (CDC), Food and Drug Administration (FDA), and manufacturers of the device and the AEWD, disinfectant, and sterilants.

Selecting Endoscopic Devices and Automatic Endoscopic Washer-Disinfectors

Issues to consider when selecting endoscopic devices and automatic endoscope washer-disinfectors (AEWDs) include the following:

- Potential risks of infection associated with the device/equipment
- Costs of equipment and reprocessing
- Space availability for storage, use, and reprocessing
- Type of disinfection/sterilization compatible with the device
- Exposure time for various disinfectants
- Ease of accessing interior channels/lumens for cleaning and disinfecting
- Use of reusable or disposable endoscope accessories
- Immersibility of all parts of the endoscope
- Type of bacteriologic sampling required
- Type and extent of training needed if the devices are to be reprocessed or transported for reprocessing
- Adverse event and outbreak readiness and reporting requirements
- Risk management/liability issues
- Use of ultrasonic cleaning versus manual cleaning
- Manual disinfection versus AEWD
- Environmental surface decontamination

Reprocessing Dialyzers for Hemodialysis

If a new dialyzer is to be reused, it must be reprocessed and tested to determine the baseline total cell volume (TCV), which is the total volume of blood that its blood compartment can hold. Before reuse, the dialyzer must be checked again to ensure that the TCV for this dialyzer is at least 80% of baseline. The dialyzer cannot be reused if the TCV is lower than 80% because the 20% drop in TCV will result in a 10% decrease in the clearance of urea. Also prior to reuse, a recirculating rinse with normal saline should be completed with a recirculating flow rate through the blood compartment (BFR) of 200 mL/min and a recirculating flow rate of 500 mL/min through the dialysate compartment (DFR) for a period of 15-30 minutes, being careful to avoid introduction of air into the arterial circuit because air may interfere with the removal of germicide. Dialyzers should be processed within 2 hours. After 2 hours, the dialyzer must be refrigerated (not frozen) because the cold helps to retard bacterial growth.

Levels of Disinfection/Sterilization

CDC's Levels of Disinfection

The CDC has set up taxonomy of germicidal disinfectant power to correspond with potential risk of infection involved in the use of various medical devices. (The EPA has another system.) The higher the risk, the greater the killing power needed.

For example, a germicide effective against *Mycobacterium tuberculosis* would be, by CDC accounting, classified at least as an intermediate-level disinfectant because it should be effective with equipment expected to come into contact with that bacillus—semicritical apparatus like endotracheal tubes and other items that may touch intact mucous membranes. Items considered critical are those introduced directly into the bloodstream or other normally sterile areas of the body; noncritical items may touch intact skin but do not otherwise ordinarily touch the patient, such as crutches.

The classification system is an aid in deciding which germicidal to use under which circumstances. The more germicidal killing power that is needed, the more toxic and (generally) expensive the agent is. There is no necessity for using a highly toxic agent when a less environmentally unfriendly one will do.

Levels of Disinfectants Used in Infection Control

Part of infection control is to identify those items and materials that should be sterilized or disinfected as well as the type of disinfectant. There are **three basic levels of disinfectants:**

- **High** kills almost all bacteria, viruses, and fungi except for large concentrations of bacterial spores and includes hydrogen peroxide and glutaraldehyde.
- **Intermediate** kills or inactivates most vegetative bacteria (including *Mycobacterium tuberculosis),* viruses (HIV and HBV), and fungi but not bacterial spores and includes sodium hypochlorite, alcohols, phenolics, and iodophors.
- **Low** kills most bacteria but only some viruses and fungi and is not effective against resistive strains or bacterial spores and includes quaternary ammonium compounds, phenolics and iodophors.

In order to meet OSHA's standards for prevention of spread of bloodborne pathogens, at least intermediate-level disinfection should be used throughout the hospital when possible, especially in labs, emergency departments, and surgery. The Environmental Protection Agency (EPA) publishes lists of registered disinfectants for different levels of disinfection.

Low- and Intermediate-Level Disinfection

Low-level disinfection kills vegetative bacteria and some fungi and viruses but does not kill mycobacteria or spores. Low-level disinfection requires liquid contact with an EPA-registered disinfectant that does not carry a tuberculocidal claim and is used for noncritical items or environmental surfaces with no visible blood. Low-level disinfectants include chlorine-based products, phenolics, improved hydrogen peroxide (2%), 70–90% alcohol, or quaternary ammonium compounds (QACs or quats) (they require 1 minute of exposure).

Intermediate-level disinfection kills vegetative bacteria and most fungi and viruses as well as mycobacteria but not spores. Intermediate-level disinfection requires liquid contact but not immersion and is used to disinfect noncritical items (such as blood pressure cuffs or environmental surfaces that are contaminated with visible blood). Disinfectants must be EPA-registered for use as a hospital disinfectant and must carry a statement about tuberculocidal activity on the label.

Disinfectants include products that are chlorine based, phenolics, or improved hydrogen peroxide (2%). Contact must be for at least 1 minute.

High-Level Disinfection

High-level disinfection (HLD) kills all pathogens, but with a high number of spores, some spores may survive. Methods include the following:

- **Heat pasteurization**: Used for heat-tolerant semicritical items (such as respiratory therapy equipment). Temperature 65-77 °C for 30 minutes.
- **Liquid immersion**: Used for heat-sensitive semicritical items (such as bronchoscopes). Chemical sterilants and HLDs include glutaraldehyde (>2%) for 10–90 minutes, glutaraldehyde (1.12%) with phenol (1.93%) for 20 minutes, ortho-phthalaldehyde (0.55%) for 12 minutes, hydrogen peroxide (7.34%) with peracetic acid (0.23%) for 15 minutes, hydrogen peroxide (7.5%) for 30 minutes, hydrogen peroxide (1%) with peracetic acid (0.08%) for 25 minutes, chlorine (650–675 ppm) for 10 minutes, hydrogen peroxide (2%) for 8 minutes, and glutaraldehyde (2.0%) with isopropanol (26%) for 10 minutes.

Peracetic Acid/Hydrogen Peroxide and Glutaraldehyde as High-Level Disinfectants

French researchers revealed, in a comparison with other high-level disinfectants, that the MSC (minimal sporicidal concentration) of the biocide combination of peracetic acid (which is already a mixture of hydrogen peroxide and acetic acid) and hydrogen peroxide was most effective even at the weakest concentration. Its effectiveness was maintained with increasing contact time. MSC could be reduced by two to eight times when compared with those of either of its two biocidal components applied individually against bacillus spore isolates found on stored membranes and collection cultures.

In addition to being used to sterilize heat sensitive medical equipment, glutaraldehyde is an embalming fluid, a component in leather tanning solutions, and an industrial chemical preservative. Though effective as a biocide, it is toxic and can result in headaches, drowsiness, dizziness, asthma, nosebleed, conjunctivitis, rash, hives, and nausea.

Peracetic Acid as a High-Level Disinfectant

Peracetic acid can deactivate a large variety of pathogenic microorganisms, viruses, and spores. Though its action is not deterred by organic compounds in water, it is affected by heat.

At a temperature of 15 °C and a pH value of 7, five times more peracetic acid is required to affectively deactivate pathogens than at a pH value of 7 and a temperature of 35 °C.

There is some indication that exposure to peracetic acid may cause adverse effects on skin or the sense organs. It is ranked as being more hazardous than most chemicals by a number of rating systems. While the acute toxicity of peracetic acid is low, it is extremely irritating to the skin, eyes, and respiratory tract. Skin or eye contact with the 40% solution in acetic acid can cause serious burns. Inhalation of high concentrations of mists of peracetic acid solutions can lead to burning sensations, coughing, wheezing, and shortness of breath.

ORTHO-PHTHALALDEHYDE (OPA) AS A HIGH-LEVEL DISINFECTANT

Ortho-phthalaldehyde (OPA), having shown superior mycobactericidal activity compared with glutaraldehyde, received clearance by FDA for use beginning in 1999. In tests, the mean time required for it to affect a 6-$\log_{10}$ reduction for *M. bovis* was 6 minutes, compared with 32 minutes using 1.5% glutaraldehyde. It also tested well against a wide range of microorganisms, including glutaraldehyde-resistant mycobacteria.

Unlike glutaraldehyde, OPA requires no activation, is not a known irritant to the eyes and nasal passages, has excellent stability over a wide range of pH and temperatures, does not require exposure monitoring, and has almost no odor. OPA does stain proteins gray (including unprotected skin), so gloves, eye protection, and fluid-resistant gowns are advisable when using it. Used solution can be neutralized with glycine for disposal in sanitary sewers.

CBIC Practice Test

Want to take this practice test in an online interactive format?
Check out the bonus page, which includes interactive practice questions and much more: **https://www.mometrix.com/bonus948/cbic**

SCAN HERE

1. When a patient is on contact precautions for MRSA, which of the following is correct?

a. Enter the room without PPE if no patient contact planned
b. Wear gown, gloves, and faceguard whenever entering the room
c. Wear gloves only if anticipating patient contact
d. Where gown and gloves whenever entering the room

2. A broad-spectrum antibiotic is usually administered for empirical therapy because:

a. it is more cost-effective than other types of antibiotics.
b. it has better prophylactic properties.
c. the pathogenic organism is not yet identified.
d. it is most appropriate for the organism.

3. Which of the following are medical intervention factors that affect risk of infection?

I. Indwelling devices
II. Staffing ratios
III. Types of disinfectants used
IV. Lengths of stay

a. I and III only
b. I, II, and IV only
c. II and IV only
d. I, II, III, and IV

4. On the first day of the month, 8 patients had CLABSI out of a total patient population of 600. What is the prevalence rate of CLABSI per 1000 patients?

a. 13.3
b. 133
c. 7.5
d. 75

5. The data used to create an affinity diagram is usually collected by which method?

a. Conducting a literature review
b. Searching databases
c. Multivoting
d. Brainstorming

6. In the Six Sigma DMAIC format, the *D* represents:

a. Develop
b. Document
c. Define
d. Demonstrate

7. When evaluating a surveillance program, the evaluators should note whether the program has effectively done which of the following?

I. Saved the facility money
II. Detected infections
III. Identified trends
IV. Identified risk factors for infections

a. II, III, and IV only
b. II, and III only
c. I, II, and III only
d. I, II, III, and IV

8. When calculating rates of CAUTI on a unit in a six-month period, the denominator must include:

a. all patients.
b. all patients with urinary catheters.
c. all patients with CAUTI.
d. all patients with urinary catheters minus those with CAUTI.

9. If an outbreak of COVID-19 occurred in a group of people who had attended a community retreat with a total of 36 participants three weeks earlier, the best method of case finding is to:

a. alert the media to the outbreak.
b. individually contact the 36 participants.
c. ask physicians to be on the alert.
d. notify laboratories to report positive findings.

10. When diagnosing an infection with *Clostridium difficile,* which type of specimen is necessary?

a. Blood
b. Skin swab
c. Solid stool
d. Liquid stool

11. Six burn patients out of 30 receiving immersion hydrotherapy (IH) developed *Pseudomonas aeruginosa* infections while 2 burn patients out of 32 receiving shower cart hydrotherapy (SCH) developed the infection. What is the relative risk of developing a *P. aeruginosa* infection if exposed to IH compared to SCH?

a. 0.31
b. 1.2
c. 1.7
d. 3.2

12. In a control chart, the central line represents the:

a. average of data points.
b. time period.
c. count/rate.
d. lower limit of data.

13. In a community outbreak of gonorrhea, out of the initial 40 cases identified, the ratio of female to male cases was 3:5. If 120 total cases are projected and the same ratio persists, how many additional cases will be female?

a. 15
b. 30
c. 45
d. 80

14. Which factor is most important in ensuring successful antimicrobial therapy?

a. Organism virulence and susceptibility
b. Patient status
c. Antimicrobial action
d. Prompt administration of the appropriate antibiotic

15. An example of active learning is:

a. analyzing a case study.
b. reading a text.
c. attending a lecture.
d. listening to an audiotape.

16. The best method to ensure compliance with the regimen for treatment of tuberculosis is:

a. keeping the patient hospitalized.
b. thoroughly educating the patient.
c. utilizing directly-observed therapy.
d. giving the patient a three-month supply of medications.

17. According to Hill's criteria for causation, when a number of studies over extended periods of time show the same association even though different research methods are utilized, this is an example of:

a. strength of association.
b. temporality.
c. coherence.
d. consistency.

18. What is the usual contact time for low-level disinfection of noncritical patient environmental surfaces and equipment?

a. 1 minute
b. 5 minutes
c. 10 minutes
d. 15 minutes

19. The second step in conducting a systematic review and meta-analysis is to:

a. develop a methodology for review.
b. select studies using predetermined criteria.
c. develop a research question.
d. conduct a review of the literature.

20. Skin testing for tuberculosis and mammography for breast cancer are examples of which type of prevention?

a. Primary
b. Secondary
c. Tertiary
d. Quaternary

21. According to the National Quality Forum's Endorsed Set of Safe Practices, Safe Practice 23, Care of the Ventilated Patient, actions should be taken to prevent which complications?

I. Ventilation-associated pneumonia
II. Dental complications
III. Venous thromboembolism
IV. Peptic ulcer disease

a. I and III only
b. I, III, and IV only
c. I, II, and III only
d. I, II, III, and IV

22. When installing alcohol-based hand rub dispensers in a 6-foot-wide hallway for use of staff and visitors, what is the minimum distance required between dispensers?

a. 4 feet
b. 6 feet
c. 8 feet
d. 10 feet

23. What is the primary limitation of qualitative research?

a. Inability to aid in development of a hypothesis
b. Inability to present participants' viewpoints
c. Lack of generalizability
d. Unsuitability for descriptive research

24. The primary element required for herd immunity is a group:

a. of homogenous people.
b. with a high proportion of immunity.
c. whose members developed immunity from receiving vaccination.
d. whose members developed immunity from having a disease.

25. What is the first link in the chain of infection?

a. Reservoir
b. Mode of transmission
c. Susceptible host
d. Causative agent

26. If an antibiotic is administered to 200 patients with SSIs attributed to *Staphylococcus aureus* with a reliability of 82%, how many patients did not respond to the drug?

a. 36
b. 18
c. 9
d. 28

27. Natural barriers to disease include which of the following?

I. Immunizations
II. Gastric acids
III. Respiratory tract cilia
IV. Tears

a. I, II, and III only
b. II and III only
c. II, III, and IV only
d. I, II, III, and IV

28. Since wide distribution of the COVID-19 vaccination, which of the following are NOT consistent with CDC guidelines regarding mask wearing?

a. Fully vaccinated individuals must still wear a mask when using public transportation (plane, trains, taxi services, etc.).
b. Fully vaccinated individuals are not required to wear masks indoors, unless the establishment or state mandates such.
c. Fully vaccinated healthcare workers do not have to wear a mask while working, unless treating patients with known or suspected cases of infectious disease.
d. Fully vaccinated individuals must still wear a mask when attending medical and dental appointments.

29. In a community of 150,000 people, 1125 people died over the course of a year. What is the crude mortality rate per 1000 population?

a. 7.5
b. 75
c. 13.3
d. 133

30. According to the Joint Commission's requirements, if a facility wants to reuse single-use medical devices, the facility must:

a. have written policy and procedures regarding reuse.
b. demonstrate cost savings.
c. have industrial-quality equipment for reprocessing.
d. apply for a reuse license.

31. The purpose of network mapping is to:

a. identify problems.
b. brainstorm ideas.
c. show flow of traffic through a facility.
d. show relationships and communication flow.

32. Which of the following medical equipment/devices routinely requires high-level disinfection, such as with chemical sterilants?

a. Surgical instruments
b. Endoscopes
c. Blood pressure cuffs
d. Bedside table

33. When large numbers of staff must be trained in utilizing PPE needed to care for Ebola patients, the best technique may be to:

a. provide one-on-one instruction.
b. provide video instruction.
c. train trainers.
d. present the information in lectures.

34. Daily environmental cleaning of COVID-19 patient rooms includes which of the following protocols?

a. Gloves, gowns, goggles, and surgical masks are to be worn.
b. Disinfectants should be EPA-approved for emerging viral pathogens, including SARS-CoV-2.
c. Trash and soiled linen should be double bagged.
d. Cleaning should be done from dirty to clean, sides to center, high to low, left to right, or clockwise.

35. What is the focus of root cause analysis during an outbreak?

a. Assigning blame
b. Identifying errors in process
c. Promoting prevention efforts
d. Reducing liability

36. If using a bleach solution to disinfect contaminated surfaces and equipment in a dialysis unit, what dilution is recommended?

a. 1:500
b. 1:10
c. 1:1000
d. 1:100

37. One method of applying the social cognitive theory to infection prevention to promote quality improvement is to:

a. ask staff members to teach other staff nurses to properly utilize PPE.
b. ask for input from staff regarding utilization of PPE.
c. convince a critical mass of staff to properly utilize PPE.
d. use peer pressure to force other staff members to properly utilize PPE.

38. A group of staff on one hospital unit cooperated to develop a plan to implement preventive strategies, resulting in a 50% decline in SSI with subsequent adoption of these strategies by other units. This is an example of:

a. social support system.
b. positive deviance.
c. modeling.
d. mentoring.

39. When choosing events to monitor for a surveillance program, which of the following will be most important for assessing the data?

a. Time periods selected for surveillance
b. Units selected for surveillance
c. Type of reports generated
d. Availability of benchmark data

40. What is the governmental agency whose mission is to improve the quality of medical care through outcomes research and development of clinical guidelines?

a. AHRQ
b. CMS
c. FDA
d. HRSA

41. When conducting a product evaluation, goals for the product should include which of the following?

I. Meeting specific clinical and financial performance criteria
II. Meeting safety requirements
III. Contributing to positive patient outcomes
IV. Supporting staff preferences

a. I and II only
b. I, II and IV only
c. I, II, and III only
d. I, II, III, and IV

42. A nurse who reports for work with a fever and cough, obviously ill, should be:

a. advised to avoid direct patient contact.
b. excluded from work.
c. provided medication to control symptoms.
d. advised to use a mask while caring for patients.

43. In a 90-day period in the ED, there were 308 cases of COVID-19 diagnosed: 112 were female and 196 were male. What is the ratio of female to male cases?

a. 2:3
b. 4:7
c. 5:7
d. 3:4

44. A patient who meets surveillance criteria for a CLABSI but does not meet the clinical diagnostic criteria for treating a CLABSI should be:

a. excluded from surveillance data.
b. re-evaluated to determine if the surveillance data are correct.
c. included as a CLABSI for surveillance data.
d. re-assigned the appropriate clinical diagnosis of CLABSI.

45. Sources of surveillance data can include which of the following?

I. Observations of staff members providing care
II. Pharmacy-generated list of medications prescribed
III. Facility-wide lists of patients on isolation precautions
IV. Incident reports

a. II and III only
b. I, II, and III only
c. II, III, and IV only
d. I, II, III, and IV

46. Fecal microbiota transplant may be indicated for which of the following diarrhea-associated infections?

a. *Escherichia coli*
b. *Clostridium difficile*
c. Norovirus
d. *Staphylococcus aureus*

47. A 340-bed acute hospital averaged a census of 300 patients per month. If 117 patients developed urinary tract infections in a one-year period, what is the annual incidence of UTIs per 1000 patients?

a. 39
b. 390
c. 325
d. 32.5

48. Which of the following procedures is excluded from SIR?

I. Procedure shorter than 5 minutes
II. Procedure longer than 250 minutes
III. Procedure with patient's age older than 109
IV. Procedure with wound class of "U"

a. I and II only
b. II, III, and IV only
c. I, III, and IV only
d. I, II, III, and IV

49. If 10 CLABSI infections occurred out of 3840 CL days, and the expected number of infections is 7.5, the SIR is:

a. 1.33
b. 0.133
c. 0.750
d. 1.75

50. What are the most common causes of healthcare-associated outbreaks?

I. Lapses in infection prevention practices
II. Contamination or defects in medical products/devices
III. Colonization/infection of healthcare personnel
IV. Intentional acts of carelessness with infection prevention

a. I, II, and III only
b. II, III, and IV only
c. I, III, and IV
d. I, II, III, and IV

51. A woman admitted for an elective Caesarean had some bleeding after surgery and 30 hours post-op developed a high fever of unknown origin and died within 6 hours. This case would be primarily classified as:

a. negative outcome.
b. adverse event.
c. complication.
d. sentinel event.

52. An increase in the number of positive microbiological cultures in the absence of clinical disease is classified as a(n):

a. aberration.
b. pseudo-outbreak.
c. outbreak.
d. cluster.

53. In an outbreak in which the case definition is primarily clinical, the most valuable resource is likely:

a. healthcare provider reports.
b. laboratory records.
c. pharmacy records.
d. census records.

54. The method of surveillance that is likely to provide the most useful information is:

a. whole-house surveillance.
b. targeted surveillance focused on defined populations.
c. combined whole house and targeted surveillance.
d. targeted surveillance focused on randomly-selected units.

55. The most important element for creating an epidemic curve during a hospital outbreak is the:

a. observations of patient care.
b. case definition.
c. methodology.
d. line list.

56. In which of the following outbreaks may community media publicity most aid in case finding?

a. *E. coli* infections linked to packaged produce
b. *P. aeruginosa* infections linked to hydrotherapy
c. AIDS infections linked to injection drug use
d. *Staphylococcus aureus* infections linked to contaminated surgical equipment

57. Which of the following are important practices in environmental sampling?

I. Sample all patient areas, including contact surfaces
II. Obtain guidelines from the microbiologic lab
III. Sample only environmental items that are suspected vectors
IV. Base environmental samples on type of organism

a. I, II, and IV only
b. I, II, and III only
c. II, III, and IV only
d. I, II, III, and IV

58. According to the second IOM report, *Crossing the Quality Chasm: A New Health System for the 21st Century,* the primary aim of the healthcare system should be on:

a. efficiency.
b. patient safety.
c. equity.
d. effectiveness.

59. If the media in the community have become aware of a hospital outbreak, the best method of dealing with this is to:

a. assign one specific person to communicate with media representatives.
b. deny that there is an outbreak.
c. send out regular printed updates.
d. ask risk management to limit media access.

60. An epidemic curve that approximates a normal distribution (Bell curve) most often results from:

a. propagated source, continuous exposure.
b. propagated source, intermittent exposure.
c. common source, intermittent exposure.
d. common source, point exposure.

61. A 45-year-old female with Guillain-Barré syndrome developed ventilation-associated pneumonia 4 days after being placed on mechanical ventilation. Which of the following is the dependent variable?

a. Guillain-Barré syndrome
b. Ventilator-associated pneumonia
c. Mechanical ventilation
d. 45-year-old female

62. The ASA rating scale is an example of which type of scale of measurement?

a. Ordinal scale
b. Nominal scale
c. Interval scale
d. Ratio

63. If the lengths of stay of 10 patients in days were 1, 29, 4, 3, 2, 4, 1, 3, 1, and 2, which measure of central tendency provides the most useful information about lengths of stay?

a. Mean
b. Mode
c. Median
d. Information is not adequate

64. In a normal distribution curve, what percentage of results should be within the first standard deviation above and below the mean?

a. 32%
b. 50%
c. 68%
d. 75%

65. If there are 25 patients with urinary catheters on a unit in a one-month period and 5 patients develop CAUTI, what is the incidence rate of CAUTI per 100 patients with urinary catheters?

a. 5
b. 8
c. 10
d. 20

66. In working with the public health department to determine if people who are HIV positive disclose this information to sexual partners, the BEST research techniques include which of the following?

I. Interviews
II. Surveys
III. Participant observations
IV. Focus groups

a. I and II only
b. I and III only
c. I, II, and III only
d. I, II, III, and IV

67. In 200 operations, the surgical staff used the surgical checklist 160 times, failing to use it 40 times. What is the projected compliance rate per 1000 operations?

a. 80
b. 800
c. 200
d. 250

68. What is the best method of reducing a type II error, accepting a null hypothesis that is incorrect?

a. Decrease sample size
b. Increase sample size
c. Increase length of rejection area
d. Decrease length of rejection area

69. What confidence interval should a researcher select to ensure that results did not occur by chance?

a. 75%
b. 80%
c. 95%
d. 100%

70. Which type of graphic display is most appropriate for communicating continuous data?

a. Pie chart
b. Bar chart
c. Scatter plot
d. Histogram

71. After determining that data collection is necessary for surveillance, the first step should be to determine:

a. who may already have the data.
b. who will review the data.
c. what resources are needed to collect the data.
d. how quickly the data can be collected.

72. Which type of epidemiological study best assesses outcomes and potential risk factors in a group at one point in time?

a. Case control
b. Cross-sectional
c. Cohort
d. Clinical trial

73. The infection preventionist (IP) knows that the organism most commonly implicated in osteomyelitis is:

a. *Pseudomonas* sp.
b. *Klebsiella* sp.
c. *Staphylococcus aureus.*
d. coagulase-negative Staphylococci.

74. Cloudy cerebrospinal fluid most likely indicates:

a. parasitic infection.
b. viral infection.
c. fungal infection.
d. bacterial infection.

75. Immunocompromised patients at risk of *Pneumocystis jiroveci* infection, such as patients with HIV/AIDS, should receive antibiotic prophylaxis with:

a. vancomycin.
b. trimethoprim-sulfamethoxazole.
c. ampicillin.
d. cephalexin.

76. Dietary restrictions that are recommended by the CDC, HHS, and USDA for neutropenic patients to prevent infection include which of the following measures?

I. Eat only cooked foods, no raw fruits or vegetables
II. Avoid raw raspberries and strawberries
III. Use only pasteurized dairy products
IV. Reheat deli meats to steaming hot before eating

a. II, III, and IV only
b. I, II, and III only
c. III, and IV only
d. I, II, III, and IV

77. A nurse has added both piperacillin/tazobactam and an aminoglycoside to the same IV infusion. This practice:

a. ensures broad-spectrum coverage.
b. follows standard protocol.
c. causes crystals to form.
d. inactivates both agents.

78. Resistance develops in microorganisms because of which of the following?

I. Point mutations
II. Cell disintegration
III. New genes
IV. Antibody failure

a. I and II only
b. I and III only
c. II and IV only
d. I, II, III, and IV

79. The CDC-recommended method of routine hand hygiene is now:

a. wearing gloves.
b. washing with soap and water.
c. using alcohol-based hand rubs.
d. using chlorhexidine scrubs.

80. In order to protect the eyes from respiratory secretions, blood, or other body fluids, which of the following PPE is adequate?

I. Face shields
II. Contact lenses
III. Eye glasses
IV. Goggles

a. I and IV only
b. I, III, and IV only
c. I, II, and IV only
d. I, II, III, and IV

81. When using steam sterilization, the sterilization process should take approximately:

a. 4 hours.
b. 60 minutes.
c. 40 minutes.
d. 2 hours.

82. Older adults who had varicella (chickenpox) as children should be advised that:

a. that have immunity to chicken pox.
b. chicken pox may recur.
c. they should have the varicella vaccination.
d. they should have herpes zoster immunization.

83. A healthcare provider who has long artificial nails should be advised that the nails increase the risk of:

a. transmission of Gram-negative and fungal organisms.
b. transmission of viral organisms.
c. personal injury.
d. no appreciable risk of transmission.

84. In order to prevent BSIs in the NICU, the CDC recommends skin antisepsis for vascular access with:

a. hydrogen peroxide.
b. isopropyl alcohol, 70 to 90%.
c. more than 0.5% chlorhexidine gluconate with alcohol.
d. povidone iodine.

85. If the water supply at a hematopoietic stem cell center is contaminated with *Legionella pneumophila*, what steps are required?

I. Decontaminating water supply
II. Drinking sterilized water
III. Removing plumbing fixtures that aerosolize water
IV. Showering only (not bathing) in contaminated water

a. I and II only
b. I, II, and III only
c. I, II, and IV only
d. I, II, III, and IV

86. In regards to reprocessing of single-use devices, the CMS recommends:

a. no reprocessing.
b. in-house reprocessing.
c. reprocessing of class I devices only.
d. use of third-party reprocessors.

87. When conducting surveillance of an ambulatory care infusion center, one observation is that the nurse has prepared infusates for multiple patients prior to their arrival. The nurse should be advised to:

a. prepare infusates immediately before use only.
b. ensure the infusates are properly labeled.
c. store the infusates in the refrigerator after preparation.
d. prepare infusates no more than two hours prior to administration.

88. What is the maximum humidity level in a cardiac cath lab?

a. 20%
b. 40%
c. 60%
d. 80%

89. A pregnant healthcare worker should be routinely screened for which of the following conditions?

a. Hepatitis C virus
b. HIV
c. Hepatitis A virus
d. Cytomegalovirus

90. An outbreak of norovirus has occurred at four daycare centers in the community. In determining the cause of the outbreak, the initial focus should be on:

a. ventilation system and air quality.
b. water system and water quality.
c. food preparation practices and environment.
d. changing tables and hand hygiene.

91. The immunization that is recommended for healthcare workers with occupational exposure to blood, blood products, or bodily secretions is:

a. hepatitis B.
b. hepatitis A.
c. hepatitis C.
d. no specific immunization.

92. When carrying out tuberculosis skin testing for long-term care residents, what extent of induration is generally considered positive?

a. 2 mm
b. 5 mm
c. 10 mm
d. 15 mm

93. The incubation period for foodborne illness caused by *Salmonella* spp. is:

a. 1 to 6 hours.
b. 1 to 3 days.
c. 12 to 48 hours.
d. 28 days.

94. If power is interrupted to the operating rooms during construction, what precaution is necessary prior to putting the HVAC system back into service?

a. No precaution necessary
b. Increased number of air exchanges to the operating rooms
c. Resuming at low activity times
d. Running the HVAC system for a period of time to flush the ducts

95. When using alcohol-based surgical hand scrub products for surgical hand antisepsis, the first step is to:

a. prewash hands and forearms with non-antimicrobial soap and water and dry.
b. prewash hands and forearms with antimicrobial soap and water and dry.
c. apply the alcohol solution and use according to manufacturer's directions.
d. scrub hands and forearms for 10 minutes with antimicrobial or non-antimicrobial soap and water and dry.

96. Which maternal host facts increase the risk of a healthcare-associated perinatal infection in both the infant and mother?

I. Immunosuppression with corticosteroids
II. BMI greater than 24
III. Low economic status
IV. Ruptured membranes

a. I and II only
b. I, II, and IV only
c. I, III, and IV only
d. I, II, III, and IV

97. According to the World Health Organization, which of the following occurs during phase 5 of the six phases of a pandemic?

a. Higher risk of human cases
b. Evidence of significant human-to-human transmission
c. Evidence of increased human-to-human transmission
d. Limited human-to-human transmission

98. The purpose of BioWatch is to collect:

a. blood samples from migratory animals to test for prion disease.
b. water samples to test for waterborne biological agents.
c. soil samples to test for environmental toxins.
d. air samples to test for aerosolized biological agents.

99. The four phases of a disaster with mass casualties include:

a. preparedness, event, interventions, aftermath.
b. preparedness, impact, response, recovery.
c. mitigation, preparedness, reaction, recovery.
d. preparedness, event, reaction, response.

100. Nonbullous impetigo is typically associated with:

a. *Staphylococcus aureus.*
b. *Pseudomonas aeruginosa.*
c. group A streptococci.
d. *Staphylococcus pyogenes.*

101. Which of the following statements regarding *Clostridium difficile* spores is NOT true?

a. Hand washing is the most effective method to prevent *C. difficile* transmission
b. Spores are noninfectious forms of the organism
c. Ingestion triggers spore activation to their disease-causing form
d. Spores can be recovered from computer keyboards and window coverings

102. Which of the following is the TRUE statement regarding enterococcal infections in the United States?

a. Most human enterococcal infections are due to Enterococcus avium
b. Enterococci are normal inhabitants of the gastrointestinal tract
c. Enterococci rarely show resistance to vancomycin
d. Gram stain typically reveals gram-negative diplococci in short chains

103. Which of the following pathogens is the LEAST likely to be associated with nosocomial wound infections?

a. *Escherichia coli*
b. *Staphylococcus aureus*
c. Coagulase-negative staphylococci
d. *Bacteroides fragilis*

104. A hospital's infection control nurse reported postsurgical wound infections by classification in a group of patients. Which was classified correctly as clean-contaminated (class II)?

a. Closed reduction of Colles fracture in 74-year-old woman
b. Emergency appendectomy and abscess evacuation in febrile 18-year-old man
c. Elective thoracotomy with right upper lobectomy in 52-year-old smoker
d. Stab wound to abdomen with intestinal perforation in 25-year-old man

105. A comparison of the incidence of lung cancer in a population of smokers compared with the incidence in a nonsmoking population defines which statistical term?

a. Relative risk
b. Incidental risk
c. Disease prevalence
d. Disease incidence

106. A large community hospital's tumor registry reports a marked decrease in cases of hepatocellular carcinoma over a 20-year period. Which of the following is LEAST likely to account for this occurrence?

a. Improved serologic screening of transfusion donors
b. Higher vaccination rates for hepatitis A
c. Higher community vaccination rates for hepatitis B
d. Decreased prevalence of seropositivity for hepatitis C over same period

107. Match the following elements of outbreak case definitions with the appropriate examples:

1) Person
2) Place
3) Time
4) Clinical features
5) Laboratory features

a. Onset during winter months December through March, 2008
b. Sputum positive for acid-fast bacilli
c. Day-shift medical technologists at tertiary-care hospital
d. Allcare Rehabilitation, Yuma, Arizona
e. Morbilliform rash

108. World Health Organization 2009 published guidelines for hand hygiene include all of the following EXCEPT:

a. after cleansing and rinsing, use a towel to turn off spigot and do not re-use.
b. use of warm or hot water for rinsing to kill off any remaining bacteria.
c. hand hygiene is needed after removing gloves used for wound dressings.
d. use of soap and water if alcohol-based hand rubs are not available.

109. What percentage of nosocomial infections is believed to be caused by bacterial contamination carried by hands of caregivers and health care workers?

a. 50%
b. 33%
c. 25%
d. 15%

110. An intensive care unit (ICU) patient in a metropolitan hospital is diagnosed with culture-positive non-acid-fast multidrug resistant bacteria (MDR). This occurs 1 week after admission to the same ICU of a homeless 46-year-old man with pneumonia and underlying COPD who was also diagnosed with MDR. Infection control surveillance should include all of the following EXCEPT:

a. masks for patient and all caregivers.
b. strict handwashing precautions.
c. decontamination procedures for all portable chest radiography.
d. surface culture samples of shared diagnostic or invasive equipment.

111. A pathogen that appears to be transmitted by airborne spread is suspected in an outbreak affecting a heavily ethnic section of a metropolitan area. Important initial public communications strategies should include:

a. early announcements with tempered reassurances.
b. delayed announcements until all information is gathered.
c. adherence to the "decide and announce" model.
d. disregard for culturally based interpretations in favor of rational explanations.

112. Proper transport protocol for blood samples drawn from an acutely ill homosexual man admitted with to the ICU with acute pneumonia and unknown serologic status for HIV requires:

a. single-compartment waterproof packaging with surrounding absorbent material.
b. double-layer waterproof packaging, absorbent material.
c. double-layer waterproof packaging, absorbent material, and appropriate documentation.
d. double-layer waterproof packaging, absorbent material, and appropriate documentation enclosed by outer packaging.

113. Infectivity risks for transmission of HIV from patients to health care workers:

a. are highest with encounters involving needles and sharps.
b. occur at about the same rate as transmission of hepatitis b given similar direct exposures.
c. are often associated with asymptomatic carriers of HIV.
d. A and C only

114. Identification of *Bacillus anthracis*:

a. shows Gram-positive diplococci in short chains.
b. shows Gram-negative diplococci in short chains.
c. shows G ram-positive nonmotile rods.
d. requires immediate quarantine precautions of index case.

115. Diseases caused by arboviruses:

a. are only associated with overt clinical symptoms and syndromes in humans.
b. include dengue and yellow fever.
c. typically involve high rates of human-to-human transmission.
d. are more frequent in winter in the United States.

116. With regard to communicable diseases, the term contamination:

a. always implies a carrier state.
b. includes noninfectious environmental pollutants.
c. describes infectious particles on body surfaces and inanimate objects.
d. does not apply to infectious agents in foods and liquids.

Questions 117 through 119 pertain to the following clinical case:

An athletic 32-year-old man is admitted with fever and convulsive episodes that have rendered him comatose. History obtained from his wife includes a prodrome of headaches and hydrophobia. She recalls he had complained about tingling around an area that had been affected by a small right shoulder wound a couple of weeks ago. She says that he had otherwise been well since his return from China 1 month ago on an adventure vacation that included visits to bat-infested caves and rural farms. She reports they have a cat and two dogs at home, all in usual apparent health. Routine blood and cerebrospinal fluid have been drawn for cell counts, cultures, and any ancillary testing.

117. Diagnostic work-up should also immediately prioritize:

a. saliva or skin testing for rabies virus nucleic acid amplification by reverse transcriptase polymerase chain reaction (RT-PCR).
b. brain biopsy to submit tissue for mouse cell culture at reference laboratory.
c. brain biopsy to identify toxoplasma cysts.
d. blood and CSF culture for rabies using vitamin-enhanced media

118. The incubation period for the primary diagnosis under consideration:

a. is within a week following ingestion of undercooked, infected meat.
b. is highly variable but often occurs within 3 to 8 weeks after exposure.
c. does not appear to be related to location of wound or protective clothing.
d. has a typical duration of 1 to 3 days.

119. Appropriate infection control measures should include:

a. quarantine of index case.
b. formal report to local health authorities.
c. post-exposure prophylaxis of intimate, mucous-membrane contacts with immune globulin.
d. B and C.

120. A male health care worker from the Philippines who is applying for a surgery scrub tech position tests positive for hepatitis B surface antibody, negative for hepatitis B e antigen (HBeAg), and negative for hepatitis B surface antigen (HBsAg). Which is the best interpretation or recommendation in light of these findings?

a. He is likely immunized to hepatitis B by prior vaccination
b. He is likely to have chronic hepatitis B infection
c. He is likely to be a carrier and should not be offered the surgical suite position
d. He is likely to be highly infectious and should receive hepatitis B immune globulin

121. Which of the following statements regarding normal flora in humans is NOT true?

a. Normal flora may be further classified into resident and transient flora
b. By definition, colonization by normal flora does not result in infection
c. Normal flora contains commensal microbes that are neither harmful nor beneficial to the host
d. Normal flora may participate in nutrient synthesis or excretion

122. Preliminary throat cultures from an 83-year-old nursing home resident are reported to you as "positive for beta-hemolytic streptococci." You are aware of two other residents of the same nursing home with new-onset fever and exudative pharyngitis this week. Initial surveillance and investigation entails all of the following EXCEPT:

a. immunization of visitors and health care personnel in contact with index cases.
b. ensure rapid antigen detection methods are available and properly used and reported by nursing home personnel.
c. isolation of index cases with staff education and implementation of precautions involving secretions and drainage.
d. investigate possible outbreak sources from possible contacts, carriers, and food contamination (milk, milk products).

123. Which of the following characterizes syndromic surveillance methodology in outbreak detection?

a. Low sensitivity and high specificity of case definitions
b. Rapid detection of outbreaks based on clinical diagnoses evidenced by laboratory findings
c. Fixed parameters of suspect case definitions over time
d. Employs broad general descriptive terms (e.g., influenza-like symptoms) and short-term statistical analysis

124. The incubation period of a transmissible disease:

a. is the time period between invasion by a pathogenic microbe and initial signs of altered tissue status or infection onset.
b. is not defined for situations in which the host organism is a vector.
c. occurs between a narrow window of days to weeks.
d. is independent of variations in host resistance and environmental factors.

Categorize the following uses of antimicrobials using the three patient scenarios below, in the order given below to answer Question 125:

Patient A is brought to the surgical suite for elective hip replacement surgery is administered an anti-infective agent active against skin flora.
Patient B begins oral antimalarials prior to travel to an endemic area.
Patient C is a kidney-transplant recipient admitted for suspected rejection. An antifungal is ordered for oral thrush noted on initial exam.

125. The categorization of the uses of antimicrobials using the three patient scenarios above in the order given above are:

a. empiric, prophylactic, and therapeutic.
b. prophylactic, empiric, and therapeutic.
c. therapeutic, empiric, and prophylactic.
d. prophylactic, prophylactic, and therapeutic.

126. Nosocomial infections include all of the following EXCEPT:

a. postsurgical wound infection identified in outpatient suture clinic 1 week following hospital discharge.
b. neonatal herpes diagnosed in newborn infant vaginally delivered from HSV-infected mother.
c. congenital malformations in newborn with positive IgM titer for rubella.
d. diagnosis of nosocomial infection made by attending surgeon.

127. A new infection control nurse seeks to revamp the infection surveillance system of a 125-patient bed community hospital. The hospital information system's (HIS) technology is old yet is highly utilized by medical staff and health care personnel. Which assessment is most accurate?

a. Passive surveillance that relies upon reporting by health care personnel and laboratory data is likely to capture and correctly classify most data
b. Active surveillance is likely to be more expensive and require more manpower but is likely to yield accurate and more comprehensive data
c. Laboratory-based plans are likely to succeed in an acceptable HIS setting, regardless of whether specific disease-monitoring protocols are in place
d. Patient-based plans should prove more time-efficient and cost-effective compared with laboratory-based plans

128. All of the following statements regarding post discharge surveillance of hospitalized patients are true EXCEPT:

a. most hospitals follow standardized post discharge surveillance guidelines.
b. decreased length of stay impedes capture of postsurgical wound infection rates.
c. telephone interviews or mailed questionnaires are two methods that can be successfully employed.
d. post discharge follow-up via physician office records may be incomplete or not timely.

129. The T-point classification system:

a. is one method of assessing risk of postoperative infection in surgical patients.
b. examines multiple variables used in assessing risk of surgical infection.
c. assigns a percentile time score based on average hours a surgical procedure is performed at the index hospital.
d. indicates a lower risk for infection when t points are exceeded.

130. The 0- to 3-point scoring system using the NNIS Risk Index:

a. assigns a score of -1 (minus 1) for no risk factors
b. assigns 1 point for clean-contaminated surgical cases.
c. assigns 2 points for exceeding a surgical procedure's t point.
d. assigns 1 point for preoperative American Society of Anesthesiologists (ASA) scores of 3 to 5.

Answer questions 131 and 132 based on the following information:

A hospital seeks to assess its overall central line infection rate. You are asked to report overall infection rates using device days based on the following data obtained:

Service	# of Patients	Total # Device Days	Total #Infections
Medical intensive care unit	12	48	2
Surgical intensive care unit	9	20	1
Oncology ward	15	72	4

131. Based on these data, the overall hospital central line infection rate per 1,000 device days is:

a. 5.
b. 7.
c. 50.
d. 257.

132. Based on device days, the service with the highest infection rate is:

a. medical intensive care unit.
b. surgical intensive care unit.
c. surgical intensive care unit, but not statistically significant.
d. oncology ward.

133. Which of the following data sets is MOST likely to meet statistical significance?

a. P value < 0.05 in study of 7 patients with uncomplicated seasonal influenza
b. P value < 0.05 in study of 100 patients with complicated seasonal influenza
c. P value > 0.05 in study of 1,000 patients with complicated seasonal influenza
d. P value > 0.05 in study of 2,000 patients with uncomplicated seasonal influenza

134. Agents and methods used to sterilize or disinfect are segregated into three tiers. Which of the following statement is NOT accurate regarding these categories?

a. Low-level agents, such as iodophors, kill most bacteria and fungi, but not viruses
b. Alcohol is an intermediate disinfectant that does not kill or inactivate spores
c. Hydrogen peroxide is an example of a high-level disinfectant
d. High disinfectants may not eradicate high concentrations of bacterial spores

135. Methods of flash sterilization:

a. employ temperatures of at least 132 °C for 10 minutes or less.
b. are not recommended for surgical equipment meant for re-use.
c. involves dry heat using oven-type equipment for as long as needed.
d. will not kill vegetative organisms or viruses, even when items are precleaned.

136. Decubiti in spinal cord injury patients:

a. are not commonly associated with spread of infection to nearby bone.
b. typically show single, dominant organisms on culture.
c. occur in about two-thirds of patients with such neurologic injuries.
d. are related to pressure and contamination.

137. Which of the following actions is NOT considered an effective infection control strategy in surgical environments?

a. Preferential use of flash sterilization
b. 15 or more air exchanges hourly
c. Hallways and nearby areas ventilated with positive pressure
d. Wet-vacuum mechanical cleaning of surgical suites at end of day

138. The role of nutritional services in a hospital's overall infection control program:

a. necessitates use of disposable materials, such as paper napkins, plates, and utensils.
b. requires delivery staff to move items such as bedpans aside so food tray can be deposited.
c. requires health care personnel to deliver trays to patients on airborne precautions.
d. includes removal of food trays contaminated by body fluids provided nutritional orderly cleanses area immediately.

139. In order to comply with the Safe Medical Devices Act of 1990, medical facilities that use medical devices associated with complications such as injury or death:

a. must report incidents requiring medical or surgical intervention within 48 hours.
b. must file semiannual and annual medical device reporting (MDR).
c. may use MedWatch forms as needed without need for written procedures.
d. must retain records related to medical device reports for 10 years.

140. While assisting in paracentesis of a patient with chronic liver failure, an emergency department nurse's aide reports a splash incident and claims he felt a drop of ascitic fluid hit his eye. According to required elements in the hospital's exposure control plan, which of the following steps must be followed?

a. Immediate post-exposure prophylaxis with hepatitis B immune globulin (HBIG)
b. Identify staff member and exposure incident to rest of hospital staff
c. Cease all paracentesis procedures in ED until investigation is complete
d. Review OSHA standards for procedure and document event compliance

141. An announcement in the hospital newsletter about a hand washing contest that involves a special glow-in-the-dark powder is MOST likely:

a. a hands-on method of promoting infection control practices to staff.
b. a waste of valuable health care worker time.
c. an educational opportunity that will only benefit students.
d. less effective than posters that show proper hand washing technique.

142. An infection control program's annual summary:

a. does not need to be filed if no incidents occurred.
b. is a document whose purpose is to summarize occupational exposures.
c. is a budgetary document used to determine cost-benefit ratios.
d. documents adherence to infection control program's goals specific to outcomes and objectives.

143. As the first dedicated infection control officer hired at a new hospital, what initial assessments should you make in designing your institution's infection control plan?

a. Determine patient population, institutional size, services, and departments
b. Request funding to hire IT consultants to upgrade hardware and software
c. Develop 30-day client satisfaction survey regarding infection control plan
d. Perform cost-benefit analysis of most frequently performed procedures

144. CDC recommendations regarding appropriate nail care for health care personnel whose duties include direct patient care or contact with food and supplies include:

a. maintaining nails to no longer than one-quarter inch length.
b. routine cultures of subungual areas of artificial nails or nail tip.
c. allowance of artificial nails or tips of any length with fresh polish applied daily.
d. routine use of double-thickness gloves for artificial-nail wearers.

145. The power to issue recalls and regulations regarding reuse issues involving medications and medical devices is held by the:

a. Occupational Safety and Health Administration.
b. The Joint Commission.
c. Food and Drug Administration.
d. Centers for Disease Control and Prevention.

146. The Shewhart cycle refers to:

a. a circular diagram used to analyze cause and effect.
b. a quality management tool for problem-solving.
c. a type of Pareto charting.
d. a schematic flow chart.

147. You are planning to educate a group of ER nurses regarding documentation for central line associated blood stream infections. Your educational planning includes a series of in-service talks with slide show presentations and handouts. To maximize effectiveness:

a. handouts are delivered by the speaker as s/he begins presentation.
b. handouts should be lengthy and use large blocks of text.
c. handouts should be legible copy of slide show presentation.
d. handouts should highlight the presentation's key points.

148. The departments of anesthesiology and surgery seek to work with infection control to increase perioperative antibiotic use within 30 minutes of skin incision. Your approach includes all of the following EXCEPT:

a. calculate compliance as number of surgical procedures divided by number of times antibiotic is given within 30 minutes of incision.
b. identify behaviors that may contribute to delay or omission of delivering antibiotic within 30 minutes of incision.
c. demonstrate appropriate perioperative time management, reinforce correct timing of dose, and monitor until desired behaviors are satisfactorily adopted.
d. use before and after data analysis of surgical infection rates as surrogate or observational marker of compliance.

149. Which of the following recommended procedures regarding pre-employment vetting of health care workers is required by the Joint Commission?

a. Testing for drugs of abuse and background check
b. Tuberculin skin testing (purified protein derivative [PPD])
c. Chest radiograph for positive PPD results
d. Vaccination against hepatitis B for nonimmune candidates

150. Which of the following health care workers who are normally involved in direct patient care should be placed on work restriction?

a. Skin rash following course of amoxicillin for otitis media
b. Latex glove skin allergy by history with no active lesions
c. Small finger lesion consistent with herpetic whitlow
d. New-onset nonproductive cough in nurse on ACE inhibitor antihypertensive

Answer Key and Explanations

1. D: When a patient is on contact precautions, especially for organisms such as MR*SA* or *C. difficile,* which can result in extensive environmental contamination, the healthcare provider should wear gown and gloves whenever entering the room because the disease may be transmitted either through direct contact with the patient or the patient's environment. If there are two patients as cohorts in the same room, then the healthcare provider must change the gown and gloves between patients.

2. C: A broad-spectrum antibiotic is usually administered for empirical therapy because the pathogenic organism is not yet identified. Often patients who have acute symptoms of infection may require treatment before culture and sensitivity results; therefore, a broad-spectrum antibiotic is usually the choice for empirical therapy in order to cover as many potential causative agents as possible. The choice of antibiotic for empirical treatment should be based on clinical symptoms and site of infection.

3. B: Medical intervention factors that affect risk of infection include indwelling devices, staffing ratio, and lengths of stay as well as type and duration of invasive procedures, medications, stays in critical care or intensive care units, number of examinations by healthcare providers, type of institution, and knowledge and experience of healthcare providers. Other factors to consider include environmental factors (including type of disinfectant used, contact with animals, compliance with hand hygiene) and anatomic/physiologic factors (including preexisting diseases, trauma, malignancies, age, gender, and nutritional status).

4. A: The prevalence rate is the number of events divided by the population. To find the prevalence rate of CLABSI per 1000 in this patient population, use the following formula:

$$\frac{\text{number of patients with CLABSI}}{\text{total patient population}} = \frac{x}{1000}$$

Plugging in the numbers given in the question yields the following equation:

$$\frac{8}{600} = \frac{x}{1000}$$

The equation can then be rearranged and solved for x as follows:

$$x = \frac{8000}{600}$$

$$x = \frac{40}{3} = 13.3$$

Thus, the prevalence rate of CLABSI in this patient population was 13.3 per 1000.

5. D: The data used to create an affinity diagram is usually collected through brainstorming. The affinity diagram utilizes language data (ideas, suggestions). Typically, participants place suggestions or ideas on sticky notes and attach them to a board. The data are then grouped according to relationships, so that categories begin to emerge. For example, one category may be suggestions for improvement and another obstacle to improvement. Redundancies can be eliminated, as there may be many repetitions.

6. C: In the Six Sigma DMAIC format, the *D* represents *define:*

- **D**: Define customers, project boundaries, and processes.
- **M**: Measure performance by developing a data collection plan and collecting data.
- **A**: Analyze data to identify causes of variation, gaps in performance, and to prioritize actions.
- **I**: Improve the process by developing by creating innovative solutions and implementation strategies.
- **C**: Control the process to prevent reverting to previous model and to document a monitoring plan.

7. A: While cost saving is always a concern for a facility, it is not a primary consideration in evaluation of a surveillance program. An effective surveillance program should be able to detect infections and injuries, identify trends, identify risk factors associated with infections or other adverse events, detect outbreaks and clusters, assess the overall effectiveness of the infection control and prevention program, and demonstrate changes in practices and procedures that lead to better outcomes for patients.

8. B: When calculating rates of CAUTI on a unit in a six-month period, the denominator must include only those at risk. In this case, the denominator would include all patients with urinary catheters and exclude all others. The numerator is the number of events or CAUTIs that occurred. Rates measure the probability of an event (such as a CAUTI) occurring and may be utilized to compare different populations. Rates include incidence, prevalence, point prevalence, and attack.

9. B: If an outbreak of COVID-19 occurred in a group of people who had attended a retreat with a total of 36 participants three weeks earlier, the best method of case finding is to individually contact the 36 participants. When an outbreak can be traced to one location or event and the number of people exposed is known and identified, then contacting and interviewing them about symptoms takes relatively little time and may facilitate identifying the source.

10. D: In order to test for infection with *Clostridium difficile,* a liquid stool specimen is required. A patient should be suspected of *C. difficile* infection with 3 or more unformed or watery stools in a 24-hour period. A number of tests are available. The microorganism may be cultured, but this takes about 7 days. The cell cytotoxicity assay may be done with a stool extract and is specific but less sensitive than culture. Nucleic amplification tests, such as PCR, have high specificity and sensitivity.

11. D: Relative risk indicates the probability that exposure will result in an adverse event (infection, disease) as opposed to those not exposed. In this situation, the risk is immersion hydrotherapy (IH), the control is shower cart hydrotherapy (SCH) and the adverse event is a *P. aeruginosa* infection. The formula:

$$\begin{aligned}\text{relative risk} &= \left(\frac{\text{IH with infection}}{\text{total IH}}\right) \Big/ \left(\frac{\text{SCH with infection}}{\text{total SCH}}\right)\\ &= \left(\frac{6}{30}\right) \Big/ \left(\frac{2}{32}\right)\\ &= 0.2/0.0625\\ &= 3.2\end{aligned}$$

Relative risk: 1.0 indicates no significant association between exposure and adverse event, above 1.0 indicates a positive association (worse outcome), and below 1.0 a negative association (better outcome).

12. A: In a control chart, the central line represents the average of the data points. The x-axis represents the time period used (days, months, years, decades) while the y-axis represents the rate or count and the data points represent the actual values. Additionally, there may an upper control limit, a line representing +3 standard deviations from the mean and a lower control limit, a line representing -3 standard deviations from the mean.

13. B: If you need to determine the actual number of people represented by one side of a ratio when the total number is known, sum the numbers on both sides of the ratio and then divide the total by that sum to determine how many people are represented by each unit in the ratio:

$$3 + 5 = 8$$

$$40 \div 8 = 5$$

Thus, each unit of the ratio represents 5 people. To find the number of females included in the total of 40, multiply the number that represents females in the ratio (3) by 5:

$$3 \times 5 = 15$$

Since a total of 120 cases are expected, with the same ratio of female to male, an equation can be set up to find the number of expected females from the 120 as follows:

$$\frac{40}{120} = \frac{15}{x}$$

$$x = 15 \times \frac{120}{40} = 15 \times 3 = 45$$

Subtract the number of females already infected to determine the number of expected additional female cases:

$$45 - 15 = 30$$

Thus, 30 more female cases are expected.

14. D: While all of these factors are important in ensuring successful antimicrobial therapy, the most important factor is prompt administration of the appropriate antibiotic as delay in treatment may result in infection that is much more difficult to treat. Other factors that are important are host factors, such as immune status and age; and site factors, such as the area of the body involved as some sites, such as heart valves and meninges, respond less effectively to antimicrobial therapy than others.

15. A: Active learning requires participation on the part of the learner so that the learner is thinking and doing as part of the learning process rather than passively receiving information, such as occurs when listening to a lecture, reading a text, or listening to an audiotape. Examples of active learning include debating, producing multimedia presentations, and problem-solving activities. Studies show that learning retention is only 5% from lectures but 90% when students are actively engaged in teaching others.

16. C: The best method to ensure compliance with the regimen for treatment of tuberculosis is utilizing directly-observed therapy (DOT). The CDC recommends this method, and it is increasingly used by health departments because even patients who seem very reliable may forget to take medications or believe it's not necessary. In DOT, a healthcare provider or other designated person watches the patient take the medication each day, with each DOT visit documented. DOT is especially important for drug-resistant TB, patients receiving intermittent therapy, and patients at high risk for noncompliance, such as drug abusers or the homeless.

17. D: Consistency: A number of studies over extended periods of time show the same association even though different research methods are utilized. Temporality: Exposure to the agent that causes the disease must occur prior to onset of the disease. Coherence: The association between the disease and the causative agent must accord with known facts regarding the disease. Strength of association: Those with more exposure to the causative agent should have higher incidence of disease.

18. A: The usual contact time for low-level disinfection of noncritical patient environmental surfaces and equipment is one minute. The CDC recommends this time period, but the EPA requires following of directions on the EPA-approved labels, so some recommend a longer time period, such as 10 minutes. However, since liquid disinfectants typically dry in 72-120 seconds, this would require repeated applications, so the one-minute timeframe is usually followed. The thoroughness of the cleaning is more important than the duration of disinfection.

19. A: Systematic reviews and meta-analysis include review of a wide range of articles related to a specific issue. The first step in conducting a systematic review and meta-analysis is to develop a research question because, without this question, the researcher has no idea how to focus research. Next, a protocol for review methodology should be developed and the literature search begun, selecting studies that address the research question and abstracting data. The last steps are analysis of data and interpretation.

20. B: Skin testing for TB and mammography for breast cancer are examples of secondary prevention. There are 3 main categories of prevention, but some have added a fourth category:

- Primary: Focused on preventing disease altogether, such as through immunizations and wellness programs.
- Secondary: Focused on early identification and treatment of disease in order to prevent increased morbidity/mortality, including smoking and drinking cessation programs.
- Tertiary: Focused on providing optimal health and prevent further progression of the disease after it has occurred, including organ transplantation and rehabilitation services.
- Quaternary: Focused on preventing healthcare-associated complications.

21. D: According to the National Quality Forum's Endorsed Set of Safe Practices, Safe Practice 23, Care of the Ventilated Patient, actions should be taken to prevent ventilator-associated pneumonia, dental complications (chipped teeth, caries), venous thromboembolism, peptic ulcer disease, and pressure sores. Ventilators should be used for the shortest time possible as increased time increases risk of pneumonia. Proper positioning, range of motion exercises, mouth care, and prevention of pressure to bony prominences are essential.

22. A: When installing alcohol-based hand rub dispensers in a 6-foot wide (or greater) hallway for use of staff and visitors, the minimum distance required between dispensers is four feet. Additionally, the volume is limited to 1.2 L in rooms, hallways and areas that open into hallways and 2 L in suites of rooms. If there is carpet, then installing dispensers directly over carpets is allowed only in smoke compartments with fire sprinklers because of the potential for fire.

23. C: The primary limitation of qualitative research is lack of generalizability; however, a positive aspect is that the participants' viewpoints are included. Qualitative research is often used for descriptive and exploratory research, especially if information about a topic is limited. A number of techniques are utilized for qualitative research, including focus groups, participant observation, interviews, and field notes.

24. B: The primary element required for herd immunity is a group with a high proportion of immunity, which can result from both natural immunity and immunizations. If many people are immune, the chain of infection is disrupted so that the pathogenic organisms lack reservoirs in which they can multiply; so eventually the organism no longer poses a threat. Herd immunity has occurred with polio and smallpox because large numbers of the population were immunized.

25. D: The chain of infection begins with the first link, the causative agent:

- Causative agent: bacteria, fungi, viruses, protozoa, parasites (such as helminths), and prions.
- Reservoir: place in which the causative agent is able to survive and sometimes multiply.
- Portal of exit: means of exiting the reservoir, such as the respiratory tract or blood.
- Mode of transmission: means of reaching a host, such as in food, water, blood, droplets.
- Portal of entry: means of entering the host, such as through the skin, mucous membranes, placenta, or blood.
- Susceptible host: host with no or insufficient immunity to causative agent.

26. A: The number of patients who did not respond to the antibiotic treatment can be found by first finding the number who did respond and subtracting that number from the total:

$$82\% \times 200 = 164$$

$$200 - 164 = 36$$

Thus, 36 of the 200 patients did not respond to the antibiotic treatment.

27. C: Natural barriers to disease are those that are innate and include various barriers and defense mechanisms:

- Barrier: Skin and mucous membranes provide mechanical barriers that prevent many organisms from entering the body.
- Transporter: Cilia in the respiratory tract move material into the upper airways where the cough mechanism can expel it.
- Flusher: Tears flush the eyes and urine flushes the genitourinary system.
- Destroyer: Gastric acid destroys or neutralizes many organisms.
- Fortifier: Good nutritional status provides improved immune response.

28. C: As the number of COVID-19 vaccinated individuals increased in the United States, and the rate of infections fell, the CDC issued new guidelines stating that fully vaccinated individuals could resume normal activities without the need to wear a mask except where mandated (such as for public transportation, and where required by state law or local regulations). The CDC continued to require masks in the healthcare facilities at all times, for patients, visitors, and employees, regardless of vaccination status.

29. A: The crude mortality rate is the number of deaths from any causes in a specified population divided by the total population. The rate per 1000 is found using this formula:

$$\frac{\text{total deaths}}{\text{total population}} = \frac{x}{1000}$$

Plugging in the numbers given in the question yields the following equation:

$$\frac{1125}{150{,}000} = \frac{x}{1000}$$

The equation can then be rearranged and solved for x as follows:

$$x = 1000 \times \frac{1125}{150{,}000}$$

$$x = \frac{1125}{150} = 7.5$$

Thus, there were 7.5 deaths per 1000.

30. A: The Joint Commission requires that facilities that want to reuse single-use medical devices have a written policy and procedures regarding reuse in place as well as a plan for reprocessing, which is often done by third-party reprocessing companies. The primary impetus for reprocessing is cost savings, but most facilities lack the equipment needed for reprocessing. The FDA provides a list of licensed reprocessors. Once a hospital authorizes reprocessing of a device, the hospital is considered the manufacturer and assumes liability if adverse events occur.

31. D: The purpose of network mapping is to show relationships and communication flow. Network maps are created by asking participants (such as staff members on a unit) questions about whom they interact with. The network map may focus on a particular process with a beginning question about whom staff members worked with initially and then since that time. To build the map, the next questions may ask about others from whom the staff members received ideas, what projects the others were working on, and whom the staff members would like to work with in the future.

32. B: High-level disinfection, which destroys all microorganisms except for high levels of bacterial spores, is required for heat-sensitive semi-critical items, such as endoscopes of all kinds, respiratory therapy equipment, and endocavitary probes. Methods of high-level disinfection include heat-automated pasteurization and liquid immersion in chemical sterilants. Time needed for high-level disinfection ranges from 10 to 90 minutes, depending on the type of sterilant used or the combination. For example, 3.4% glutaraldehyde with 26% isopropanol requires 10 minutes and 2% glutaraldehyde requires 90 minutes.

33. C: When training needs require one-on-one instruction, but there are large numbers of staff that need trained, then the best solution is often to train trainers so that they can take over some of the instruction or assist with instruction. Because proper use of PPE when caring for Ebola patients is critical to the safety of the healthcare workers, lecture and video instruction are not adequate because someone needs to observe the staff members as they practice and ensure that they complete each step.

34. A: Daily environmental cleaning of COVID-19 patient rooms requires the following: PPE (N95 [not a surgical mask], gown, gloves, shield, or goggles) must be worn during cleaning. Disinfectants should be EPA-approved for emerging viral pathogens, including SARS-CoV-2. All surfaces and dedicated equipment in the room and bathroom must be wiped clean and disinfectants left in place or wet for required time. Cleaning should be done from dirty to clean, sides to center, high to low, left to right, or clockwise. Trash and linen must be double bagged.

35. B: While a root cause analysis may indicate the cause of an outbreak, the purpose is not to assign blame but to identify errors in process that led to the outbreak, such as failure to use proper hand hygiene, so that proactive steps can be taken to reduce risk. RCA is a retrospective analysis that may include interview, surveys, reviews of medical records, and observations. The Ishikawa (fishbone) diagram is frequently used as a tool for analysis of the data.

36. D: If using a bleach solution to disinfection contaminated surfaces and equipment in a dialysis unit (after first cleaning them of residue), the recommended bleach dilution is 1:100. Other options for disinfection include an EPA-approved disinfectant with tuberculocidal properties or EPA-registered disinfectant effective against HBV and HIV. Disposable items that are contaminated with blood or peritoneal fluid should be disposed of according to federal and state requirements, which may vary somewhat from one state to another.

37. C: One method of applying the social cognitive theory to infection prevention to promote quality improvement is to convince a critical mass of staff to properly utilize PPE. The social cognitive theory is based on the interaction of the individual, the person's behavior, and the environment. When a critical mass—a sufficient number to constitute a noticeable group—of staff persons act in a particular way, the environment changes, and others are more likely to carry out similar behaviors.

38. B: Positive deviance is a behavioral approach to change that is based on the fact that some individuals or groups develop methods that results in better outcomes than others and that others can learn from these deviations. Positive deviance is based on four steps:

1. Define the problem.
2. Determine the presence of positive deviance.
3. Discover the practices or behaviors the deviants use.
4. Design a program based on those practices.

When another unit utilizes the practices developed by the group exhibiting positive deviance, this is referred to as "scaling up."

39. D: When assessing data from a surveillance program, the availability of benchmark data, such as that provided by NHSN, is especially important as it allows comparisons with national rates. Systems for benchmarking have been developed for a number of different types of healthcare facilities and setting, including acute hospitals, hemodialysis units/centers, home health care, long-term care, and ambulatory/outpatient surgery. Using benchmark data from NHSN allows an organization to utilize z-tests and SIR to compare rates.

40. A: The Agency for Healthcare Research and Quality (AHRQ) has the mission to improve the quality of medical care through outcomes research and development of clinical guidelines. AHRQ coordinates federal quality improvement initiatives and aims to make healthcare safer and more accessible and affordable. AHRQ sends email updates to those who register regarding patient safety, quality improvement, and national healthcare quality and disparities. Additionally, AHRQ provides research tools and data, funding and grants, and information for consumers and professionals.

41. C: A product evaluation is conducted when a need is identified. When conducting a product evaluation, the committee members should avoid being biased toward staff preferences but should consider more important factors, including ensuring that the product meets specific clinical and financial performance criteria, that it meets safety requirements, that it contributes to positive patient outcomes, and that it is cost effective, not only from the perspective of the facility but also from the patients' perspective.

42. B: Although staff members frequently report to work when ill because of lack of sick time, concern about job security, or inadequate staffing, doing so puts both patients, who are especially vulnerable, and other staff members at risk for infection; so the person who is ill should be excluded from work and advised to stay home until symptoms subside. Both Medicare and Medicaid require that those who participate in these programs actively screen and report staff members who may contact patients, food, or laundry and have a program in place to prevent patient contact.

43. B: There are few different ways to solve a problem like this. Given the limited number of answer choices, simply comparing the value of each ratio to the two totals may be feasible. However, the approach we recommend is to proportionally reduce the total numbers until the simplest expression of the ratio is found. There are 112 female patients and 196 male patients, so begin there:

$$112 \div 2 = 56 \qquad 196 \div 2 = 98$$
$$56 \div 2 = 28 \qquad 98 \div 2 = 49$$
$$28 \div 7 = 4 \qquad 49 \div 7 = 7$$

These two numbers no longer have any common factors, so 4:7 is the simplest way to express the ratio.

44. C: Diagnostic criteria and surveillance criteria are not necessarily the same, and surveillance criteria must be utilized for surveillance activities. Surveillance criteria are based on epidemiological principles and not diagnostic, so it's important to apply the surveillance criteria exactly as defined without consideration of diagnosis. The surveillance criteria should be carefully defined as part of the development of a surveillance program. Surveillance criteria that are most commonly utilized in the United States are those developed by NHSN.

45. D: Data may be obtained from a wide range of sources, which can include direct observations of staff members providing care, pharmacy-generated lists of medications prescribed, facility-wide lists of patients on isolation precautions, and incident reports as well as the commonly utilized laboratory reports, medical records, census data, and injury (such as needlestick) reports. Valuable information may be gained from reports from healthcare providers so a staff well trained in surveillance techniques and surveillance criteria is essential.

46. B: Fecal microbiota transplant (fecal transplant) is increasingly used to treat *Clostridium difficile* infections, although usually not as a first-line treatment. This may change, however, as the fecal material is now available in capsule form so it can be ingested easily. Traditional modes of administration include per nasogastric tube and colonoscopy with stool often obtained from family members. Fecal microbiota transplants replace the normal flora found in the intestines and have high rates of cure.

47. D: The annual incidence is the number of events divided by the number of patients for the entire year. To find the annual incidence of UTIs per 1000 in this patient population, use the following formula:

$$\frac{\text{number of patients with UTI}}{\text{total patients for the year}} = \frac{x}{1000}$$

This problem gives the average monthly census, so it will necessary to calculate the total for the year before plugging any numbers in. Since there was an average of 300 patients per month, multiply this by 12 to find the number for the entire year:

$$300 \times 12 = 3600$$

This number can now be used along with the numbers given in the question to yield the following equation:

$$\frac{117}{3600} = \frac{x}{1000}$$

The equation can then be rearranged and solved for x as follows:

$$x = 1000 \times \frac{117}{3600}$$

$$x = \frac{1170}{36} = 32.5$$

Thus, the annual incidence of UTIs in this patient population was 32.5 per 1000.

48. C: A number of factors may exclude a procedure from SIR data, including procedures that are fewer than five minutes in duration and procedures in which the patient's age is equal to or greater than 109 or the wound class is "U." Exclusion also applies if one or more of the defined risk factors as indicated for each procedure are missing, the procedure exceeds the IQR5, and the date of the procedure is prior to the date of the patient's birth.

49. A: The SIR is a very simple value to calculate. It is simply the number of infections divided by the expected number of infections:

$$\text{SIR} = \frac{10}{7.5} = 1.33$$

If the SIR is 1.0, then the number matches those expected. A number higher than 1.0 indicates the rate of infection exceeds that expected, and a number lower than 1.0 indicates it is less than that expected.

50. A: While intentional acts of carelessness with infection prevention may occur, they are not primary causes of healthcare-associated outbreaks. The three most common causes include contamination or defects in medical products or devices, colonization or infection of healthcare personnel who then transmit the infection to others, and lapses in infection prevention practices, such as forgetting to carry out hand hygiene or doing so inadequately.

51. D: If a woman was admitted for an elective Caesarean and developed a high fever of unknown origin 30 hours post-op and died within 6 hours, this case would be classified as a sentinel event because it was unanticipated and resulted in death. Sentinel event are those unexpected events that result in death or severe injury (physical or psychological) to a patient. Sentinel events can also include infant abduction, suicide (in a continuous care setting or within 72 hours of discharge), and surgery on the wrong patient or body part.

52. B: An increase in the number of positive microbiological cultures in the absence of clinical disease would be classified as a pseudo-outbreak. For example, a patient's airway may be contaminated with an endoscope so that a culture may be positive, but the patient may not have or develop active disease. Mistakes can also be made in conducting or interpreting tests, leading to the conclusion that an outbreak is occurring when it is not.

53. A: In an outbreak in which the case definition is primarily clinical, the most valuable resource is likely healthcare provider reports because the healthcare providers are in the best position to note symptoms in patients and to identify further cases, especially if the causative agent is unknown and so cannot be readily confirmed by laboratory testing. Medical records may also be helpful in identifying symptoms that fit the case definition. Once the possible pathogen is identified, then the case definition may expand.

54. C: While the NHSN system focused on targeted surveillance of defined populations, and overall rates of infection based on whole house surveillance provide little useful information, a combination strategy that includes targeted surveillance and some whole-house monitoring, such as lab-monitoring for multi-drug resistant organisms or MR*SA*, is likely to provide the most useful information, as targeted surveillance alone may miss small outbreaks or breaches of infection control and prevention in non-targeted areas.

55. D: The most important element for creating an epidemic curve during a hospital outbreak is the line list, which is a valuable tool during the investigation. The line list may contain demographic information as well as a description of the signs and symptoms, the environment, risk factors, date of onset, and laboratory findings, if appropriate. Line lists are created so that the cases are numbered on the vertical axis and variable are listed on the horizontal axis.

56. A: An outbreak of *E. coli* infections linked to packaged produce may most benefit from media publicity to aid in case finding as mild cases may be occurring within the community that have not come to the attention of healthcare providers, and the publicity may encourage those affected to notify the health department or healthcare providers. Additionally, the media publicity may help to curb the outbreak by providing notice to consumers to avoid contaminated products.

57. C: Environmental sampling often provides little information, as isolating the surface that is contaminated may be very difficult, so mass environmental sampling of all patient areas is not recommended. Before beginning environmental sampling, the IP should seek guidance from the microbiologic lab regarding appropriate sampling. Only suspected vectors should be sampled and the sampling should be based on the type of organism. For example, if a pathogen is water-borne, then sampling dry patient contact surfaces cannot provide useful information.

58. B: While all of these are important, the IOM states that the primary aim of the healthcare system should be on patient safety with safe care provided in a safe environment. While errors may occur, the goal is to prevent harm to the patient as well as the harm to the healthcare provider. The IOM stresses the importance of patient-centered approaches that consider the values and needs of the patient, effectiveness that relates to use of evidence-based care, efficiency, and equity.

59. A: If the media in the community have become aware of a hospital outbreak, the best method of dealing with this is to assign one specific person to communicate with media. This person may be part of the publicity department in a large hospital or may be a member of the medical staff, but the person should be knowledgeable about the outbreak and able to provide clear information. While hospitals may want to avoid the negative publicity associated with outbreaks, denying that there is an outbreak will likely generate worse publicity.

60. D: An epidemic curve that approximates a normal distribution (Bell curve) most often results from a common source, point exposure. This means that all of the identified cases were infected from the same reservoir (item, person, material). If the exposure from the common source were intermittent, then instead of a normal distribution, there would be a number of irregularly spaced peaks evident. Common source cases usually occur over a shorter duration that propagated source cases in which the infection goes from person to person.

61. B: The dependent variable is that which occurs as the result of something else. In this scenario, the dependent variable is the ventilator-associated pneumonia. The independent variable, on the other hand, is the cause of or influence on the dependent variable. Mechanical ventilation, for example, is an independent variable. In a 2x2 table, the dependent variable in on the X-axis (horizontal), and the independent variable is on the Y-axis (vertical).

62. A: The ASA rating scale is an example of an ordinal scale, which organizes things into distinct categories that have a relationship to each other. Other examples include staging cancer or classifying something according to degrees of satisfaction. Nominal scale involves categorizing by naming, such as gay and straight or male and female. Interval scales have exact distance between observations, such as the temperature scale. Ratio is not a scale of measurement.

63. C: These data contain an outlier (29 days), which skews the average to 5, so mean is not useful. The mode is 1 because that number occurs 3 times, but this provides almost no information about the range of lengths of stay. The median is calculated by reordering the data into rank order: 1, 1, 1, 2, 2, 3, 3, 4, 4, 29. Because there is an even number, the two central numbers, 2 and 3, are averaged, with the result of 2.5, which provides the most useful information about lengths of stay.

64. C: In a normal distribution curve, also described as a Bell curve, 68% of the results should be within the first standard deviation above and below the mean. The interval from two standard deviations below the mean to two standard deviations above the mean should contain 95% of the results. When extended to 3 standard deviations, the results should contain 99.7% of the results with outliers constituting a negligible percentage of results.

65. D: The incidence rate is the number of events divided by the number of patients under consideration. To find the incidence rate of CAUTI per 100 in this patient population, use the following formula:

$$\frac{\text{number of patients with CAUTI}}{\text{total patient population}} = \frac{x}{100}$$

Plugging in the numbers given in the question yields the following equation:

$$\frac{5}{25} = \frac{x}{100}$$

The equation can then be rearranged and solved for x as follows:

$$x = 100 \times \frac{5}{25} = 20$$

Thus, the incidence rate of CAUTI per 100 patients in this period is 20.

66. A: In working with the public health department to determine if people who are HIV positive disclose this information to sexual partners, the best research techniques include both personal interviews and surveys. While solutions to the problem on non-disclosure may be explored in focus groups, and the groups may have opinions about disclosure, the members can only speak for themselves and can't provide useful data. Participant observations are not appropriate for the data needed.

67. B: The projected compliance rate is the number of events in which staff are compliant divided by the total number of events. To find the projected compliance rate per 1000 operations, use the following formula:

$$\frac{\text{number of compliant events}}{\text{total number of events}} = \frac{x}{1000}$$

Plugging in the numbers given in the question yields the following equation:

$$\frac{160}{200} = \frac{x}{1000}$$

The equation can then be rearranged and solved for x as follows:

$$x = 1000 \times \frac{160}{200}$$

$$x = 800$$

Thus, the projected compliance rate is 800 per 1000 surgeries.

68. B: The best method of reducing a type II error, accepting a null hypothesis that is incorrect, is to increase the sample size because the larger the sample size, the more the data follow a normal distribution, and analysis is easier. However, sample size cannot always be controlled when using infection data, so it may not always be clear when a type II error has occurred, so the IP must remain aware of this when analyzing data.

69. C: The most commonly used confidence interval is 95%, which means that the researcher can be 95% sure that the results did not occur by chance. The confidence interval is the range of possible values, taking into account the margin of error. Confidence intervals are always described in percentages but cannot predict that a value will fall within the parameters established by the confidence interval. The confidence interval may be affected by sample size.

70. D: The type of graphic display that is most appropriate for communicating continuous data is a histogram, frequency polygon, or ogive (line chart). The ogive is a line chart that indicates data over time. Histograms use vertical bars to show the number of data points in a range of different values. A frequency polygon is constructed similarly to a histogram except points are used to show values rather than bars. For this reason, the frequency polygon is a better choice than a histogram when comparing sets of data.

71. A: After determining that data collection is necessary for surveillance, the first step should be to determine who may already have the data. Data are collected in various areas for different purposes. For example, if the data collection involves multi-drug resistant organisms, then a logical place to begin the search for data would be in the laboratory, which likely maintains records of cultures and sensitivities or can provide easy access to the information with the help of the IT department.

72. B: The type of epidemiological study that best assesses outcomes and potential risk factors in a group at one point in time is the cross-sectional study. Because both risk factors and outcomes are assessed at the same time, cross-sectional studies are not helpful in determining cause and effect. Cross-sectional studies may be used to determine prevalence and correlations but not incidence. The researcher should be careful to avoid selection bias that may skew results. Cross-sectional studies can be done quickly and are generally easier than cohort studies.

73. C: The most common organism associated with osteomyelitis is *Staphylococcus aureus,* which is also associated with empyema, endocarditis, septic arthritis, septicemia, sinusitis, and cellulitis. Less commonly, *S. pneumoniae* and *S. pyogenes* may be causative agents for osteomyelitis. *Klebsiella* sp. is commonly associated with septicemia and urinary tract infections. *Pseudomonas* sp. is associated with healthcare-associated pneumonia, and coagulase-negative staphylococci with device-related infection.

74. D: Cloudy cerebrospinal fluid most likely indicates bacterial meningitis as the cloudiness occurs because of purulent material. Cerebrospinal fluid is normally clear and colorless. Both viral infections and fungal infections can result in cerebrospinal fluid that ranges from clear to hazy. Other important factors in diagnosis, such as protein, glucose, and white blood count, may vary according to the type of pathogen and the patient characteristics, such as immune status and age.

75. B: Immunocompromised patients at risk of *Pneumocystis jiroveci* infection, such as patients with HIV/AIDS, should receive antibiotic prophylaxis with trimethoprim-sulfamethoxazole. They should receive the prophylaxis for the entire duration of risk. Patients who are unable to tolerate TMP/SMX because of allergies may take oral dapsone or atovaquone or inhaled pentamidine. Generally, studies have varied regarding the efficacy of other patients with compromised immune systems and neutropenia receiving prophylaxis with some studies showing no benefit.

76. A: Dietary restriction that are recommended by the CDC, HHS, and USDA for neutropenic patients to prevent infection include avoiding sprouts and rough-skinned raw fruits, such as raspberries and strawberries; using only pasteurized dairy products; and reheating deli meats and hot dogs to steaming hot before eating. While some physicians still advise patients to avoid all raw fruits and vegetables and eat only cooked foods, this practice is not supported by evidence-based research.

77. D: Adding piperacillin/tazobactam and an aminoglycoside to the same IV infusion inactivates both agents when they interact. Co-administration of antimicrobials may result in either inactivation, as in this case, or antagonism, in which the co-administered antimicrobials are both less effective than when they are administered individually. However, synergy, increased effectiveness, may occur with co-administration of some antibiotics; so, the healthcare should always check the literature for information about interactions when administering more than one antimicrobial.

78. B: Resistance develops in microorganisms because of point mutations in pre-existing genes or acquisition of new genes. Point mutations are random and result from errors in DNA replication. When these mutations cause a change in structure of a drug-receptor or target site, then resistance may occur. These types of point mutations occur rarely. Most resistance is caused by newly acquired genes that interfere with the action of the drugs.

79. C: The CDC-recommended method of routine hand hygiene is now using alcohol-based hand rubs. This can be done relatively quickly, and compliance tends to be better than washing hands with soap and water. However, if the hands are visibly soiled or have come into contact with bodily fluids, then they must be thoroughly washed with soap and water to remove all residue. Additionally, if the healthcare provider is exposed to spore-producing microbes, such as *B. anthracis* or *C. difficile,* or norovirus, then washing with soap and water is required.

80. A: In order to protect the eyes from respiratory secretions, blood, or other body fluids, only face shields and goggles are adequate. Contact lenses do not provide protection, and protection is minimal with eye glasses because of open spaces about the eye. Patients who wear eye glasses may continue to wear them when using face shields but they must be removed to apply goggles. PPE to protect the face and eyes should be used whenever there is a possibility of splashes or sprays of body fluids and always if caring for an Ebola patient.

81. C: When using steam sterilization, the sterilization process should take approximately 40 minutes. Steam sterilization is a high temperature procedure that destroys all microorganisms, including bacterial spores, and is used for heat-tolerant items, such as surgical instruments. Other sterilization processes include dry heat, which takes 1 to 6 hours, depending on the temperature. Low temperature sterilization for heat resistant items includes the use of ethylene oxide gas, hydrogen peroxide gas plasma or hydrogen peroxide vapor. Liquid immersion in various chemical sterilants may also be used.

82. D: Older adults who had varicella (chickenpox) as children should be advised that they should have the herpes zoster (shingles) immunization because the virus may reactivate in the presence of immunocompromise, disease, or some drugs. Herpes zoster is common in older adults and usually begins with a prodrome of tingling pain for up to 7 days, followed by a papular rash that becomes vesicular and is extremely painful. Some people develop post-herpetic neuralgia, with severe pain that may persist for months or years.

83. A: A healthcare provider who has long artificial nails should be advised that the nails could result in transmission of gram-negative and fungal organisms. Even long natural nails may increase risk of transmission, so nails should be kept trimmed. If nail polish is allowed, it should be removed if chipped as the chipped area may harbor pathogenic agents. Additionally, long nails may make caring for the patient more difficult and increase risk of injury to the patient from scratches.

84. C: In order to prevent BSIs in the NICU, the CDC recommends skin antisepsis for vascular access with greater than 0.5% chlorhexidine gluconate with alcohol. A solution of 2% chlorhexidine gluconate in 70% alcohol is often used for IV insertion in neonates, but alcohol may burn the friable skin of premature infants (less than 28 weeks or less than 1000 g) so solutions with lower levels of alcohol should be used for these neonates. Povidone iodine is safe for use for mature infants but may be absorbed in premature infants, resulting in thyroid dysfunction.

85. B: If the water supply at a hematopoietic stem cell center is contaminated with *Legionella pneumophila,* the water supply must be decontaminated and sterilized water used for drinking, brushing teeth, and treatments. Patients should not be allowed to shower or bathe or have any contact with the contaminated water supply because of their immunocompromised status. Hematopoietic stem cell centers should avoid any plumbing fixtures that aerosolize water or water systems that allow water to stagnate, as these are risk factors for legionellosis.

86. D: In regards to reprocessing of single-use devices, the CMS recommends use of third-party reprocessors because of the stringency of the regulations by the FDA for reprocessing and the type of equipment needed. The trend is toward increased reprocessing of single-use devices because of the costs of medical care. The FDA categorizes medical devices as class I, II, or III with class I posting the lowest risk to the patient and class III the highest. Requirements for reprocessing of class III devices are more stringent than for class I or II.

87. A: When conducting surveillance of an ambulatory care infusion center, if one observation is that the nurse has prepared infusates for multiple patients prior to their arrival, the nurse should be advised to prepare infusates immediately before use only. Preparing multiple infusates ahead of time not only increases the risk of infection but also the risk of giving the wrong infusate to a patient. The IP should ensure that a mechanism to track positive blood cultures is established as part of surveillance.

88. C: The maximum humidity level in cardiac catheter lab is 60%. American Institute of Architects' requirements include a minimum floor space of 400 square feet, temperature in the range of 70-75 °F (21-24 °C) maximum, and 15 air exchanges per hour with 3 of those fresh air. Materials used in the catheter lab must be nonporous and easily cleanable, so no wood materials (shutters, doors, shelves) or carpeting is allowed.

89. B: Pregnant healthcare workers should be routinely screened only for HIV unless other risk factors are identified. Immunizations that are recommended for pregnant healthcare workers include influenza (inactivated) and Tdap. Immunizations that are not recommended include HPV. Those that are contraindicated include influenza (LAIV), MMR, varicella, and herpes zoster. Hepatitis A and B vaccines may be indicated in some situations. Pregnant workers should be made aware of the risks of infectious diseases and potential harm to the fetus.

90. D: Since norovirus is spread per the fecal-oral route, the initial focus should be on the changing tables and hand hygiene. Environments in which toddlers and infants play or receive care (such as diaper changing) are frequently contaminated with fecal material, which is easily transmitted from one child to another on the hands of caregivers and other children. Environmental cleaning and disinfecting and strict hand hygiene are critical elements to controlling a norovirus outbreak.

91. A: The immunization that is recommended for healthcare workers with occupational exposure to blood, blood products, or bodily secretions is hepatitis B. Hepatitis A is recommended for laboratory workers. Other recommended immunizations include influenza, MMR, Td, Tdap, and varicella, depending on immune status. While healthcare workers have no increased risk over the general public of developing tetanus, they should follow general recommendations of Td every 10 years. Tdap should be taken one time and may replace a dose of Td.

92. C: When carrying out tuberculosis skin testing for long-term care residents, the extent of induration that is generally considered positive is 10 mm unless residents have added risk factors and meet the criteria for positive findings at 5 mm or greater. Tuberculosis (TB) is more common in the elderly than in younger populations and this is represented by higher rates in long-term care facilities, which have primarily elderly patients. TB control plans and plans for housing TB patients (in the facility or elsewhere) should be in place.

93. B: The incubation period for foodborne illness caused by *Salmonella* spp. is 1 to 3 days, and the infection persists for 4 to 7 days. Symptoms include fever, abdominal cramping, and diarrhea. *S. typhi* and *S. paratyphi* result in more severe symptoms and typhoid fever. Infection often results from contaminated poultry, eggs, unpasteurized milk products or juices, and raw fruits and vegetables. Outbreaks may occur if the water supply becomes contaminated. Antibiotics are usually contraindicated except for *S. typhi* and *S. paratyphi.*

94. D: If power is interrupted to the operating rooms during construction, the HVAC system should be run for a period of time to flush the ducts prior to ventilating the operating rooms because the HVAC system can carry airborne infectious agents. Construction projects, especially, increase the risk of *Aspergillus* infections. The HVAC system includes all air handling elements: heating, ventilation, and air conditioning. Generally centralized HVAC systems have an air-handling unit (AHU), which is typically located on the roof or in a separate room.

95. A: When using alcohol-based surgical hand scrub products for surgical hand antisepsis, the first step is to prewash hands and forearms with non-antimicrobial soap and water and dry. Then, the alcohol scrub is applied and massaged thoroughly into the hands and forearms for the duration specified by the manufacturer. After the alcohol is applied to the skin it should be allowed to air dry completely prior to the person's donning sterile gloves. When surgical hand scrubs are done with antimicrobial soap, the scrub should be completed in 2-6 minutes.

96. C: The maternal host facts that increase the risk of a healthcare-associated perinatal infection in both mother and infant include immunosuppression from corticosteroids or other reasons, low economic status, and ruptured membrane. Other risk factors include uncontrolled diabetes mellitus, BMI under 19 or over 30, ASA score of 3 or greater, smoking, colonization (HIV, GBS, HSV, chlamydia, gonorrhea, syphilis), preterm labor, and extended stay in the hospital.

97. B: According to the WHO, the six phases of a pandemic include:

- Phase 1: Low risk of cases in humans.
- Phase 2: Higher risk of cases in humans.
- Phase 3: Human-to-human transmission is nonexistent or low.
- Phase 4: Some human-to-human transmission is evident.
- Phase 5: Significant human-to-human transmission is occurring.
- Phase 6: Efficient/Sustained human-to-human transmission is occurring.

Pandemics usually hit communities in waves that last 6-8 weeks, so it may take a long period for a full pandemic to become evident.

98. D: The purpose of BioWatch is to collect air samples to test for aerosolized biological agents. BioWatch is a program jointly coordinated by the CDC, EPA, and Homeland Security. BioWatch collects air samples from various places in the United States and monitors air quality around the clock. Air samples are examined for various biological agents by the Laboratory Response Network, and reports, referred to as BioWatch Actionable Results (BARS), are sent to emergency personnel and public health officials if biological particles are found.

99. B: The four phases of a disaster with mass casualties include:

- Preparedness: Time prior to the disaster, which may include a warning phase (tornado, hurricane) or not (earthquake, airplane crash).
- Impact: Mass casualty event occurs. May be sudden or with slow onset and may or may not be evident at onset.
- Response: May begin with the impact phase or later, depending on the type of disaster and recognition that the disaster is occurring.
- Recovery: The event is declared over, and no additional victims are likely to be recovered.

100. C: Impetigo may be bullous, commonly associated with *Staphylococcus aureus,* or nonbullous, commonly associated with group A streptococci. Generally, these two types of organisms (*S. aureus* and group A streptococci) are responsible for most common skin infections, including folliculitis, furuncles and carbuncles, erysipelas, cellulitis, and paronychia although streptococcus groups B, C, and G may be implicated in erysipelas. Skin infections with MR*SA* have become more common and are more difficult to treat.

101. A: In a manner similar to the spores of Bacillus anthracis, an outermost layer of Clostridium difficile spores called the exosporium renders these microbes sticky, which enables them to adhere to health care workers' hands or environmental surfaces, such as computer keyboards, window coverings, and telephones, used by clinical staff. The most effective prevention strategy is barrier protection, as in rigorous adherence to glove use, which should always be followed by thorough hand washing. Although many commercial products claim to rid hands of spores, their success rates are less than that of barrier methods. Spores are the noninfectious forms of the organisms, which are activated following ingestion to their disease-causing form.

102. B: The ubiquity and increasing antimicrobial resistance patterns among Enterococcus spp. is an infection control challenge for health care facilities worldwide. Vancomycin-resistant strains are frequently reported in the United States. These enteric, facultative gram-positive cocci grow in short chains. They are normal inhabitants of the gastrointestinal tract (large bowel) and female genitourinary tract. While E. faecalis causes the majority of infections and shows emerging resistance to many antibiotics, E. faecium isolates demonstrate a high degree of vancomycin resistance. Because many nosocomial enterococcal infections are transmitted by contact, these organisms are also found on skin and wounds, often as a result of hand carriage by health care workers.

103. D: The bacterial species most commonly responsible for surgical site infections (SSI) is Staphylococcus aureus. In one study, this species accounted for 20% of all SSI. Given this microbe's increasing rates of antimicrobial resistance, as in methicillin-resistant S. aureus (MRSA), these infections represent a formidable foe in terms of mortality, morbidity, and increasing health care costs. Following S. aureus in frequency are those infections caused by coagulase-negative staphylococci (14%), as in S. epidermidis, frequently found on skin and mucous membranes as normal bacterial flora. These organisms are often associated with infections related to indwelling devices and catheters, and in endocarditis. Following staphylococci in frequency are wound infections involving enterococcus (12%) and E. coli (8%). Although infections involving anaerobic Bacteroides fragilis are worrisome, these organisms accounted for only 2% of all SSI in the study noted, following other more frequently occurring infections related to pathogens such as Pseudomonas, Klebsiella, Proteus, and Enterobacter species.

104. C: Clean-contaminated or class II surgical wounds may involve entry into parts of the body that normally contain flora, such as the respiratory or urinary tracts; however, in order to qualify as class II, such procedures must be elective and not violate aseptic technique nor show evidence of an infectious process. By definition, the closed wrist fracture reduction does not involve a break in skin and would be a class I procedure. The emergency appendectomy with evidence of abscess implicates perforation and infection, and is thus a class IV wound. The elective thoracotomy with right upper lobe resection involves the respiratory tract, a potential source of contamination. However, surgery was elective and did not note infection or break in technique, so it is correctly classified as clean-contaminated.

105. A: Relative risk (RR) is a useful statistical term in infectious epidemiology as well as noninfectious disease surveillance. Although a noninfectious example is used here, the concept remains important to understanding risk of disease transmission in certain populations. Relative risk is a ratio that shows the risk of developing a disease or infection in a population exposed to a causative agent compared with the risk for developing the same entity in a population that is not exposed to that agent. Because RR involves two ratios, that of the event probability in the exposed group divided by that in the unexposed group, it is also known as the risk ratio. Disease prevalence references the number of cases of a disease in a given population at a set time; disease incidence represents the frequency or rate at which new cases of a disease are seen in a given population during a specified time frame. Disease incidence is often used in epidemiologic investigations.

106. B: The greatest risk factor for the development of hepatocellular carcinoma (hepatoma) worldwide is infectious. Hepatitis B is a viral infection endemic in much of the non-Western world for which an effective vaccine has been available since the 1980s. Hepatitis A, for which there is also an effective vaccine delivered in two doses spaced 6-12 months apart, does not show strong statistical correlation with development of hepatocellular carcinoma, in contrast to data involving hepatitis B and C viruses. Twinrix, a vaccination against both hepatitis A and B, is administered in three doses, similar to that given against hepatitis B alone. Increased rates of hepatocellular carcinoma in Western countries have paralleled increased rates of hepatitis C, and appear likely due to increased use of blood products, growing populations of intravenous drug users, and chronicity of infections caused by hepatitis C–tainted blood products administered in the past. Serologic screening improvements have helped decrease the number of transfusion-associated nosocomial infections caused by these viruses.

107. 1-C, 2-D, 3-A, 4-E, 5-B. Essential data that must be collected during the investigation of an outbreak reference person, place, time of event, and its clinical and laboratory features. In this match, the person can represent a defined group as in the day-shift technologists of choice C. The place is the facility in Arizona. The time can be a reference period, as in the winter months of choice A. Clinical features include signs and symptoms, as in the morbilliform rash of choice E, and other clinical findings or comments regarding disease transmission. Laboratory features include those diagnostic findings such as results of cultures, special serology, or specialized testing as in polymerase chain reaction (PCR), immunofixation, or other techniques that specify the nature of the infection.

108. B: Hand hygiene remains an opportunity area for increased compliance and improved technique. Warm or hot water is not recommended for rinsing off soap or other disinfectant materials because of the increased risk for skin irritation or dermatitis that may be caused by higher water temperatures combined with topical chemicals. Rather, use of a towel or disposable napkin is recommended following cleansing before handling spigots or other community-soiled areas with prompt disposal of said item, not to be reused again. Even use of gloves is not fail-safe. In fact, hand washing is recommended after gloves are removed as in the wound-dressing example here. Alcohol-based hand rubs are effective when used around all surfaces of hands and fingers until dry; however, soap and water can be effective when such agents are not available.

109. D: Many studies attribute about 15% of nosocomial infections to contamination caused by hand carriage of pathogens by health care workers. These incidents may occur via direct patient-to-patient contact or with intermediary static objects that may be contact-contaminated, from computer keyboards, pens, or even radiologic equipment. The latter is a common occurrence in ICU settings where portable radiography is employed. Many health care workers erroneously believe (or become complacent through years of clinical practice) that the use of gloves trumps the need for meticulous hand hygiene, or do not understand or follow the need for proper hand washing even after gloves are removed. Particularly in settings where gloved health care workers come into contact with potentially devastating pathogens (e.g., C. difficile, antibiotic-resistant strains, MRSA), it is imperative that hand washing and other infection-control strategies be ingrained in staff, with appropriate reminders, surveillance, and continuing education as necessary.

110. A: Cross-contamination or cross-colonization may occur even with strict infection control precautions in place. Laxity in adhering to IC guidelines increases the likelihood of breaching IC standards, which may be especially hazardous with multidrug resistant organisms, particularly those that require long periods of complex antimicrobial therapy, as in multidrug-resistant tuberculosis (MDR-TB). With isolation of a non-acid-fast organism, contact transmission appears more likely than airborne transmission that would indicate mask precautions for patient and caregivers. Surface cultures of shared equipment may help isolate the infectious culprit while rigorous decontamination procedures may halt the spread of infection to new unit admissions. As in any outbreak occurrence, increased vigilance to hand washing techniques should be enforced because suboptimal compliance by health care workers in multiple settings is frequently reported.

111. A: Transparency is at the core of effective communications strategies during outbreaks, which promotes trust among the public and aids in acceptance of the information conveyed. Even when all information has not been gathered and analyzed, early announcements are appropriate and may be tempered by accurate reassurances as more information emerges or recommendations shift. Communication delays until all information is known not only hinders trust but may increase public fear. Such delays also appear to show lack of leadership or inhibit outbreak containment. Failures of the expert-centered *decide and announce* model have caused strategists to largely abandon this one-way method. Instead, successful communications have shifted towards listening to public concerns, including cultural considerations, and a more open, two-way dialogue guided by organized operational planning.

112. D: The sample described fulfills criteria for a category A specimen, one that has the potential to cause permanent disability, life-threatening morbidity or death in immunologically intact, otherwise healthy humans or animals because of infectious agents the specimen may harbor. Proper transport for category A specimen dictates the use of triple packaging as described in option D. In addition, packaging must be documented as having met performance criteria whereby adequate resistance has been shown to stresses by gravity, puncture, and pressure. Enclosed absorbent material must be of sufficient volume and absorbance capacity to take up all escaped fluids should breakage occur.

113. D: Even with improved infection control practices and heightened awareness, transmission of HIV from patients to health care workers remains an area of concern. The highest risk for exposure occurs in settings involving sharps and needles. Although there is a higher chance of knowing the HIV serologic status of patients today than in the past, there is a greater risk of infectivity of HIV to health care workers from patients with unknown or uncertain serologic status. Given similar exposures, the rate of seroconversion following exposure to infectious hepatitis B particles in the health care setting is about 25%, much greater than the 0.5% seroconversion rate for HIV. Such statistics underscore the need for a robust program of hepatitis B vaccination for health care workers and strict precautions in settings where hepatitis B is likely to occur, as in hospital populations from endemic areas, those with large numbers of intravenous drug abusers, dialysis units, and in endemic areas abroad.

114. C: Infection control personnel are often the first individuals notified of preliminary results, particularly when there is a high index of suspicion for a worrisome pathogen or one that involves a patient with an aggressive clinical course. IC staff must have working familiarity with the ways in which preliminary results are communicated, and understand differential diagnostic considerations and implications for action. Laboratories report results of preliminary Gram-stain results, some of which help narrow diagnostic possibilities, as in the typical "tennis racket" appearance of *Clostridium tetani*, the infectious agent of tetanus. Here, *Bacillus anthracis* is a Gram-positive rod associated with environmental flora in settings that involve livestock, such as sheep and cattle.

Because it is transmitted via inhalation or breaks in intact skin or mucous membranes, quarantine precautions of the index are not indicated, while further investigations are certainly warranted.

115. B: Viruses are classified by many characteristics that may include their ribonucleic acid (DNA vs RNA), protein coat structure, virus size or shape, envelope coating (if any), and method of replication. Arboviruses are a taxonomic class of viruses that involve transmission by an arthropod insect vector that is required for human infection to occur. The prototypical arboviral infection is malaria, spread by vector transmission by the Plasmodium falciparum mosquito species. Mosquitoes and ticks are common arbovirus vectors. Arboviruses are capable of causing acute and chronic infections; however, most acute infections are asymptomatic. In the case of malaria, disease may not manifest until a decade or more following initial exposure in extreme cases. Human-to-human transmission is not a factor in spread of these diseases. The vector of the dengue fever flavivirus is the Aedes aegypti mosquito; Aedes spp. mosquitoes also harbor the yellow fever flavivirus. In the Northern hemisphere, most cases of arboviral-associated encephalitis are reported in the warmer months, typically June through September.

116. C: Contamination is a term whose nuanced meanings must be thoroughly understood and properly communicated by infection control personnel. While a disease carrier may be contaminated by an infectious agent, the converse is not true and, therefore, contamination does not necessarily imply a carrier state. Materials that are considered contaminated by infectious agents include foods, liquids such as water or milk, or objects/substances that may harbor infectious agents on their surfaces or that may contain the infectious particles. These latter categories can include contaminated toys, bedding, or even items commonly found in health care settings such as surgical supplies. Noninfectious environmental pollutants are not considered contaminants for the purpose of infection control monitoring and surveillance, even though they may be irritating, offensive, or even noxious.

117. A: Symptoms of hydrophobia, headaches, and altered mental state progressing to coma should alert clinicians to rabies, particularly following travel to an endemic area and a history of a wound with paresthesia. Bites or scratches involving rabid animals closer to the head and neck area are of particular concern and may shorten the incubation period to disease manifestation. Choices B and C are unsuitable as brain biopsy is not an immediate diagnostic test choice but useful as postmortem confirmation. Rather, saliva or skin, especially the latter sampled from the hairline of the posterior neck region, may be tested by fluorescent antibody or RT-PCR for rabies. Cultures are not indicated for this viral disease. China has seen increased numbers of confirmed rabies cases, while rabies has decreased in other parts of Asia, particularly in Thailand.

118. B: The primary diagnosis under consideration is rabies, a disease in which the incubation period may vary depending on factors such as the proximity of the bite or scratch to the head and neck area; the depth of the wound; infectivity of the index animal; the virulence and concentration of virus delivered into the wound; and amount of protection offered by clothing or other protective coverings, such as backpacks. Because of these and other animal vector and host factors, the incubation period may fall between a few days or many years. Many rabies cases occur following incubation periods of 3 to 8 weeks. Choice A does not relate to the disease in question, nor would these symptoms appear typical for acute infection with toxoplasma, which is more typically asymptomatic or presents with a viral-type illness that might suggest infectious mononucleosis rather than the cataclysmic events in this case.

119. D: Quarantine of the human index case is not an appropriate action for suspected rabies as the incidence of person-to-person transmission is exceedingly rare, particularly in a controlled hospital setting. Rather, had this patient been bitten by a dog, cat, or other animal that remained in contact with humans, it would be appropriate to quarantine and observe the animal, perform appropriate diagnostic tests, and euthanize it as indicated. A formal report to local health authorities is required, and is likewise obligatory in many countries worldwide. In an attempt to neutralize viral load, efforts should be made to deliver passive prophylaxis with rabies immune globulin (human or equine) as soon as possible after the rabid attack. In addition, close contacts of the infected patient who have had mucous membrane exposure to the index case should also receive post-exposure prophylaxis with immune globulin.

120. A: Following completion of the full, three-dose immunization schedule for hepatitis B, immune-competent vaccine recipients will show positive results for hepatitis B surface antibody but will have negative serology for the markers of current or past hepatitis B infection. HBeAg positivity is associated with a high degree of potential infectivity while positive results for hepatitis B surface antigen (HBsAg) indicate a potentially infectious carrier state. HBsAg may be detected any time within a wide time frame, from initial acute infection to years later when the disease enters a chronic phase. The chronic active carrier state for hepatitis B would be expected to show positive serologic markers for HBsAg and HBcAb. The diagnosis of chronic hepatitis requires additional marker seropositivity, elevation of liver enzymes, biopsy confirmation, or other ancillary studies.

121. B: Up to a thousand different microbial species live on or inside our bodies. Because these microbes do not normally cause disease or infections, they are termed normal flora. Some normal flora is present at all times while the presence of other transient microbes ebbs and flows. As normal flora multiply, the expanded microbial population colonizes the host, provided they remain nonpathogenic and do not invade tissues or cause infections or disease. However, in cases of immune compromise, colonizing organisms can take advantage of host defense weaknesses to cause disease as pathogens, which can result in infections. Commensal organisms that neither benefit nor harm the host organism also represent subsets of normal flora. Some normal flora function to mutual benefit, such as E. coli that feed off contents of their intestinal tract home, and where they benefit the host organism through their actions in nutrient synthesis (e.g., Vitamin K) or elimination.

122. A: In the laboratory, group A streptococci cause a visible clear zone of beta-hemolysis on sheep's blood agar culture plates. Group A strep are causative organisms in a wide variety of disease from sore ("strep") throat to the potentially lethal toxic shock syndrome (TSS). The organism is also capable of attacking heart valves, as in rheumatic heart disease that may ensue days or weeks following acute strep pharyngitis. There is no vaccine for group A streptococcal disease. All other steps B to D should be initiated while the outbreak is investigated. Milk and milk products have been identified in food-associated streptococcal outbreaks in which the food contamination is caused by transfer from humans infected with streptococci. Rapid antigen detection methods are handy and useful, provided they are made available in a timely fashion to staff and they are used and interpreted properly.

123. D: To investigate the source and scope of a potential outbreak, infection control professionals use syndromic surveillance to gather situational information and review broad clinical descriptions and impressions, rather than data from diagnostic testing. Because it acts as a large net, such surveillance should be designed for high sensitivity in order to capture data from as many patients who are actually positive for the disease in question. Low specificity is also desired, as specificity identifies the true negatives in such a study, such as patients who do not have a disease and their test results or assessment also shows that they do not appear to have the disease. Because parameters may need to be refined and adapted as more information is gathered, a surveillance system should also offer the flexibility to shift case definitions, clinical descriptors, such as "influenza-like symptoms," or other parameters over time.

124. A: An incubation period is defined as the time between invasion by a pathogenic microbe and initial signs of altered tissue status or onset of infection. When the host organism is a vector, the incubation period falls from vector invasion by the microbe to the next step in vector transmission, that is, when the vector spreads infection to other hosts, as in the bite of an infected mosquito. Diseases caused by some microbes involve longer incubation periods that may extend over years while other transmissible diseases can require mere hours before invasion is manifested as defined. Differences in incubation time length may be affected by variations in host factors, such as immune status, the virulence or type of microbial pathogen, microbial load, and environmental factors, such as sanitation, pest control, and weather patterns.

125. D: Prophylactic antimicrobials are used to prevent infections before they occur. Although overuse of this preventive strategy has contributed to increased resistance to antimicrobials, evidence of its usefulness in many clinical scenarios is strong. One is in elective orthopedic reconstructive surgery, as in example A, wherein anti-infectives active against skin flora are typically used, often within 30 to 60 minutes of skin incision. Prophylaxis is also used with travel to areas of endemic illness, such as malaria, as in Patient B. Empiric antimicrobials are given when there is cause to suspect an infectious etiology but the specific microbe(s) has yet to be determined, as in a patient admitted with fever, cough, and purulent sputum. Patient C clinically shows oral thrush and is immune-suppressed. Therapeutic antimicrobials are given based on diagnosis, infective microbial identify, results of sensitivity tests as indicated, and relative cost factors. The clinical diagnosis of thrush in this case indicates therapeutic care. Routine culture and sensitivities are not generally performed in cases of this type.

126. C: Nosocomial infections encompass those hospital-acquired illness caused by pathogenic microbes that were not present in the index case when the patient entered the facility, whether the diagnosis is made during that stay or after discharge. Because infections categorized as nosocomial in nature may involve clinical as well as laboratory diagnoses, the diagnosis may also be made based on appropriate clinical data by an attending physician. The surgical site infection of Patient A occurred after discharge but is nosocomial in origin. The vaginal delivery in case B is the likely source of the neonate's herpes infection and is likewise nosocomial. However, the malformations and positive rubella titer in case C results from placental transfer of the rubella virus, which is not considered nosocomial.

127. B: Surveillance systems come in many types. When feasible, active surveillance is preferred over passive systems for completeness, accuracy, and consistency over time. Active programs require trained infection control staff and, thus, may be more costly. However, they are designed to root out hospital-acquired infections and involve proactive interventions. The accuracy and completeness of unmonitored passive systems rely upon reporting by health care personnel that may be incomplete or vary from one department to another. All plans, whether laboratory- or patient-based, require clear and well-constructed protocols to ensure timely and accurate reporting, regardless of the sophistication or version of HIS in place. Patient-based plans require more time for interviews and data collection and input, and therefore tend to be more costly than laboratory-based systems.

128. A: Decreased length of hospital stay may account for nearly half of missed cases of postdischarge, postoperative wound infections. Many different methods have been employed for postdischarge surveillance, in part because there is no standardized procedure that is universally accepted or that applies to the variety in health care settings, personnel, technology adaptation, and other factors. Telephone interviews, mailed questionnaires, and follow-up using physicians' postdischarge records and reports have all been used. The latter is prone to incompleteness and requires a dedicated effort to root out specific results that many office practices may not easily access, especially if the practice does not employ an efficient electronic health record system.

129. A: The T-point system is a method of assessing an institution's variations in average time length of surgical procedures compared with the database of the National Healthcare Safety Network (NHSN). T-point baseline scores are not based on length of surgery as performed at the index hospital. The T-point number assigned to a procedure reflects a percentile (e.g., a T-point of 2 for hernia repair means that 75% of herniorrhaphies in the database were completed within 2 hours). This classification system looks at one variable and does not take into account other factors that may increase or decrease risk of surgical infection. Operative times that exceed any given T-point are associated with a greater chance of postoperative complications and risk of infection.

130. D: The NNIS Risk Index is scored from 0 (zero) to 3 (three) based on total points assigned as measured by four variables: wound classification (1 point if satisfies criteria for contaminated or dirty only); ASA preoperative score (1 point if ASA 3, 4, or 5); and T-point classification (1 point if procedure exceeds the T-point). Zero points are assigned if the patient has no risk factors. No single variable is assigned more than 1 point and none of the subscores are assigned a negative value. The correct answer is D, wherein 1 point is assigned for a preoperative ASA score of 3, 4, or 5 representing, respectively, severe systemic illness(es), life-endangering systemic disease(s), or a potentially preterminal state in which the patient is not expected to survive without surgical intercession.

131. C: Medical progress in this century moves in step with increased use of invasive testing and therapeutics. Despite their many benefits, devices must be regularly monitored for their associated risks and rates of infection. Specific and comparable measurements are useful for quality improvement, detection of unintended injury, and many other factors, included cost/benefit ratios and cost-effectiveness. To calculate overall infection rate for central line devices, divide the total number of infections by the total number of device days:

$$\text{Infection rate per 1000} = \frac{\text{total number of infections}}{\text{total number of device days}} = \frac{x}{1000}$$

$$\text{Infections} = 2 + 1 + 4 = 7$$

$$\text{Device days} = 48 + 20 + 72 = 140$$

Plugging in these numbers yields the following equation:

$$\frac{7}{140} = \frac{x}{1000}$$

The equation can then be rearranged and solved for x as follows:

$$x = 1000 \times \frac{7}{140} = 50$$

Thus, the overall hospital infection rate is 50 per 1000.

132. D: Use the same calculation above to arrive at infection rates on each service.

$$\text{Medical ICU infection rate} = 2 \div 48 = 0.0417 = \frac{41.7}{1000}$$
$$\text{Surgical ICU infection rate} = 1 \div 20 = 0.05 = \frac{50}{1000}$$
$$\text{Oncology ward infection rate} = 4 \div 72 = 0.0556 = \frac{55.6}{1000}$$

Therefore, the oncology ward has the highest rate of infection expressed in device days. The 9 surgical ICU patients in this survey may not lend statistical significance to the result obtained but this service does not have the highest infection rate. The data obtained may still provide useful comparison information. These findings may alert the infection control team about variations in technique, patient selection, device preferences, or other early indicators that can be tracked or investigated in an effort to improve patient care.

133. B: Many different variables are used to determine statistical significance. No measurement is ideal nor should it be used without other supportive or challenging analyses. The P value is an accepted statistical method used to assess the likelihood that a statistical result resulted due to chance. A P value of 0.05 indicates a 5% probability that the result was caused by chance, or a 95% probability that it was not a random or chance event and is more likely a statistically sound occurrence. In statistics, P values less than (<) 0.05 are used to indicate higher probability of statistical significance. Statistical power can be increased by other variables, such as study design, number of subjects or events in the cohort studied, bias, and fulfillment of Hill's criteria. Here, the P values > 0.05 are not likely to fulfill statistical significance despite the larger cohort groups. Choices A and B have P values < 0.05, but choice A only measured 7 patients in an uncomplicated illness, leaving choice B as MOST likely to represent statistical validity.

134. A: Hospitals seeking to fulfill OSHA regulations for prevention of illnesses spread by bloodborne pathogenic microbes employ intermediate-level agents for disinfection, particularly in critical areas such as the emergency department, surgical suites (and related-use areas as in pre- and post-op recovery), and laboratories. Iodophors are examples of low-tier agents that kill most bacteria but may not kill certain strains of fungi or viruses. Their lack of activity against resistant microbial strains and spores makes use of more effective agents imperative, especially in higher risk areas. A greater range of microbial kill or inactivation is seen with intermediate agents such as alcohol and sodium hypochlorite (bleach). This broader kill or inactivation range extends to vegetative organisms such as M. tuberculosis, viruses such as HBV and HIV, and fungi. High-level disinfectants additionally kill most bacterial, viral, and fungal strains, but may not fully eradicate areas, equipment, or surfaces contaminated by high concentrations of bacterial spores.

135. A: Flash sterilization is a method of heat sterilization that generally requires 3 to 10 minutes at 132 °C to eradicate microbes, including most vegetative forms (i.e., mycobacteria) and viruses, given appropriate and adequate pre-sterilization cleaning. These techniques are commonly used for reusable surgical equipment, especially when time and supply constraints demand rapid turnaround. Dry heat that uses oven-type equipment typically takes much longer and is not useful when sterilized materials are needed in short order. By definition, flash-sterilized items that have been appropriate precleaned will be rendered free of pathogens, including viruses, fungi, and vegetative microbes.

136. D: Decubiti develop in about one-third of patients with spinal cord injury. Given this high occurrence rate, decubitus ulcers present management issues that call for appropriate actions to prevent their development or hasten resolution in a timely manner by a well-educated clinical staff. Pressure and contamination combine to create a setting in which decubiti may develop. These factors underscore the role of active infection surveillance and interaction with clinical staff to ensure that patients are kept clean and that all available methods are employed (e.g., turning, special mattresses) to prevent excessive pressure and breaching of healthy, intact skin. Colonizing organisms are typically mixed, comprising aerobic and anaerobic flora. What may appear to be a small decubitus on the skin surface may instead represent more profound damage to subjacent soft tissue. Underlying osteomyelitis, or spread of infection to nearby bone, is commonly traced to a preexisting decubitus ulcer in these and other at-risk patient groups.

137. A: Surgical suite infection control practices must be known, assessed, and regularly revised to improve outcome measures. Routine sterilization procedures are preferable to flash sterilization, which may be incomplete because of inadequate precleaning, timing, or temperature considerations. Air exchange is also important, with at least 15 hourly air exchanges recommended, of which at least three should be using fresh air. Horizontal laminar air flow, air filtering, and positive pressure ventilation of hallways and areas adjacent to the surgical theatres should also be employed. Mechanical cleaning should be considered essential to proper postcleaning sterilization and should include daily wet vacuuming after the last procedure has been performed.

138. C: Nutrition service staff are an integral part of the health care team. They should be included in ongoing infection prevention and control strategies. They are permitted to deliver and remove trays from all patients with exception of those on precautions related to airborne pathogens. Although some institutions may choose disposables for their food service, paper and one-use items are not necessary. Food service staff should never move potentially contaminated items on a flip tray or surface so that food trays can be deposited. Instead, they must notify medical personnel so the item(s) can safely be disposed of and the tray or surface area properly cleansed. They should not remove trays that have been contaminated by medical equipment or body fluids, and should instead notify health care personnel rather than touch or cleanse an area themselves.

139. B: The FDA's MedWatch program provides a wealth of information related to drug and device recalls, safety updates, adverse event reporting, medical device reporting (MDR), and forms for detailing required events and voluntary case reports. Device-related incidents that require medical intervention must be reported within 10 days. Facilities that use medical devices must issue MDR every 6 and 12 months. Although such facilities are encouraged to use MedWatch forms, they must also develop written procedures that detail what types of incidents must be reported using an MDR, how cases should be evaluated, and protocols for filing MDR. Records related to MDR must be kept for a minimum of 2 years.

140. D: Infection control coordinators are involved in occupational exposures to potential infectious agents that involve contact with skin, eyes, or mucous membranes, or a parenteral breach involving blood during execution of duties. IC staff consults and reports to hospital management regarding compliance with the institution's exposure control plan, appropriate interventions, investigations, and education to help minimize risk for event recurrence, protect patient and staff, and strengthen prevention measures. OSHA standards regarding precautions for this type of procedure must be reviewed and documentation of the event must include compliance with such standards. Postexposure prophylaxis with HBIG may not be indicated in this case, regardless of perceived benefit of immediacy. The staff member should not be individually identified in communicating the incident to the rest of the staff, similar to patient privacy regulations. Exposure control plans do not dictate cessation of procedures that may be medically necessary while investigations are underway.

141. A: Participatory events such as hand washing contests that use materials designed to demonstrate technique efficacy in ridding hands of microbes are highly effective tools for staff education. As opposed to passive or didactic learning through posters, pamphlets, and other written materials, hands-on learning is a teaching tool associated with better penetration and retention of instructive material and, often, better recall and adherence to best-practices recommendations. While some medical personnel might say these activities are a waste of time, the effectiveness of these methods has been shown to be worthwhile. Students tend to be more receptive towards new information but they are not the only group likely to benefit from activities that reveal how each individual's habits may or may not be in step with regulations and best practices. All provider levels should be encouraged to improve handwashing habits through specific methods that can be easily learned and incorporated into new behaviors.

142. D: The infection control program annual summary is only as useful and the information it contains. Thus, specific information related to the goals and procedural guidelines of the institution's infection control program general plan must be included for maximal usefulness in future planning and assessment of adequacy of current procedures. Numerical and statistical examples, as applied to specific objectives such as surgical infection rates, are extremely helpful in this regard. Even if no incidents occurred, summaries must be filed with each goal and objective of the infection control program plan addressed. Occupational exposures are included in the exposure control plan and while they may be included in the infection control program annual summary, the report is not limited to these events. Financial summaries of cost-benefit and/or cost-effectiveness may be highlighted as part of the summary, but the document is not designed as an accounting or budgetary vehicle.

143. A: Even without ingrained old behaviors that may need to be revised, a new hospital presents its own set of challenges. Top priority in the development of an infection control program plan is to determine a profile of the institution (i.e., patient base [sociodemographic profile, number of hospital beds], client needs [including that of patients, clinical staff, administrators, regulatory bodies, environmental engineers], size of health care personnel staff, types of services offered). While hardware and software may need to be upgraded at some point, initial efforts should not be directed towards costly endeavors without first assessing the strengths, limitations, needs, and expectations of the primary institution and its personnel. Assessment of client satisfaction is an important part of the final infection control program plan document but is not an initial priority, and will be incompletely assessed at a brief 30-day interval. Similarly, cost-benefit analysis comes into play once initial assessments are underway and the IC officer/team begins to analyze problem areas or procedures in need of quality improvement.

144. A: Health care workers have specific responsibilities in overall infection control practices, particularly regarding their personal hygiene and habits. Nails, particularly when long or artificially enhanced, are a reservoir of potentially transmissible microbes, such as *Staphylococcus*, other skin flora, yeast, and pathogenic gram-negative rods such as *Pseudomonas* spp. Large numbers of potential pathogens can be recovered from the subungual areas of personnel who wear artificial nails, even in those who practice prudent handwashing techniques or use of surgical scrubs. While one-quarter inch length is the maximum recommended fingernail length, most bacteria are present within the first (most proximal) 1 mm of nail adjacent to subungual skin. Artificial nails present an infection hazard, even when fresh polish is applied daily. Chipped polish appears to harbor greater numbers of potentially infectious microbes, as can decorative flourishes such as sequins. Longer nails, whether natural or artificial, may predispose health care workers to injuring patients through inadvertent scratching or palpation that causes patient discomfort, whether physical or emotional. Longer nails may also tear through surgical gloves, potentially exposing health care workers to infectious materials. Because they interfere with precision during palpation, longer nails may interfere with proper clinical patient assessment, procedural performance, or handling of medical equipment.

145. C: The Food and Drug Administration (FDA) is the federal agency charged with the regulation of medications and medical devices. Their strict procedural guidelines outline regulations for preapproval of all prescription drugs and, through the Center for Devices and Radiologic Health (CDRH), medical devices. This also includes issuance of drug recalls and issues regarding safe reuse of medical equipment. Through the MedWatch program, FDA offers safety information and an avenue for reporting of adverse events. OSHA is a federal body whose regulatory powers include exposure to infectious agents in the workplace, as well as general and specific aspects of safety in the workplace. The Joint Commission is an accreditation body that sets standards for health care facilities, such as hospitals and outpatient surgical centers. The Centers for Disease Control and Prevention acts as a preventive and monitoring body that issues recommendation procedures for infectious disease control, hygiene, infection control practices, vaccination scheduling, and population-specific guidelines.

146. B: A Shewhart cycle is a problem-solving tool that employs four steps: Plan, Do, Check, Act. The method enables a systems approach to quality management. In this cycle, a process is identified and analyzed for problem or faulty processes, and root-cause analysis is done prior to developing a trial plan of action; followed by a check phase of analysis and determination of efficacy; and then to implementation and monitoring. Choices B to D are also used in performance improvement and educational efforts. A fishbone or Ishikawa diagram is used to help identify and illustrate cause and effect. A Pareto chart integrates two types of schematics: vertical bar graph and superimposed linear graph. Pareto charts help identify the greatest contributor to a given problem, as in 70% of all central lines that became infected were inserted by 10% of all residents. A flow chart is by definition a diagram or schematic that illustrates a process with directionality or flow, and input points to pictorially represent how a process unfolds or where problems and bottlenecks may occur.

147. D: Everyone wants handouts but they often go unused or filed next to the unread handout from last time. To be effective, handouts should not be distributed just as a presentation begins; an audience is likely to miss large parts of the presentation while flipping through the notes. Lengthy handouts with small font or smudged print, or those that incorporate difficult-to-read blocks of uninterrupted text are less likely to be considered useful. Bullet points are handy teaching tools, as are handouts that do not merely recapitulate the presentation material but highlight key points of the talk and underscore practical teaching points.

148. A: Compliance is calculated by measuring degree of fulfillment of a desired behavior or procedure. Traditionally expressed as a fraction or percentage, it is calculated by dividing the number of times a desired event occurs (numerator) by the total number of eligible procedures (denominator). When setting out to modify health care personnel behavior, it is important to observe, understand, and analyze in-place behaviors that may impede the desired behavioral change, whether by force of habit or conflicting rules, hierarchical concerns, and other factors. A useful technique is to demonstrate, reinforce, and then monitor as steps are taken to institute the desired change. Data may also be used to assess compliance, particularly when the effect of a desired change, such as the lowered infection rate in this case, can be easily measured and act as a surrogate marker for successful behavioral adaptation.

149. A: Policies and procedures for screening, vetting, and placing of candidate health care workers in medical facilities are developed along guidelines provided by four federal bodies: OSHA, CDC, the

Joint Commission, and the American Hospital Association. The Joint Commission requires choice A, testing for drugs of abuse and background check, which may include criminal checks or some degree of financial/credit investigation as appropriate. OSHA recommends a tuberculin skin test performed in two stages. The standard Mantoux test involves intradermal purified protein derivative (PPD) injection. The injection site is read by a trained professional after 48 to 72 hours. TB testing is recommended to be performed at 1- and 3-week intervals to identify true negatives. A positive result necessitates a follow-up chest radiograph. While vaccination against hepatitis B is strongly recommended for health care workers, particularly those who work in higher risk areas, they are not required. However, employers may opt to engage nonimmune personnel in patient-care endeavors that involve lower risk of exposure to patients likely to harbor hepatitis B virus.

150. C: Herpetic whitlow is a type of herpes simplex infection of the skin that may manifest as blisters or vesicles on the finger, often at the tip. Virus may be shed from these lesions even when gloves are worn. Health care workers should be restricted from work until the lesions are fully healed. Latex allergy that manifests as dermatitis would qualify for work restriction but is noted in the example by history with no active lesions. This health care worker should be offered nonlatex gloves in his/her work station and advised of the need to have nonallergenic gloves on hand for situations where no nonallergenic gloves are immediately accessible. The nurse on ACE inhibitors with a new onset of nonproductive cough may be experiencing a common side effect of such drugs and does not require work restriction. However, health care workers with cough due to suspected viral or bacterial infection should be restricted from work until their symptoms clear.

How to Overcome Test Anxiety

Just the thought of taking a test is enough to make most people a little nervous. A test is an important event that can have a long-term impact on your future, so it's important to take it seriously and it's natural to feel anxious about performing well. But just because anxiety is normal, that doesn't mean that it's helpful in test taking, or that you should simply accept it as part of your life. Anxiety can have a variety of effects. These effects can be mild, like making you feel slightly nervous, or severe, like blocking your ability to focus or remember even a simple detail.

If you experience test anxiety—whether severe or mild—it's important to know how to beat it. To discover this, first you need to understand what causes test anxiety.

Causes of Test Anxiety

While we often think of anxiety as an uncontrollable emotional state, it can actually be caused by simple, practical things. One of the most common causes of test anxiety is that a person does not feel adequately prepared for their test. This feeling can be the result of many different issues such as poor study habits or lack of organization, but the most common culprit is time management. Starting to study too late, failing to organize your study time to cover all of the material, or being distracted while you study will mean that you're not well prepared for the test. This may lead to cramming the night before, which will cause you to be physically and mentally exhausted for the test. Poor time management also contributes to feelings of stress, fear, and hopelessness as you realize you are not well prepared but don't know what to do about it.

Other times, test anxiety is not related to your preparation for the test but comes from unresolved fear. This may be a past failure on a test, or poor performance on tests in general. It may come from comparing yourself to others who seem to be performing better or from the stress of living up to expectations. Anxiety may be driven by fears of the future—how failure on this test would affect your educational and career goals. These fears are often completely irrational, but they can still negatively impact your test performance.

Review Video: 3 Reasons You Have Test Anxiety
Visit mometrix.com/academy and enter code: 428468

Elements of Test Anxiety

As mentioned earlier, test anxiety is considered to be an emotional state, but it has physical and mental components as well. Sometimes you may not even realize that you are suffering from test anxiety until you notice the physical symptoms. These can include trembling hands, rapid heartbeat, sweating, nausea, and tense muscles. Extreme anxiety may lead to fainting or vomiting. Obviously, any of these symptoms can have a negative impact on testing. It is important to recognize them as soon as they begin to occur so that you can address the problem before it damages your performance.

Review Video: 3 Ways to Tell You Have Test Anxiety
Visit mometrix.com/academy and enter code: 927847

The mental components of test anxiety include trouble focusing and inability to remember learned information. During a test, your mind is on high alert, which can help you recall information and stay focused for an extended period of time. However, anxiety interferes with your mind's natural processes, causing you to blank out, even on the questions you know well. The strain of testing during anxiety makes it difficult to stay focused, especially on a test that may take several hours. Extreme anxiety can take a huge mental toll, making it difficult not only to recall test information but even to understand the test questions or pull your thoughts together.

Review Video: How Test Anxiety Affects Memory
Visit mometrix.com/academy and enter code: 609003

Effects of Test Anxiety

Test anxiety is like a disease—if left untreated, it will get progressively worse. Anxiety leads to poor performance, and this reinforces the feelings of fear and failure, which in turn lead to poor performances on subsequent tests. It can grow from a mild nervousness to a crippling condition. If allowed to progress, test anxiety can have a big impact on your schooling, and consequently on your future.

Test anxiety can spread to other parts of your life. Anxiety on tests can become anxiety in any stressful situation, and blanking on a test can turn into panicking in a job situation. But fortunately, you don't have to let anxiety rule your testing and determine your grades. There are a number of relatively simple steps you can take to move past anxiety and function normally on a test and in the rest of life.

Review Video: How Test Anxiety Impacts Your Grades
Visit mometrix.com/academy and enter code: 939819

Physical Steps for Beating Test Anxiety

While test anxiety is a serious problem, the good news is that it can be overcome. It doesn't have to control your ability to think and remember information. While it may take time, you can begin taking steps today to beat anxiety.

Just as your first hint that you may be struggling with anxiety comes from the physical symptoms, the first step to treating it is also physical. Rest is crucial for having a clear, strong mind. If you are tired, it is much easier to give in to anxiety. But if you establish good sleep habits, your body and mind will be ready to perform optimally, without the strain of exhaustion. Additionally, sleeping well helps you to retain information better, so you're more likely to recall the answers when you see the test questions.

Getting good sleep means more than going to bed on time. It's important to allow your brain time to relax. Take study breaks from time to time so it doesn't get overworked, and don't study right before bed. Take time to rest your mind before trying to rest your body, or you may find it difficult to fall asleep.

Review Video: <u>The Importance of Sleep for Your Brain</u>
Visit mometrix.com/academy and enter code: 319338

Along with sleep, other aspects of physical health are important in preparing for a test. Good nutrition is vital for good brain function. Sugary foods and drinks may give a burst of energy but this burst is followed by a crash, both physically and emotionally. Instead, fuel your body with protein and vitamin-rich foods.

Also, drink plenty of water. Dehydration can lead to headaches and exhaustion, especially if your brain is already under stress from the rigors of the test. Particularly if your test is a long one, drink water during the breaks. And if possible, take an energy-boosting snack to eat between sections.

Review Video: <u>How Diet Can Affect your Mood</u>
Visit mometrix.com/academy and enter code: 624317

Along with sleep and diet, a third important part of physical health is exercise. Maintaining a steady workout schedule is helpful, but even taking 5-minute study breaks to walk can help get your blood pumping faster and clear your head. Exercise also releases endorphins, which contribute to a positive feeling and can help combat test anxiety.

When you nurture your physical health, you are also contributing to your mental health. If your body is healthy, your mind is much more likely to be healthy as well. So take time to rest, nourish your body with healthy food and water, and get moving as much as possible. Taking these physical steps will make you stronger and more able to take the mental steps necessary to overcome test anxiety.

Mental Steps for Beating Test Anxiety

Working on the mental side of test anxiety can be more challenging, but as with the physical side, there are clear steps you can take to overcome it. As mentioned earlier, test anxiety often stems from lack of preparation, so the obvious solution is to prepare for the test. Effective studying may be the most important weapon you have for beating test anxiety, but you can and should employ several other mental tools to combat fear.

First, boost your confidence by reminding yourself of past success—tests or projects that you aced. If you're putting as much effort into preparing for this test as you did for those, there's no reason you should expect to fail here. Work hard to prepare; then trust your preparation.

Second, surround yourself with encouraging people. It can be helpful to find a study group, but be sure that the people you're around will encourage a positive attitude. If you spend time with others who are anxious or cynical, this will only contribute to your own anxiety. Look for others who are motivated to study hard from a desire to succeed, not from a fear of failure.

Third, reward yourself. A test is physically and mentally tiring, even without anxiety, and it can be helpful to have something to look forward to. Plan an activity following the test, regardless of the outcome, such as going to a movie or getting ice cream.

When you are taking the test, if you find yourself beginning to feel anxious, remind yourself that you know the material. Visualize successfully completing the test. Then take a few deep, relaxing breaths and return to it. Work through the questions carefully but with confidence, knowing that you are capable of succeeding.

Developing a healthy mental approach to test taking will also aid in other areas of life. Test anxiety affects more than just the actual test—it can be damaging to your mental health and even contribute to depression. It's important to beat test anxiety before it becomes a problem for more than testing.

Review Video: Test Anxiety and Depression
Visit mometrix.com/academy and enter code: 904704

Study Strategy

Being prepared for the test is necessary to combat anxiety, but what does being prepared look like? You may study for hours on end and still not feel prepared. What you need is a strategy for test prep. The next few pages outline our recommended steps to help you plan out and conquer the challenge of preparation.

Step 1: Scope Out the Test

Learn everything you can about the format (multiple choice, essay, etc.) and what will be on the test. Gather any study materials, course outlines, or sample exams that may be available. Not only will this help you to prepare, but knowing what to expect can help to alleviate test anxiety.

Step 2: Map Out the Material

Look through the textbook or study guide and make note of how many chapters or sections it has. Then divide these over the time you have. For example, if a book has 15 chapters and you have five days to study, you need to cover three chapters each day. Even better, if you have the time, leave an extra day at the end for overall review after you have gone through the material in depth.

If time is limited, you may need to prioritize the material. Look through it and make note of which sections you think you already have a good grasp on, and which need review. While you are studying, skim quickly through the familiar sections and take more time on the challenging parts. Write out your plan so you don't get lost as you go. Having a written plan also helps you feel more in control of the study, so anxiety is less likely to arise from feeling overwhelmed at the amount to cover.

Step 3: Gather Your Tools

Decide what study method works best for you. Do you prefer to highlight in the book as you study and then go back over the highlighted portions? Or do you type out notes of the important information? Or is it helpful to make flashcards that you can carry with you? Assemble the pens, index cards, highlighters, post-it notes, and any other materials you may need so you won't be distracted by getting up to find things while you study.

If you're having a hard time retaining the information or organizing your notes, experiment with different methods. For example, try color-coding by subject with colored pens, highlighters, or post-it notes. If you learn better by hearing, try recording yourself reading your notes so you can listen while in the car, working out, or simply sitting at your desk. Ask a friend to quiz you from your flashcards, or try teaching someone the material to solidify it in your mind.

Step 4: Create Your Environment

It's important to avoid distractions while you study. This includes both the obvious distractions like visitors and the subtle distractions like an uncomfortable chair (or a too-comfortable couch that makes you want to fall asleep). Set up the best study environment possible: good lighting and a comfortable work area. If background music helps you focus, you may want to turn it on, but otherwise keep the room quiet. If you are using a computer to take notes, be sure you don't have any other windows open, especially applications like social media, games, or anything else that could distract you. Silence your phone and turn off notifications. Be sure to keep water close by so you stay hydrated while you study (but avoid unhealthy drinks and snacks).

Also, take into account the best time of day to study. Are you freshest first thing in the morning? Try to set aside some time then to work through the material. Is your mind clearer in the afternoon or evening? Schedule your study session then. Another method is to study at the same time of day that you will take the test, so that your brain gets used to working on the material at that time and will be ready to focus at test time.

Step 5: Study!

Once you have done all the study preparation, it's time to settle into the actual studying. Sit down, take a few moments to settle your mind so you can focus, and begin to follow your study plan. Don't give in to distractions or let yourself procrastinate. This is your time to prepare so you'll be ready to fearlessly approach the test. Make the most of the time and stay focused.

Of course, you don't want to burn out. If you study too long you may find that you're not retaining the information very well. Take regular study breaks. For example, taking five minutes out of every hour to walk briskly, breathing deeply and swinging your arms, can help your mind stay fresh.

As you get to the end of each chapter or section, it's a good idea to do a quick review. Remind yourself of what you learned and work on any difficult parts. When you feel that you've mastered the material, move on to the next part. At the end of your study session, briefly skim through your notes again.

But while review is helpful, cramming last minute is NOT. If at all possible, work ahead so that you won't need to fit all your study into the last day. Cramming overloads your brain with more information than it can process and retain, and your tired mind may struggle to recall even previously learned information when it is overwhelmed with last-minute study. Also, the urgent nature of cramming and the stress placed on your brain contribute to anxiety. You'll be more likely to go to the test feeling unprepared and having trouble thinking clearly.

So don't cram, and don't stay up late before the test, even just to review your notes at a leisurely pace. Your brain needs rest more than it needs to go over the information again. In fact, plan to finish your studies by noon or early afternoon the day before the test. Give your brain the rest of the day to relax or focus on other things, and get a good night's sleep. Then you will be fresh for the test and better able to recall what you've studied.

Step 6: Take a Practice Test

Many courses offer sample tests, either online or in the study materials. This is an excellent resource to check whether you have mastered the material, as well as to prepare for the test format and environment.

Check the test format ahead of time: the number of questions, the type (multiple choice, free response, etc.), and the time limit. Then create a plan for working through them. For example, if you have 30 minutes to take a 60-question test, your limit is 30 seconds per question. Spend less time on the questions you know well so that you can take more time on the difficult ones.

If you have time to take several practice tests, take the first one open book, with no time limit. Work through the questions at your own pace and make sure you fully understand them. Gradually work up to taking a test under test conditions: sit at a desk with all study materials put away and set a timer. Pace yourself to make sure you finish the test with time to spare and go back to check your answers if you have time.

After each test, check your answers. On the questions you missed, be sure you understand why you missed them. Did you misread the question (tests can use tricky wording)? Did you forget the information? Or was it something you hadn't learned? Go back and study any shaky areas that the practice tests reveal.

Taking these tests not only helps with your grade, but also aids in combating test anxiety. If you're already used to the test conditions, you're less likely to worry about it, and working through tests until you're scoring well gives you a confidence boost. Go through the practice tests until you feel comfortable, and then you can go into the test knowing that you're ready for it.

Test Tips

On test day, you should be confident, knowing that you've prepared well and are ready to answer the questions. But aside from preparation, there are several test day strategies you can employ to maximize your performance.

First, as stated before, get a good night's sleep the night before the test (and for several nights before that, if possible). Go into the test with a fresh, alert mind rather than staying up late to study.

Try not to change too much about your normal routine on the day of the test. It's important to eat a nutritious breakfast, but if you normally don't eat breakfast at all, consider eating just a protein bar. If you're a coffee drinker, go ahead and have your normal coffee. Just make sure you time it so that the caffeine doesn't wear off right in the middle of your test. Avoid sugary beverages, and drink enough water to stay hydrated but not so much that you need a restroom break 10 minutes into the test. If your test isn't first thing in the morning, consider going for a walk or doing a light workout before the test to get your blood flowing.

Allow yourself enough time to get ready, and leave for the test with plenty of time to spare so you won't have the anxiety of scrambling to arrive in time. Another reason to be early is to select a good seat. It's helpful to sit away from doors and windows, which can be distracting. Find a good seat, get out your supplies, and settle your mind before the test begins.

When the test begins, start by going over the instructions carefully, even if you already know what to expect. Make sure you avoid any careless mistakes by following the directions.

Then begin working through the questions, pacing yourself as you've practiced. If you're not sure on an answer, don't spend too much time on it, and don't let it shake your confidence. Either skip it and come back later, or eliminate as many wrong answers as possible and guess among the remaining ones. Don't dwell on these questions as you continue—put them out of your mind and focus on what lies ahead.

Be sure to read all of the answer choices, even if you're sure the first one is the right answer. Sometimes you'll find a better one if you keep reading. But don't second-guess yourself if you do immediately know the answer. Your gut instinct is usually right. Don't let test anxiety rob you of the information you know.

If you have time at the end of the test (and if the test format allows), go back and review your answers. Be cautious about changing any, since your first instinct tends to be correct, but make sure you didn't misread any of the questions or accidentally mark the wrong answer choice. Look over any you skipped and make an educated guess.

At the end, leave the test feeling confident. You've done your best, so don't waste time worrying about your performance or wishing you could change anything. Instead, celebrate the successful completion of this test. And finally, use this test to learn how to deal with anxiety even better next time.

Review Video: 5 Tips to Beat Test Anxiety
Visit mometrix.com/academy and enter code: 570656

Important Qualification

Not all anxiety is created equal. If your test anxiety is causing major issues in your life beyond the classroom or testing center, or if you are experiencing troubling physical symptoms related to your anxiety, it may be a sign of a serious physiological or psychological condition. If this sounds like your situation, we strongly encourage you to seek professional help.

Tell Us Your Story

We at Mometrix would like to extend our heartfelt thanks to you for letting us be a part of your journey. It is an honor to serve people from all walks of life, people like you, who are committed to building the best future they can for themselves.

We know that each person's situation is unique. But we also know that, whether you are a young student or a mother of four, you care about working to make your own life and the lives of those around you better.

That's why we want to hear your story.

We want to know why you're taking this test. We want to know about the trials you've gone through to get here. And we want to know about the successes you've experienced after taking and passing your test.

In addition to your story, which can be an inspiration both to us and to others, we value your feedback. We want to know both what you loved about our book and what you think we can improve on.

SCAN HERE

The team at Mometrix would be absolutely thrilled to hear from you! So please, send us an email at tellusyourstory@mometrix.com or visit us at mometrix.com/tellusyourstory.php and let's stay in touch.

Additional Bonus Material

Due to our efforts to try to keep this book to a manageable length, we've created a link that will give you access to all of your additional bonus material.

Please visit https://www.mometrix.com/bonus948/cbic to access the information.

Made in the USA
Middletown, DE
23 May 2023

31214528R00203